Clinical
Computing
Competency
for Speech-Language
Pathologists

Clinical
Computing
Competency
for Speech-Language
Pathologists

by

Paula S. Cochran, Ph.D., CCC-SLP
Truman State University

with contributions by

Christine L. Appert, Ed.D., ATP
University of Virginia Children's Medical Center

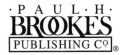
·P·A·U·L·H·
BROOKES
PUBLISHING CO.®

Baltimore • London • Sydney

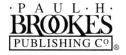

Paul H. Brookes Publishing Co.
Post Office Box 10624
Baltimore, Maryland 21285-0624

www.brookespublishing.com

Typeset by A.W. Bennett, Inc., Hartland, Vermont.
Manufactured in the United States of America by Versa Press, East Peoria, Illinois.

All of the cases in this book are composites of the author's actual experiences. In all
instances, names have been changed and identifying details have been altered to
protect confidentiality.

Author royalties from the sale of this book are donated to the American Speech-
Language-Hearing Foundation and the Truman State University Foundation.

Library of Congress Cataloging-in-Publication Data

Cochran, Paula.
   Clinical computing competency for speech-language pathologists/by Paula
Cochran, with contributions by Christine L. Appert.
      p.   cm.
   Includes bibliographical references and index.
   ISBN 1-55766-685-7 (paperback)
   1.   Speech therapy–Data processing.   2.   Medical informatics.
[DNLM: 1.   Communication Aids for Disabled.   2.   Communication Disorders–
rehabilitation.   3.   Computer-Assisted Instruction–methods.   4.   Language
Development Disorders–rehabilitation–child.   5.   Speech-Language Pathology–
methods.   6.   Telemedicine–methods.]   I.   Cochran, Paula.
II.   Appert, Christine L.   III.   Title.

   RC423.C576 2005
   616.85′503–dc22   2004022711

British Library Cataloguing in Publication data are available from the British
Library.

Contents

Section V   Using a Computer as a Feedback Device

Section VI   Getting Connected: Telepractice, the Internet, and PDAs

Section VII   Using a Computer as a Diagnostic Tool

Section VIII   Adapted Access to Computers: Assistive Technology

About the Author

Paula S. Cochran, Ph.D., CCC-SLP, is a professor of communication disorders at Truman State University, Kirksville, Missouri. She received her bachelor's in English from the College of Wooster, a Diploma in Linguistics from the University of Cambridge, England, her master's in communication disorders from Ohio University, and her doctorate from the University of Virginia. In addition to clinical computing and assistive technology, Dr. Cochran focuses her teaching and research on child language development and disorders. Dr. Cochran has published and presented extensively about the clinical uses of computers and how to effectively integrate computer-based activities into teaching and intervention.

About the Contributor

Christine L. Appert, Ed.D., ATP, is an assistive and instructional technology specialist and education consultant at the University of Virginia Children's Medical Center, Charlottesville, Virginia. She earned an educational specialist degree in learning disabilities and reading disorders from Teachers College, Columbia University, and a doctorate from the Curry School of Education, University of Virginia. Her extensive experience in early childhood and special education has included classroom teaching and interdisciplinary diagnostics and rehabilitation. A credentialed Assistive Technology Practitioner, Dr. Appert presents frequently at professional conferences and teaches courses on instructional and assistive technology for pre-service and practicing special educators and speech-language pathologists.

Foreword

It's been almost two decades since the idea of using computers in speech, language, and hearing was introduced. That was an exciting time. I was in my doctoral program, learning several new procedures for analyzing phonology and other aspects of language. Although these new methods yielded important and interesting data, they were very time-consuming. I spent close to 50 hours working on an assessment project that incorporated these new approaches. Of course that was fine for an eager doctoral student, but I wondered whether it could actually be feasible for working clinicians.

Enter the microcomputer. One of my first research projects was to determine whether I could figure out a way to have the computer help with those interesting, but arduous, analyses. I discovered that Jon Miller and Robin Chapman had already developed a computer-based system for language analysis, *Systematic Analysis for Language Transcripts* (see Topics 31 and 32), so I focused my efforts on phonological analysis. The early program that I wrote was so large and cumbersome that I feared the university would place restrictions on when I could execute it on their mainframe! Nevertheless, it could analyze and return the requested statistics on a large speech sample in mere minutes rather than hours (or days or weeks).

At the same time I was thrilled with how generic applications, such as word processing and spreadsheets, were making my daily tasks not only much easier but also much better. The need for multiple revisions, which is part of any dissertation experience, was far more palatable because I had access to the computer-based "cut and paste," instead of actually having to re-type each draft. Although I was sold on the use of technology to aid linguistic analyses and perform writing, statistical analyses, and graphing, I really didn't see much potential for its use in treatment of children with language disorders. All of the software developed for that purpose was based on a behavioral stimulus-response model for treatment, and that was not consistent with my theoretical orientation regarding child language acquisition. That all changed when I heard Paula Cochran speak at the 1985 ASHA Convention. She talked about the computer providing a "context for conversation," and that it should be viewed as any other "resource" or "tool" under the control of an expert clinician who would manipulate the environment to set up conditions for the child to have a desire to communicate. I was hooked, and I wanted to learn more about how clinicians and researchers could use the computer in their everyday work. I met others in the field with similar interests, and these visionaries established a special organization, Computer Users in Speech and Hearing (CUSH), to facilitate the encouragement and exchange of ideas regarding how computers might be best used. I was amazed that

I now had access to this wonderful tool that could perform analyzes in a small fraction of the time it took me by hand.

I share this personal story with you to emphasize an important point. *My computer use resulted naturally from the discovery that technology could allow me to do something that I was already doing with so much more speed and accuracy.* Shortly after, I realized that technology did more than that—it allowed me to do things that I simply could not have done without it. I'm not sure I would have had the energy for one more revision of a dissertation section—those additional follow-ups on what the child was doing with velars surrounded by back vowels—if it were necessary for me to do those things by hand. I shudder to think about the important characteristics about so many children's phonological or spelling systems that I would have missed had I not employed these analyses.

CUSH was disbanded in the early 1990s because the sentiment was that "computer users" were no longer a distinctive, unique group. Instead, we felt that everyone would soon be a computer user because it would be natural, somewhat self-preserving, to do so. Where are we today with this notion? Unfortunately, it seems that technology use for clinical applications lags behind my hopes and expectations. Few professionals continue to insist on writing a report via pen and paper first and later entering it into word processing software. Simply put, we all understand that it is simply easier and faster to produce a quality report when we use a computer. Why is it that this notion has not transferred to other clinical applications such as linguistic or voice analysis? Dr. Cochran explores this notion in the current volume, and I am grateful that she does.

The knowledge base underlying speech-language pathology is exploding. We have ever-increasing responsibilities in meeting the challenges of our broad scope of practice. Technology offers us a way to successfully address those challenges, but we need to acknowledge that the standard has been raised. I remember having to consult an actual hard copy (i.e., catalog) to review the literature available on a specific topic. Today, technology allows almost instant access to a listing of articles on a topic of interest and in many cases a few more clicks result in the actual papers appearing on the computer screen or printing right there in your office. We no longer have to play endless telephone tag with our colleagues about important issues because we can gain virtually instant access to them via email. The flip side of these wonderful privileges is that they carry increased expectations. Certainly one can no longer use a lack of time to get over to the library as an excuse to not keep up with current literature. Similarly, I think today's clinicians should be hard pressed to justify the use of only cursory testing and analyses in assessment when the computer can make additional analyses quite feasible. Will we take advantage of these resources in an effort to offer optimal services to our clients? Will clinicians have an adequate understanding of what the resources are? *Clinical Computing Competency for Speech-Language Pathologists* can serve as a jump start for both students and professionals in gaining such an understanding.

Finally, it will likely be necessary for some individuals to commit to making some changes. As with all areas of professional practice, we can't be content to continue to do things the way we do just by tradition. We must evolve professionally, and some of the enhancements that may be necessary include increased use of appropriate instrumentation. Clinicians must be willing to experiment with current software and read the associated reviews. Just as they do with any tool, they must ensure that the underlying approach to assessment or treatment is consistent with their theory regarding development of abilities and skills in the pertinent areas. The current certification standards include expectations regarding appropriate use of instrumentation. Just as faculty are responsible for providing current research data in their courses and activities to meet other clinical standards, they also must be conscientious to first ensure their own competency and then ultimately their students' in the responsible use of clinical technology. It's important because it's best for our students and ultimately their clients. I believe my students would likely find it somewhat odd that anyone would choose to do an analysis of a child's phonological, linguistic, or spelling systems by hand. They are being taught in an atmosphere in which necessary analyses are expected and are feasibly completed because of access to technology tools. I am hopeful that students in educational programs across the country are having similar experiences.

Clinical Computing Competency for Speech-Language Pathologists is the culmination of Dr. Cochran's work to emphasize optimal, desirable uses of the computer while also cautioning potential users to beware of simple bells and whistles. I've been anticipating the completion of this book for some time. I predict that it will be a wonderful resource for faculty, students, and practicing clinicians.

Julie J. Masterson, Ph.D.
Southwest Missouri State University

Acknowledgments

This book is based on research, teaching, and clinical experiences developed over nearly 20 years. In that time, many people inspired, supported, and encouraged me as well as the work. I never would have pursued the idea of clinical applications of technology if it were not for the inspiration and instruction of my mentor and friend, Glen L. Bull. Many thanks to him, Gina, and Stephen for adopting me as an honorary member of their family and sharing many happy technology-enmeshed summers with me.

Thank you to Mom, Sheila, and the doggies for endless inspiration and support, and much patience especially during the final throes of book writing. Thanks for always knowing I could do it. My special appreciation goes to my university family: the students, faculty, clients, and staff of the Truman State University communication disorders program and the Truman State University Speech and Hearing Clinic. Dozens of student clinicians bravely tried new computer applications with their clients under the watchful eyes of equally game clinical supervisors. They generously shared the results with me, for which I can never thank them enough. Sixteen years' worth of student volunteer researchers helped me explore new applications of technology through a group we called Top Secret Research (TSR). I thank them for their help and their tolerance while I fooled around and tried to figure out how to do at least some of the things I was so sure were possible. I learned so much from them and with them! Thanks to John Applegate, Carl DeFosse, Sheila Garlock, Janet Gooch, Connie Ikerd, M. Barbara Kline, Kees Koutstaal, Melissa Passe, and Amy Wilson for their interest and support. I would also like to thank my colleagues for the opportunity to include assistive technology and clinical computing in a crowded curriculum, for the essential space and time to play and experiment, and for your unflagging cooperation.

I was enormously influenced by my work with an outstanding group of innovators involved in the UVA/IBM Institute on Learner-Based Tools for Special Populations, 1986–1987. With Glen Bull, I co-directed this project, which included several dedicated experts from IBM and 20 carefully chosen clinicians and special educators from around the country. Together, among other things, we began the first online discussion group regarding technology and special populations, on the CONFER II system at the University of Michigan. These interactions led to life-long associations that I continue to treasure.

Early in my academic career I was the co-recipient of a development grant co-sponsored by Apple Computer, Inc., and the American Speech-Language-Hearing Foundation (ASHF). It would be hard to over-estimate the importance of this support at that time. I remain grateful to Nancy Minghetti and the Foundation for their investment and their enthusiastic fostering of technology leadership.

I am indebted to many early technology adopters and innovators in our field. Several of them were founding members of an influential if short-lived national organization called Computer Users in Speech and Hearing (CUSH). Some of their work inspired me, and many of them personally encouraged me when I was first deciding to pursue the use of technology in communication disorders in the late 1980s. My hat is off to:

Barbara Allen	Richard McGuire
David Beukelman	Laura Meyers
Sarah Blackstone	Russ Mills
Glen Bull	Gary Moulton
Betsy Calvert	Bonnie Nelson
David Cartmell	Jack Pickering
Mike Chial	Teresa Rosegrant
Richard Dean	Gary Rushakoff
James Fitch	William Seaton
Ed Garrett	Julie Scherz
Richard Katz	Art Schwartz
Judith Kuster	Lawrence Shriberg
Nick Lape	Joe Smaldino
Steven Long	Robert Volin
Tom Lough	Cheryl Wissich
Bruce Mahaffey	Mike Wynne
Doug Martin	Kendall Young
Julie Masterson	

Several people have contributed specifically to this book. My appreciation goes to the many student assistants who vainly tried to keep me and my office organized. A special thanks to experts who commented on earlier versions of sections of the book, including Linda Evans, Jennifer Garrett, Janet Gooch, M. Barbara Kline, Steven Long, Julie Masterson, Richard McGuire, Jon Miller, and Amy Wilson. I'm grateful for the expertise and patience of the staff of Paul H. Brookes Publishing Co., especially Elaine Niefeld. And, last but not least, the biggest thanks of all to Christine Appert, who has read and reread the manuscript almost as many times as I have, for being a determined coach and a constant friend.

Introduction

REPORTS FROM THE TRENCHES

The deliberate use of new technologies to improve communication skills is happening in all educational and rehabilitation settings. Everywhere, computers are being used at the instigation of a wide variety of professionals and consumers—speech-language pathologists (SLPs), teachers, occupational and physical therapists, parents, spouses, physicians, and persons with communication impairments themselves. Each year at state and national conferences, clinicians make presentations about their clients' successes resulting from technology-based procedures. Occasionally, experimental data-based research is presented, usually confirming the positive effect of a new technique based on a new technology. But how much has the widespread availability of computers actually affected routine intervention with persons who have speech or language disabilities? Is the innovative and effective use of technology happening as frequently and as skillfully as we might have predicted that it would be by now?

Clearly, many clinicians are finding technology applications that serve their students and clients well and that facilitate improvement in communication. A former student sent me the following e-mail.

> I am working in the local school district. I work solely with preschoolers and am in the classroom most of the time. You are welcome to come visit! I use the computer mostly as a language context setting tool. With children who have severe disabilities I use it to initiate pointing, etc. With children who are more advanced I take turns being mouse operator and we describe what we want the other person to click on. I also live and breathe *Boardmaker* [Mayer-Johnson, 1993]. I use it to make communication boards and recipes, sequence games, etc. Next year I will be in a new building with just early childhood (kindergarten & preschool). We will have 4 SLPs under the same roof! My principal is really into technology and I will be the "technology resource person." I know we will have a [new] scanner and printer!

This clinician has a clear view of how computer applications contribute to her work with preschoolers. She is using the technology directly with children at all ability levels, who have a variety of strengths and impairments. In addition, she develops individualized materials to meet a range of therapy needs with the help of her computer. She sounds flexible and confident about the technology she has now, as well as what might be coming her way in the future.

I would love to claim that this is the typical scenario reported by students who have taken my clinical computing course, worked in my technology research group or practiced using computers in therapy in the university clinic where I supervise. However, the truth is that there is no typical scenario so far. Newly graduated speech-language pathologists continue to encounter a wide range of realities regarding the clinical use of new technologies.

Some, especially the ones who asked about computers during their job interviews, find themselves in high-tech surroundings in which staff members are issued their own handhelds or laptops, technical support is competent, and in-service education is readily available. Others encounter a technological wasteland, where computers are still barely available for administrative paperwork, let alone instructional or clinical purposes. Some clinicians have developed innovative technology applications and are very successful in the complete absence of good training or support—they are just determined, creative individuals. It can be a mistake to judge the many by the few—whether the few are the cutting edge leaders or stragglers, they may not be representative of the profession at large. Although there are many clinicians and educators successfully using new technologies to promote speech and language skills, there is ample evidence of a persistent need for more technology training opportunities, more access to relevant technology in clinical work settings, and more technical support.

WHY I WROTE THIS BOOK

The rapid rate of change in technology combined with the slow rate of change in university curricula has resulted in a sizable gap between the state-of-the-art and the typical experience of student clinicians. Naturally some lag time is to be expected between the advent of a new technology and its adoption by the majority of a professional group. Studies in the diffusion of innovation suggest that even a gap of a decade or more is not unusual between the time an innovation becomes available and the time that adoption is common among members of a target population (Rogers, 1995). Even though I know this is true, the adoption and dissemination of clinical computing technologies within university speech-language pathology programs is not happening fast enough for me.

Through no fault of their own, new clinicians as well as veterans may find themselves with what they perceive as a serious need for more technology expertise. A decade ago, surveys of university programs and school clinicians indicated an extensive need for more and better opportunities to acquire such skills (McRay & Fitch, 1996; Walz & Cochran, 1996). School clinicians continue to report that instructional use of computers with students is an area in which they feel inadequately prepared (U.S. Department of Education, 2004). Clinicians want help learning to use computers effectively with the children and adults whom they serve. I hope this book addresses that need and inspires many clinicians to take the plunge into clinical computing.

WHAT THIS BOOK IS AND IS NOT

This book is designed to help pre-service and in-service clinicians learn how to use new technologies effectively in speech and language assessment and intervention activities.

The people who will benefit most from this book are speech-language pathologists, student clinicians, and people designing standards and educational opportunities related to technology skills for SLPs. Readers with intermediate word processing skills probably have enough computer expertise to be successful with the majority of clinical applications described in this book. There is no attempt here to provide a technical introduction to computers or administrative applications of computers. There are many excellent resources already widely available for getting such generic information and experience. I highly recommend the local library and an evening course at a local community college or vocational school for those who need an introduction to computers, word processing, and the Internet.

In fact, the focus of this book is not technology at all; the focus of this book is *how to use* technology. The distinction is as important as the difference between a book about cars and a book about how to drive. Surprisingly little understanding of car mechanics is prerequisite to being a good driver. Likewise, surprisingly little technical understanding is prerequisite to making effective use of technology for many clinical purposes. As clinical successes occur, a clinician's motivation and need to know increases, and that is the best time to acquire more technical expertise. So, this book isn't about which key to press or how much RAM to buy or where to click in a particular piece of software. That kind of information is short-lived and better acquired through direct instruction, online tutorials, and personal exploration. Instead, this book will help readers understand *why* clinicians should want to use computers in assessment and intervention, and *how* clinicians can use computers effectively in assessment and intervention.

Although issues related to augmentative and alternative communication (AAC) are discussed, especially in the assistive technology sections, the principles of good practice and the technical information needed by professionals implementing AAC are beyond the scope of this book. There are many outstanding resources available for developing expertise in AAC. Some recommendations are mentioned in Section VIII.

SOME LINGUISTIC CONCERNS

In an attempt to deal with the problem of gender and English pronouns, I have used "he" and "she" back and forth throughout the book to refer to clinicians, people in therapy, and so forth. This prevents the awkward he-or-she and him-or-her business, but means that in a particular sentence or example, only one gender will be represented. I would also like to draw attention to a few of the other linguistic conventions that have been employed.

In 1980, the World Health Organization defined *impairment* as "the loss or abnormality of psychological, physical, or anatomical structure or function." It went on to contend that a *disability* results "when an impairment leads to an inability to perform an activity in the manner or within the range considered normal for a human being." The third in this trio of terms, *handicap*, results "when an individual with an impairment or disability is unable to fulfill his or her normal role." In this sense, then, a handicap is a description of the relationship between a person and the environment and not a characteristic of a person. A person with an impairment might be handicapped in some circumstances and not in others, depending on the presence of aides and other factors. This seems to be a reasonable way to employ these terms and this is how they are used in this book. Note, however, that when these words appear within a law or regulation, they usually do not carry such nuances.

Professionals who help people improve their communication skills include speech-language pathologists, teachers, special educators, and other health care providers. In this book, I use *speech-language pathologist* and *clinician* interchangeably to refer to professionals whose specialty is communication disorders and who work in all settings.

Now we come to labels for persons who receive the services of a speech-language pathologist. Clinicians who work in schools refer to them as "students," clinicians who work in clinics say "clients," and clinicians in medical settings usually refer to "patients." Please think of your own students, clients, or patients as you read this book, and substitute the term that seems most natural to you. The principles of clinical management and the clinical applications of computers presented herein should be useful to clinicians in all settings.

The discretionary time of working clinicians and student clinicians is scarce and valuable. I hope that every minute spent with this book is worth it and that it inspires many clinicians to try using new technologies with clients. Together we will spread the word about clinical computing.

For my grandmother, Marguerite Peacock Slagle, who loved books

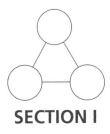

SECTION I

Clinical Computing Competency

The Big Picture

Clinical Computing Competency versus Computer Literacy

Early in the history of educational computing, Seymour Papert wrote *Mindstorms: Children, Computers, and Powerful Ideas* (Papert, 1980). It became a best seller because it described a vision of the future focused not on technological details, but on the philosophy of putting the power of computers into the hands of young minds. At the time, "small" computers were the size of refrigerators and the price of luxury automobiles. Nevertheless, Papert made what was a startling prediction: some day every classroom would have a computer, if not every child. People would have access to computers as tools for their own mental explorations, the way they had long used pencils for doodling. The notion of widespread access to computing power was mind-boggling a generation ago; with the advent of hand-held computers, we are seeing Papert's prediction come true, the way our parents and grandparents saw the technologies of telephones, automobiles, and televisions become ubiquitous.

The story of computers infiltrating our personal and professional lives is not finished; on the contrary, it has barely begun. Describing a set of skills related to tools that continue to change so rapidly may seem premature. However, our clients have needs now, some of which can be uniquely addressed by available technology. Clinicians must become aware of the many possibilities, and competent at using the best available assessment and intervention tools.

HOW IS CLINICAL COMPUTING COMPETENCY DIFFERENT FROM COMPUTER LITERACY AND COMPUTER PROGRAMMING?

Usually lists of computer-related skills developed to guide "computer literacy" courses and workshops focus on the technology itself. For example, a typical computer literacy checklist might include being able to identify and label parts of the computer, turn it on and off, "boot" or load software, save files, copy files, and print documents. Alternatively, some early introductions to computers ignored all such practical matters and focused exclusively on theory and technical knowledge such as binary code, programming languages, flow-charts, and data structures.

Although it may seem surprising now, word processing was primarily a mainframe computer activity when discussions of computer competencies for clinicians began. At the 1985 *Leadership Conference in Technology* sponsored by the American Speech-Language-Hearing Foundation, many acknowledged the importance of clinicians learning to encode their own computer programs. In fact, clinicians might be very surprised to learn that a hot topic was which computing language should be taught first as an introduction to programming: BASIC, Logo, PILOT, or FORTRAN. The focus on computer programming at that time was partly in response to extremely limited software availability. Some computer enthusiasts still believe that computing competencies for speech-language pathologists and audiologists should include, at least, principles of basic software design and knowledge of an authoring language.

Computer programming for clinicians is beyond the scope of this book. The skills that a clinician would require in order to independently design new computer applications or make significant modifications in the code for existing ones are beyond those required for basic clinical computing competency. Consider the following analogy: some clinicians find advanced musical training and singing ability clinically useful. Some clinicians hone their drawing skills and employ them in the design and development of original therapy materials. This does not mean that all effective clinicians must develop advanced musical or artistic skills. Similarly, some clinicians will pursue and enjoy advanced technical understanding and computer programming skills. Although they are beneficial, such skills are not prerequisite for making effective clinical use of a computer.

The clinical computing competencies outlined in this book emphasize the importance of learning how to use technology and applications to meet professional needs, rather than merely acquiring information about computers in the abstract. In particular, the emphasis is on how to use computers during assessment and intervention activities with a wide variety of clients. Excellent applications exist for use in articulation therapy, voice therapy, fluency therapy, language therapy, and diagnostic activities. Clinical computing competence involves much more than just knowing how to run such software (Cochran, 1989). Ten recommended competencies for clinicians are outlined in Topic 2.

If a clinician working with a student or patient forgets which key to press or how to hook up the printer (a failure of *computer literacy*), what is the worst possible consequence? Potentially, some therapy time will be wasted while the client and clinician try again or joke about the error; at worst, the activity might be abandoned for that day. All in all, the consequences are unfortunate, but relatively minor.

Compare this to the situation that results if a clinician operates a software program perfectly but misunderstands the limitations or advantages inherent in the computer application he is using with a student or patient. In other words, the role of the computer in the session is not clearly understood (a failure of *clinical computing competence*). For example, imagine that a clinician presents a software game during which a child is supposed to practice /r/ production. The child loves the game and seems to enjoy therapy sessions more than ever. The child, however, is so busy thinking about how to spell words for the game that very few oral /r/ productions occur. What if this low response rate persists for an entire activity, a session, or possibly a week or two of sessions? This scenario presents more serious potential for underutilizing resources, wasting time, inaccurately judging client performance, or failing to meet the goals of therapy.

CLINICAL COMPUTING COMPETENCY AS AN ESSENTIAL PROFESSIONAL SKILL

A national survey of 452 public school speech-language pathologists found that 31% made use of computers at least weekly, especially for administrative purposes such as word processing reports (McRay & Fitch, 1996). Many respondents, however, noted that they felt ill prepared to make effective use of computers and other new technologies for evaluation and treatment of their students and clients. More than 95% of the respondents indicated that they needed more technology training, with 71% considering their training needs to be from moderate to extensive (McRay & Fitch, 1996). Other surveys in education suggest that although computers and Internet access are available in virtually all schools and most classrooms, fewer than 30% of educators feel well prepared to integrate technology into instruction (CEC Today, 2002; Cradler, Freeman, Cradler, & McNabb, 2002).

Because most clinicians and teachers are already making extensive use of applications such as word processing and e-mail, sufficient traditional computer literacy content has presumably been mastered. In other words, most clinicians have access to computers and few require basic information about how a computer works or how to accomplish basic functions such as saving or printing a document. Instead, many clinicians still need models of how to use computers with their clients and students. With the advent of Internet-based health care services (telepractice), understanding the strengths and limitations of computer-based therapy activities becomes even more essential.

It is the purpose of this book to inform clinicians about research regarding clinical computer applications, to provide examples and models of how others have used new technologies effectively, and to encourage clinicians to explore new ways of using computers for the benefit of their clients. Minimal information about computers in general is included here. Many clinicians will be relieved to know that they will not be required to become technology experts in order to achieve clinical computing competency. In fact, clinical computing competency depends more on clinical judgment than technical expertise. Certainly, good clinicians who have minimal technical skills will achieve clinical computing competency more easily than computer experts who have minimal clinical skills.

That said, it should not be assumed by training programs and credentialing agencies that appropriate clinical use of computers is intuitive. Although advanced technical knowledge about computers is not required for most applications, there is much to be learned about legal and ethical considerations that apply to the clinical use of technology, various roles that computers can play in clinical practice, the important functions of assistive technology, and how clinicians can facilitate the success of their clients while using computer-based therapy activities.

In its requirements for professional certification, technology competency is encouraged by ASHA. The words "assistive technologies" are included under Communication Modalities in the Knowledge and Skills Acquisition summary used to document the competence of certification candidates. The term "assistive technology" in ASHA documents, however, refers primarily to augmentative and alternative communication (AAC) and assistive listening devices (e.g., ASHA, 1997). From 2001 through 2003, ASHA declared the Internet and telepractice to be a "focused initiative" of the association, which helped to acknowledge the ways that clinicians use on-line technology. To date, however, no specific technology-related skills or knowledge have been recommended or required of clinicians receiving a Certificate of Clinical Competence from ASHA. Many accredited programs in communication disorders do not yet regularly offer or require coursework or practicum opportunities specifically related to computer use, assistive technology, or AAC. It is interesting to compare this situation to the stronger emphasis on knowledge and expertise in the areas of computer use and a much more broadly defined notion of "assistive technology" promoted by other education and rehabilitation professions and organizations.

Nearly a decade ago, a task force of the American Occupational Therapy Association (AOTA), developed a hierarchy of technology competencies for occupational therapists (Hammel & Angelo, 1996). The competencies emphasized improvement of client function and included knowledge of "basic and complex levels" of technology and service delivery issues related to evaluation, implementation, and resource coordination.

Subsequently the NASDSE Research Institute for Assistive and Training Technologies (RIAT) developed a series of on-line courses that could be taken to earn Competency Certificates, continuing education units (CEUs), or undergraduate and graduate credit from universities around the country. A basic technology competency certificate was complemented by eight specialty area certificates, including a "Communication Certificate," targeted for school-based speech language pathologists. The Rehabilitation Engineering and Assistive Technology Society of North America (RESNA) web site maintains a listing of professional development opportunities and courses for rehabilitation professionals across areas of expertise, such as physical therapists, occupational therapists, educators, engineers, and speech-language pathologists. One example is the California State University at Northridge ATACP certificate program described in Topic 41. Completion of a certificate program paired with professional experience may contribute to an individual's preparation for undertaking RESNA's ATP, ATS, or CRE/CRET credentialing process.

The *2001 Council for Exceptional Children (CEC) Performance-Based Standards for Accreditation and Licensure* of special educators include specific knowledge and skill standards regarding the use of technology. Examples of standards that beginning special educators are expected to meet include the following: "Use appropriate adaptations and technology for all individuals with disabilities;" "Select, design, and use technology, materials and resources required to educate individuals whose disabilities interfere with communication;" and "Use technology to conduct assessments" (CEC, 2004).

The International Society for Technology in Education (ISTE) has prepared standards for students and instructional personnel in schools. The National Education Technology Standards for Teachers (NETS)(ISTE, 2000) has presented a comprehensive profile of performance indicators for teachers that goes well beyond traditional training models focused on computer mechanics and productivity software. The NETS profiles serve as a model for teacher preparation programs and state education agencies that have stipulated technology literacy standards for licensure or teaching certification. In many cases, school-based speech-language pathologists and occupational and physical therapists must satisfy these requirements. It would be desirable if comparable but specialized competencies, incorporating reference to assistive technology, were implemented for all related service personnel. Toward this end, this book presents an introduction to clinical computing competencies for speech-language pathologists. Clinical computing competency is an ideal professional goal for both student clinicians and in-service clinicians. As is seen in Topic 2, competency can be achieved by choosing specific objectives that can be tailored to match a clinician's individual needs and technology resources.

SUMMARY

The notion of clinical computing competency presented in this book stresses the importance of adding technology to a firm foundation of good clinical practice. All clinicians forget which key to press now and then. But clinicians with clinical computing competence always know why they brought the computer into the therapy room in the first place.

Many technology training standards and computer literacy checklists have placed undue emphasis on hardware-specific procedures and computer technology in the abstract. For more than 20 years, professionals, organizations, and university training programs related to communication disorders have been exploring the potential clinical applications of computers. Nevertheless, according to surveys of working professionals, there remains a critical need for more training and practicum opportunities involving the use of computers to enhance clinical practice. The purpose of this book is to help preservice and in-service clinicians identify and obtain the clinical computing competencies that will best serve their clients and their careers.

REVIEW FOR TOPIC 1

1. What kinds of topics are usually included in computer literacy checklists and workshops?
2. At this point, how would you define (briefly) clinical computing competency?
3. Explain the relationship between computer programming and clinical computing competency.
4. List three other professions for whom assistive technology, or the use of computers with persons who have special needs, is an important area of expertise.

QUESTIONS FOR DISCUSSION

1. Consider Papert's notion about using the computer as a tool with which to think. What do you think this experience would be like?
2. When you have to write something important, what is your method of creating a first draft? Do you use traditional pencil and paper, or do you compose at a computer? How has this changed during your life as a writer? Why?
3. How is it possible for a clinician to be highly computer literate and not possess clinical computing competency? Is the reverse also possible?

RESOURCES FOR FURTHER STUDY

American Speech-Language-Hearing Association. (1997). *Maximizing the provision of appropriate technology services and devices for students in schools: Technical report.* Rockville, MD: Author. (Also available online at ASHA's web site in Volume IV of the Online Desk Reference. www.asha.org.)

Cochran, P.S., & Masterson, J.M. (1995). NOT using a computer in language assessment/intervention: In defense of the reluctant clinician. *Language, Speech, and Hearing Services in Schools, 26*(3), 213–222.

International Society for Technology in Education. (2000). *National educational technology standards for teachers.* Eugene, OR: Author. (Also available: http://cnets.iste.org/.)

Masterson, J.J. (1995). Computer applications in the schools: What we *can* do—what we *should* do. *Language, Speech, and Hearing Services in Schools, 26*(3), 211–212.

Masterson, J.J. (1999b). Preface: Technological advances for speech-language interventions. *Seminars in Speech and Language, 20*(3), 201–202.

Ten Recommended Clinical Computing Competencies

The clinical computing competencies outlined here reflect the current state of technology in speech-language pathology and may be used to guide curriculum revisions, software and hardware acquisition, continuing education events, or personal learning plans. Hardware-related information is de-emphasized not because hardware-related knowledge is entirely unimportant, but because operation and maintenance of computer components is brand-specific and tends to change with each product generation. Opportunities for acquiring an introduction to computers and basic business applications are available through local community colleges, vocational-technology programs, public libraries, and public schools and universities. However, help learning how to use computers for their specific professional needs is not readily available to many clinicians.

The competencies that follow are divided into two types. The first six deal with delivery of speech-language services directly to clients. This book emphasizes these six competencies, because resources to help clinicians learn about using computers in assessment and intervention are most needed at this time. The last four competencies deal with speech-language-hearing program development and management. These competencies benefit clinicians in any work setting, and are even appropriate goals for audiologists and others in fields related to health care or education.

These ten competencies require clinicians to evaluate and understand the various roles that computers can play in their professional activities. Most clinicians will be surprised at the diversity and efficacy of computer applications that are available for their use. It is crucial for clinicians to have a framework or model of clinical computing in mind as new technologies appear. With a clear idea of what roles the computer might play, especially in assessment or intervention, clinicians are better able to evaluate the merits of new applications and new efficacy research.

It is important to note the omission of augmentative and alternative communication (AAC) from the recommended competencies. Many of the competencies and activities discussed in this book are useful to clinicians in the practice of providing AAC. However, direct consideration of the principles of good practice and the technical information needed by professionals implementing AAC are beyond the scope of this book. Clinicians will find extremely helpful related information in Section VIII. Section VIII is designed to help clinicians achieve competency number 7, and includes the basic information about assistive technology across work settings that all clinicians should know.

WHAT IF I DON'T HAVE ACCESS TO THE LATEST TECHNOLOGY?

Establishing guidelines for technology-related skills is like shooting at a moving target. The ten clinical computing competencies that follow, however, have already stood the test of time. It is unlikely that they will quickly become outdated because they are based on good clinical practice, not on the details or idiosyncrasies of today's computers. Therefore, clinicians can and should aspire to these competencies even if they lack access to cutting-edge computer technology or technical support. Any clinician with regular access to any computer can work on these competencies. Each competency can be accomplished through the attainment of more specific objectives. Objectives guiding specific skill development must be developed individually, because the use of technology depends on available resources in the form of hardware, software, and technical expertise. Sample objectives for each competency are provided that reflect a range of resources. These specific skills are meant only as examples of objectives that clinicians can define locally or individually and modify as their resources change.

TEN CLINICAL COMPUTING COMPETENCIES FOR SPEECH-LANGUAGE PATHOLOGISTS

1. Using a Computer as an Instructor

Competency: The clinician will demonstrate the ability to choose, configure, and evaluate appropriate computer-assisted instruction (CAI) activities for independent use by clients.

Examples of specific objectives that should be modified to reflect local circumstances and resources:

- The clinician will choose appropriate drill-and-practice or tutorial software for client use, based on the abilities of the client and previously established communication goals.

- By changing default options in the software (e.g., speed of presentation, number of trials, type or content of stimulus, availability of hints, method of input), the clinician will personalize a computer-based lesson to be used independently by a client.

- The clinician will evaluate the success of a CAI lesson not only according to the performance of the client during the computer activity, but also according to evidence of generalization, carryover, or functional use of new skills.

2. Using a Computer as a Context for Conversation

Competency: The clinician will demonstrate ability to use computer-based materials to form a shared context for communication with clients.

Examples of specific objectives that should be modified to reflect local circumstances and resources:

- The clinician will select appropriate software and plan an appropriate activity based on intervention goals previously established for the client.

- The clinician will integrate a computer application effectively into therapy sessions by planning related pre- and post-computer activities.

- The clinician will provide appropriate language models and communication opportunities for the client as they use the computer together to accomplish a shared goal such as making a greeting card, writing a story, or playing a game.

- The clinician will plan and implement a computer-based activity for children who need to practice verbal negotiation and clarification skills.

3. Using a Computer as a Clinical Materials Generator

Competency: The clinician will take advantage of computer capabilities to generate personalized clinical materials to enhance intervention with specific clients.
Examples of specific objectives that should be modified to reflect local circumstances and resources:

- Using a software template designed to generate calendars, the clinician will create a calendar showing suggested daily homework activities for a client (e.g., carryover of /r/ sounds).

- From a collection of clip art or a symbol library, the clinician will create a symbol worksheet for use with a client who has limited literacy skills.

- Using a digital camera or scanner, the clinician will illustrate a class field trip book or bulletin board.

- Using graphical organization software, the clinician will help a client understand the "main idea" of a paragraph by developing a semantic web or concept map.

4. Using a Computer as a Feedback Device

Competency: The clinician will demonstrate the ability to plan and implement activities in which performance feedback to the client from the clinician is supplemented by feedback (visual and/or auditory) from the computer.
Examples of specific objectives that should be modified to reflect local circumstances and resources:

- The clinician will plan and implement procedures for helping a client establish appropriate pitch, using computer-based visual biofeedback.

- The clinician will plan and implement procedures for helping a client establish correct production of /s/ in isolation, using computer-based visual feedback.

- The clinician will plan and implement a series of activities using computer-based feedback to teach typical English intonation patterns to a speaker of English as a second language.

- The clinician will plan and implement activities for teaching long and short syllable contrasts to a child with a hearing loss, using visual feedback from computer-based speech analysis.

- The clinician will plan and implement activities for helping a dysfluent client establish easy onset using computer-based feedback.

- The clinician will be aware of the limitations of computer-based feedback and the importance of correct configuration and adjustment of computer-based therapy tools.

5. Using a Computer as a Clinical Data Assistant

Competency: The clinician will demonstrate the ability to use computer-assisted data management tools to document and facilitate client improvement.

Examples of specific objectives, which should be modified to reflect local circumstances and resources:

- With 95% accuracy, the clinician will use a computer-based record-keeping program to track the articulation behavior of a client during a 20-minute speech therapy activity.

- Using software designed to present stimuli at pre-set intervals, the clinician will evaluate and record responses during rate-reduction exercises with a client.

- The clinician will use computer-assisted graphing capabilities to chart the progress of a client.

- The clinician will help a client understand and use a computer-based reminder system to increase personal independence.

6. Using a Computer as a Diagnostic Tool

Competency: The clinician will make appropriate use of computer-based instruments designed to assist in the evaluation or diagnosis of communication disorders.

Examples of specific objectives that should be modified to reflect local circumstances and resources:

- The clinician will be aware of the strengths and weaknesses of computer-assisted speech or language sample analysis software.

- The clinician will correctly interpret the results of a computer-assisted test scoring protocol.

- The clinician will transcribe, enter, and code a language sample for computer-assisted analysis with at least 95% accuracy.

- The clinician will obtain a comprehensive analysis of a client's phoneme production skills through the use of a computer-based speech analysis program.

- The clinician will demonstrate correct implementation of a protocol for estimating habitual pitch using a computer-based voice analysis system.

7. Basic Computer Operations and Assistive Technology

Competency: The clinician will demonstrate the ability to complete basic computer operations, troubleshoot common problems, and use various assistive technology options to provide adapted computer access.

Examples of specific objectives that should be modified to reflect local circumstances and resources:

- The clinician will demonstrate the ability to access and operate software programs for administrative and/or clinical use.

- The clinician will demonstrate the ability to operate common peripheral devices, such as a printer, a scanner, and a digital camera.

- The clinician will use recommended practices in the care of and back-up of electronic storage media.

- The clinician will be familiar with a wide range of low-tech and high-tech assistive technology tools.

- The clinician will be aware of common adaptive access solutions and alternatives to regular keyboard and mouse control, such as speech recognition, keyguards, touch windows, and switches.

- The clinician will demonstrate the ability to operate standard software utilities (that come with system software), that make computer access easier for users with special needs.

8. Awareness of Technology-Related Legal and Ethical Issues

Competency: The clinician will demonstrate familiarity with legal and ethical considerations that apply to assistive technology and the use of computers in the management of communication disorders and will adhere to appropriate standards.

Examples of specific objectives that should be modified to reflect local circumstances and resources:

- The clinician will take equivalent, reasonable precautions to ensure the confidentiality of client records that are developed or maintained on any medium, including paper, personal computers, CD-ROM, networks, or any other format.

- The clinician will describe the technical and legal distinctions between copy-protected, copyrighted, licensed, shareware, and public domain software.

- The clinician will abide by current federal, state, and local laws, regulations, and policies governing the provision of assistive technology devices and services.

- The clinician will be aware of ethical considerations that pertain to providing services via electronic conferencing or other non–face-to-face configurations.

- The clinician will present a rationale for a policy pertaining to billing for time that clients spend in continuously supervised versus partially supervised or independently implemented computer activities.

9. Awareness and Use of Technology Resources

Competency: The clinician will demonstrate awareness of resources that provide continuing education, research results, technical support and information about availability, funding, efficacy, and efficiency of new clinical computing products as well as assistive technology devices and services.

Examples of specific objectives that should be modified to reflect local circumstances and resources:

- The clinician will be familiar with at least three regularly published sources for reviews of software and new technologies related to communication disorders and other special needs.

- The clinician will maintain a list of web sites and toll-free telephone numbers of technical assistance centers that focus on the needs of special populations.

- The clinician will make use of a web site or on-line database to obtain information about an assistive technology product.

- The clinician will use technologies such as e-mail, electronic journals, on-line discussion groups, video-conferencing, or other Internet resources as a means of continuing education and updating professional knowledge.

10. Using a Computer as a Productivity Tool

Competency: The clinician will increase and maintain personal productivity by using a computer for administrative purposes.

Examples of specific objectives that should be modified to reflect local circumstances and resources:

- The clinician will develop and revise computerized templates for generating diagnostic reports, cover letters, and treatment plans.

- The clinician will develop and maintain computer-based records of one or more of the following: billable hours, budget expenditures, or business expenses for tax purposes.

- The clinician will develop and maintain computer-based records of one of the following: locally available therapy materials and tests, possible short-term and long-term clinical objectives, client caseload information and re-evaluation schedule, or personal library of professional resources.

- The clinician will use a computer to access an electronic mail system, newsgroup, or web-based discussion group in order to interact with other professionals about clinical practices.

- The clinician will generate an individualized education program for a school-age client, using specialized software.

USING THESE COMPETENCIES AND THIS BOOK AS A BLUEPRINT

Clinicians should not be intimidated by the number or variety of clinical computing competencies. Of course it is desirable for clinicians to be knowledgeable about many computer applications, aware of ethical issues related to computer use, and familiar with technology-related professional resources. But these ten competencies represent an *ideal*, which may be attainable only for clinicians who have access to the entire range of computer applications and technical support. A particular clinician could have a much smaller subset of skills and resources and still have great success with particular software and a particular client.

Clinicians in some work settings may face professional certification or continuing education regulations that encourage or require them to obtain and document technology-related competencies. In many states, for example, public school personnel are being required to demonstrate certain computer skills in order to maintain their teaching certification. Working clinicians and student clinicians are encouraged to use the ten competencies as a guide for establishing and pursuing technology standards that are both appropriate and useful for professionals in speech-language pathology.

Table 2.1 shows where each competency is emphasized throughout the text. Using this table, clinicians may choose to focus on particular competencies in the order that best suits their needs and interests. Individual working clinicians could consider using the sections of this book as the basis for obtaining ASHA continuing education units (CEUs)

Table 2.1. Where to find content focused on each of the ten recommended clinical computing competencies

Competency	1	2	3	4	5	6	7	8	9	10
Topic 4	X									
Topic 5	X									
Topic 6	X									
Topic 7		X								
Topic 8		X								
Topic 9		X								
Topic 10		X								
Topic 11		X								
Topic 12		X								
Topic 13									X	
Topic 14								X		
Topic 15			X							
Topic 16			X							
Topic 17			X							
Topic 18			X							
Topic 19			X							
Topic 20								X		
Topic 21				X						
Topic 22				X						
Topic 23				X						
Topic 24				X						
Topic 25				X						
Topic 26									X	
Topic 27					X				X	
Topic 28					X					X
Topic 29									X	
Topic 30						X				
Topic 31						X				
Topic 32						X				
Topic 33						X				
Topic 34						X				
Topic 35								X		
Topic 36							X			
Topic 37								X		
Topic 38							X			
Topic 39							X			
Topic 40							X			
Topic 41								X	X	
Topic 42								X	X	
Topic 43								X	X	

through the Independent Study option. This option requires the participant to propose an independent study experience that is approved by a registered ASHA Continuing Education Provider (e.g., a university or agency). Each Independent Study proposal can be awarded up to .2 CEUs. The ASHA web site explains this procedure and lists approved CE providers.

The format of the book facilitates its use as a framework for a series of independent studies or workshops. For example, a clinician could use the title and competency at the beginning of each topic as the title and goal for her independent study, and the exercises and discussion questions at the end as part of her study's evaluation. It is recommended that the clinician add a hands-on component that matches his or her individual access to resources and technical support. The clinician should try some of the activities described in the topic and have the opportunity to demonstrate competency. As topics are completed, additional independent study plans can be proposed (note that plans must be approved and submitted in advance to obtain ASHA CEUs).

A similar approach could be adopted by small groups of clinicians, school systems, or even state organizations. The framework for a strong continuing education program focused on technology is provided. A committee might choose to focus CE efforts for the year, for example, on using computers to assist with diagnostics (Section VII). The topics in Section VII could be divided among participants for them to "present" at later meetings, guest speakers could be invited, a panel discussion could be organized, demo discs and videotapes could be requested from software publishers, or hands-on workshops could be sponsored to help clinicians get the information and experience they need.

SUMMARY

Ten clinical computing competencies for speech-language pathologists are proposed. The competencies address the awareness of relevant legal and ethical issues; awareness of technology resources, basic hardware functions; and assistive technology; use of computers to increase personal productivity; use of the computer as a diagnostic tool, as a context for conversation, as an instructor, and as a feedback system; use of a computer to generate clinical materials; and use of a computer to record and track clinical data. These competencies can be accomplished in a number of ways, the specifics of which depend on each clinician's clinical opportunities and access to technology resources.

In pursuit of clinical computing competency, clinicians (or course instructors) will need to develop more individualized or focused objectives based on their own access to resources and technical support. The competencies outlined in this topic are accompanied by multiple examples of such focused objectives. Each of the remaining topics in this book is organized to illustrate the competencies by looking at particular applications of computers in more depth.

REVIEW FOR TOPIC 2

1. In the clinical computing competency list, why are the specific objectives listed under each goal intended only to be examples rather than the actual skills every clinician should work on?

2. Why are goals related to AAC not included in this competency list?
3. Why does this book focus on the first six competencies?

QUESTIONS FOR DISCUSSION

1. Rank the ten major competencies in order according to your personal goals and interests at this time.
2. What will you need to obtain or do in order to make sure that you achieve the top three competencies on your list?
3. Look through the latest convention program preview or schedule for the annual convention of the American Speech-Language-Hearing Association (ASHA). List the titles of 5–10 computer-related presentations or workshops. Which competencies could you work on if you attended this ASHA convention?

Author's note: The competencies described in this topic are adapted from those initially proposed in *Asha* magazine (Cochran, Masterson, Long, Katz, Seaton, Wynne, Lieberth, & Martin, 1993). They have held up well, but examples and specific objectives have been updated to reflect technology changes. I repeat my thanks to the many early technology innovators who inspired this framework for thinking about clinical computing competency, especially Glen L. Bull.

RESOURCES FOR FURTHER STUDY

Cochran, P.S., & Bull, G.L. (1992). Computer-assisted learning and instruction. In J. Rassi & M. McElroy (Eds.), *The education of audiologists and speech-language pathologists* (pp. 363–386). Timonium, MD: York Press.

Cochran, P.S., Masterson, J.J., Long, S.H., Katz, R., Seaton, W., Wynne, M., Lieberth, A., & Martin, D. (1993). Computing competencies for clinicians. *Asha, 35*(8), 48–49.

International Society for Technology in Education. (2002). *National educational technology standards for teachers: Preparing teachers to use technology.* Eugene, OR: Author.

Getting Started

Principles for Integrating Computers Into Intervention

Some readers will want immediate advice about using computers with clients. That is the purpose of this topic. Specific clinical examples and strategies for particular kinds of applications and clients are discussed in later topics. The principles that follow are at the heart of the view of clinical computing competency described throughout this book.

USE COMPUTER-BASED ACTIVITIES FOR MORE THAN JUST A REWARD

Many clinicians use a computer activity as an after-you-do-the-real-work reward. The fact is, such bribery often works—the lure of the computer is strong enough to keep a child or adult with a communication disorder participating through less interesting therapy routines until finally the clinician declares "Enough!" The positive effect of computers on the motivation of learners with and without special needs has often been described (Bull, Cochran, & Snell, 1988; Lepper, 1985; Meyers, 1984; Shriberg, Kwiatkowski, & Snyder, 1989). However, although the use of a computer as a simple reward is not a sin, it is a waste. Why not use the computer for the "real work" and let that be a motivating and interesting experience, too?

Plan for Success

Any clinician who has been using administrative software for tasks such as word processing, already knows enough to be technically proficient with 90% of the software recommended for most diagnostic and therapy purposes. This is *not* to say that there is little to learn about computer applications in communication disorders or that appropriate use of computers is usually intuitive. However, to get started using a computer activity with most clients, very little understanding about computers is required. What predicts the success of such an activity is not the clinician's *computer* expertise, but rather her *clinical* expertise.

The most important guidelines for planning effective computer-based therapy activities will sound familiar to most clinicians, regardless of whether they use computers (see Table 3.1). The impact of these three guidelines cannot be overemphasized. Failure to follow through on one or more of these tenets of good clinical practice is responsible for most of the problems with computer activities that novice clinicians or computer users experience.

Table 3.1. Guidelines for planning computer-based activities

Choose appropriate therapy objectives based on the client's current communication abilities and other developmental factors such as motor control or academic skills.

Preview software and plan how specific speech or language target behaviors will be modeled and practiced during the activity.

Plan for carryover to contexts and situations beyond the initial activity.

Avoid Common Pitfalls

To ensure that a computer-based language therapy activity is effective, it is important not only to prepare the activity, but also to plan specifically how the activity will address the client's communication needs. Computer activities excite and motivate many children and adults. However, it is important to remember that just because a client enjoys a computer activity and asks to do it again does not mean that target communication goals are successfully being addressed.

It is fairly easy to lose track of therapy objectives, especially when using software that is flexible and open-ended. For example, it can be all too easy to let a speech or language therapy activity accidentally turn into a silent hunt-and-peck session (*"Which letter comes next?"* or *"Can you find the first letter in your name?"*). There is nothing inherently wrong with having a client find the letters in his name if such literacy skills are established goals; however, there may be a problem if this task becomes time-consuming and is irrelevant to the primary goal of practicing velar sounds in the initial position of words. In the course of an enjoyable computer-based activity, attention may unintentionally focus on typing, spelling, or computer literacy (*"This is the CD-ROM. That is the enter key."*).

The following strategies will help prevent instruction from going astray:

- Set therapy objectives before choosing materials (choose computer-based materials only when they are appropriate for the language level and abilities of the client).

- Plan pre- and post-computer activities that facilitate generalization.

- Thoroughly preview software before attempting to use it in therapy; consider any special configuration or modifications that will help maintain the focus on your goals.

- Periodically video and/or audiotape sessions that include computer activities, or have another experienced clinician observe the session and make recommendations.

Clinicians are encouraged to give computer-based activities a try, even if the outcome is uncertain. At first, try something with an "easy" client who is comfortable with new experiences and procedures in therapy. After some experience at that level, go on to more challenging applications for less predictable clients.

The emphasis on planning may sound like using a computer in therapy will take too much preparation time for most clinicians. Although previewing software and planning therapy activities may seem time-consuming at first, clinicians soon find they are saving time with computer activities. Computer-based activities can instantly put hundreds of words or pictures sorted by target sound at the fingertips of the clinician. Once the software is familiar, clinicians often think of many activities and clinical applications, so the initial time investment pays off several times over. And, computer activities can compare favorably to traditional activities that are equally interesting and beneficial for clients, but

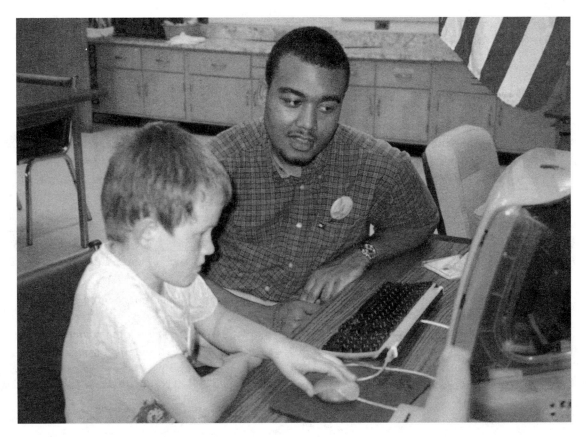

Figure 3.1. Example of three-way interaction between client, computer, and clinician.

have high overhead in time or resources. Computer-based language therapy activities can be engaging and motivating for clients.

SUMMARY

Clinicians who want to get started using computers with clients are encouraged to use the computer for the substantive activity of the session, not just as a reward. More about how to do this is presented throughout the remainder of this book. Planning is the key to the success of computer-based activities, especially for inexperienced clinicians or novice computer users. Common pitfalls to avoid include failing to choose appropriate therapy objectives before choosing a computer activity, getting distracted from therapy goals during a computer activity, and failing to preview software sufficiently. These problems can be minimized with planning and objective evaluation of sessions where new computer-based activities are attempted.

REVIEW FOR TOPIC 3

1. Is it wrong for clinicians to use computer activities as rewards? Why or why not?
2. How can common pitfalls be avoided?

3. How can clinicians get objective information about how their computer-based therapy activities are going?

QUESTIONS FOR DISCUSSION

1. A clinician new to using computers in therapy comes to a colleague and asks, "Do you have any good software for 4-year-olds?" What is wrong with this question?
2. A clinician starts a software program while her client watches. A demo automatically begins which takes several minutes and which loses the client's interest. The clinician decides to skip using a computer for that session. What advice would you give this clinician for future planning?

RESOURCES FOR FURTHER STUDY

Cochran, P.S., & Bull, G.L. (1991). Integrating word processing into language intervention. *Topics in Language Disorders, 11*(2), 31–48.

Musselwhite, C., & King-DeBaun, P. (1997). *Emergent literacy success: Merging technology with whole language for students with disabilities.* Park City, UT: Creative Communicating.

Steiner, S., & Larson, V.L. (1991). Integrating microcomputers into language intervention with children. *Topics in Language Disorders, 11*(2), 18–30.

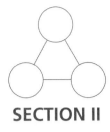

Using a Computer as an Instructor

Introduction to Using a Computer as an Instructor

Clinical computing competency #1: The clinician will demonstrate the ability to choose, configure, and evaluate appropriate computer-assisted instruction (CAI) activities for independent use by clients.

This competency requires clinicians to choose software that is appropriate for their individual clients. Clinicians who are competent will know how to preview the software, notice features or characteristics that might interfere with or facilitate client success, and understand how to assess the effectiveness of the client's work with the computer serving as an instructor. Competent clinicians will select communication goals for the client and then seek software appropriate for addressing those goals, recognizing the limitations that may be inherent in programs that control the sequence and structure of therapy activities.

In the early years of educational computing, people who were developing "programmed instruction" dominated the field. Their intent was to use the computer as a means of delivering instruction that previously had been conveyed by teachers or workbooks (hence, *computer-assisted instruction* or CAI). This is still the way most people envision using a computer in education, even though many effective alternatives exist. The image of the computer as a "teaching machine" is so strong that it continues to influence the design of much of the software developed for use during speech and language therapy. This topic introduces two common formats of CAI: tutorials and drill-and-practice. The essential features of CAI, the role of the clinician using CAI, and special considerations important to effective use of CAI are discussed in the following sections.

USING CAI AS A TUTORIAL

Before personal computers were available, attempts were made to produce programmed instruction on mainframe computers. Enormous investments of time, energy, and funds were dedicated to creation of "teaching machines" for college students. Although some projects claimed moderate success, the main goal—providing a stand-alone alternative to classroom instruction—was never widely achieved. The notion of a personal "tutor" that would be a learning partner for each student never fully evolved, even with the advent of more sophisticated technologies. On a smaller scale, some successful tutorial software has been developed for educational and business settings. At one time, it was estimated that one hour of good tutorial software required at least 1,000 hours to develop.

In a computer-based tutorial, the computer is in control of what is happening. New content is explained to the learner, and then learning is assessed. In tutorials designed for education, the learner is often required to pass a quiz at certain levels of proficiency before progressing to the next level in the tutorial. If the student is unsuccessful, the tutorial may be repeated as many times as needed. Individual performance records are kept by the computer and may contribute to a student's grade.

Many computer users are familiar with CAI from experience with the on-line tutorials that accompany complex software programs. Sometimes the user can control which part of a tutorial to view or skip or repeat, but otherwise there is generally little user control. Highly interactive tutorials—those which frequently require the learner to respond—are deemed more desirable than those that force the learner into a more passive role.

A popular example of software that includes a tutorial component is *A.D.A.M. The Inside Story*. *A.D.A.M.* is an award-winning CD-ROM that provides a general overview of the anatomy of the human body. Only certain parts of the CD have the traditional characteristics of a CAI program. Learners hear lecture material, view diagrams and animated examples, and then take optional quizzes to assess their learning. For example, a student chooses to learn about the respiratory system. Adam and Eve, the on-line guides, then present basic information in an amusing way and even demonstrate the effects of smoking and snoring.

Although there have been a few software tutorials especially related to communication disorders, most have been developed for university students rather than clients. They have included such content as speech and hearing anatomy, hearing aids, audiological testing and masking, the concept of decibel, and sign language. Most of these programs have failed to survive the frequent revolutions in hardware capabilities that occur. It is hard to recoup the investment in excellent small market CAI before the technology has changed so much that the format of the product—if not the content—renders it obsolete.

USING CAI AS DRILL-AND-PRACTICE

Practice makes perfect, or so we say. Researchers and software distributors evaluating tutorial software eventually realized that there was a great deal of overhead in developing computer programs that could actually provide instruction. The way learners acquire new information is highly individualized and often unpredictable. Software filling the role of an instructor must anticipate common errors and branch to provide review if necessary and informative feedback at the very least. Even if a perfect tutorial was developed, new information or technology changes could quickly date it. Developers of tutorials realized that the process of software development could easily become perpetual rather than profitable.

A less costly alternative is to focus on a single, isolated skill—such as adding 2-digit numbers—and just let the computer provide practice. Most often, such practice opportunities have a stimulus-response-reinforcement format. Always there is a clearly focused objective (e.g., identifying letters, punctuating sentences, identifying parts of speech). Usually there is a strong performance-tracking component. A clear advantage to drill-and-practice over tutorials is that such specific skills are rarely subject to theoretical revolutions, and the computer programming is easier—one branch for correct answers, one branch for wrong ones!

CASE EXAMPLE: Drill-and-Practice on Vocabulary Items

Computer display: Three numbered pictures showing a cow, a chair, and a truck.

Computer voice: *Which one is an animal? Show me the animal.*

Learner: (says nothing, but presses the #1 key or uses touch screen to select cow)

Computer display: Picture of cow blinks and a happy cartoon character appears.

Computer voice: *Yes, a cow is an animal.*

Note that in the example just described there is no explanation of the characteristics of animals versus vehicles versus furniture. In classic drill-and-practice software little or no effort is spent on teaching new information in a coherent context (Nippold, Schwarz, & Lewis, 1992). The focus is on practicing what has presumably been taught previously. It is important for teachers, parents, and clinicians to be aware of the limited intent of such software.

There have been many drill-and-practice programs developed especially for use by children and adults with communication disorders. Usually, the language content and objectives of such software are narrow in focus (e.g., labeling common objects, opposites, synonyms, noun categorization, or word associations). The specific instructional objectives are determined in advance by the software designers. The most frequently employed tasks come directly from common workbook and test formats. They include matching, multiple choice, and fill-in-the-blanks. Further discussion of the characteristics of CAI compared to other categories of instructional software can be found in Topic 13.

ROLE OF THE CLINICIAN

What is the role of the clinician while a client is using CAI? By design, drill-and-practice and tutorial software puts the computer in control of the activity. The clinician may be required to choose the initial settings of the program so that the client is working at the appropriate difficulty level, with the optimal stimulus type, number of trials, feedback conditions, and so forth. Then, however, the computer proceeds with its standard instructional sequence: present a stimulus, wait for a response, evaluate the response, and provide positive reinforcement or correction.

Determining how the clinician fits into this interaction is one of the challenges presented by CAI software when used during a therapy session. Typically, CAI promotes

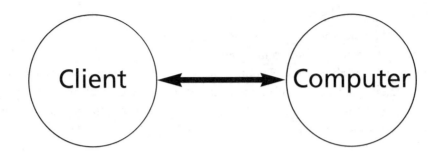

Figure 4.1. Traditiona CAI promotes two-way interaction between a c ient and the computer, without the input of a c inician.

two-way interaction between a client and the computer, rather than three-way interaction that includes the clinician (see Figure 4.1). It can be difficult for a clinician to participate in or guide this interaction within the constraints of pre-programmed questions, answers, and reinforcements.

Deciding Whether CAI Is Right for the Client

In order to use CAI effectively in a therapy situation, each clinician must work through the following questions:

1. Does this CAI focus exactly on the skill my client needs to practice?

2. If this is a drill-and-practice program, has my client received enough previous instruction about this content or skill?

3. Am I expecting this stimulus-response-reinforcement exercise to provide practice for my client that will carry over to real communication situations with people? Is this a reasonable expectation?

4. Can I provide motivation or reinforcement or feedback during this kind of an activity that is helpful and not just confusing when combined with what the computer is doing?

5. Is it easy for my client to talk during such activities? If not, are nonspeaking tasks congruent with my goals for this client?

6. If I elect to have my client use this software independently (without a qualified professional present) what improvements in communication can I reasonably expect?

Obviously, integrating CAI software into a long-range intervention plan presents significant challenges. Some clinicians will choose to explore alternative ways to use computers with their clients instead, because the nature of CAI does not match their clients' needs or their personal therapy style. Other clinicians may find that CAI gives their clients a much needed sense of independence, and that a good match between learning style and software is possible after all.

SUMMARY

Communication disorders have inherited the conceptual framework of computer-as-instructor or computer-assisted instruction (CAI) from educational computing. CAI may include tutorials or drill-and-practice software. Developing excellent tutorials that teach new content to a diverse group of users is time-consuming and expensive. A less costly, and therefore more common, alternative is drill-and-practice, in which a specific, narrowly-defined skill is rehearsed and tracked.

The use of CAI during therapy imposes a two-way interaction structure on the clinical activity. The client and the computer are interacting, but it can be difficult for a clinician to participate in or guide an activity in which the computer is controlling what will happen next. For this reason and others, many clinicians choose alternatives to CAI when using computers in speech and language therapy.

EXERCISES FOR TOPIC 4

1. What does the common abbreviation "CAI" mean?
2. What are the key features of tutorial software?
3. How do drill-and-practice and tutorial programs differ?
4. Why are there so few tutorials specific to communication disorders?
5. List three of the questions that a clinician must answer in order to ensure that using the computer as an instructor is a good choice for the client.

QUESTIONS FOR DISCUSSION

1. Recall any personal experiences you have had with CAI (independent use of a computer tutorial or drill-and-practice program). What were your feelings about this experience as a learner? How successful was CAI in meeting your needs?
2. Before reading this topic, if you heard the phrase "computer-assisted instruction" what would have come to mind? Draw a scene or model or diagram of what "CAI" should be in your view, if you were allowed to re-define the term.
3. In your experience, can people learn better *from* computers or *with* computers? Be prepared to discuss an example to support your opinion.

RESOURCES FOR FURTHER STUDY

Cochran, P.S., & Masterson, J.M. (1995). NOT using a computer in language assessment/intervention: In defense of the reluctant clinician. *Language, Speech, and Hearing Services in Schools, 26*(3), 213–222.

Katz, R.C., & Wertz, R.T. (1997). The efficacy of computer-provided reading treatment for chronic adult aphasics. *Journal of Speech and Hearing Research, 40,* 493–507.

Schwartz, A.H., Brogan, V.M., Emond, G.A., & Oleksiak, J.F. (1993). Technology-enhanced accent modification. *Asha, 35*(8), 44–45, 51.

Using Computer-Assisted Instruction (CAI) with Children

Clinical computing competency #1: The clinician will demonstrate the ability to choose, configure, and evaluate appropriate computer-assisted instruction (CAI) activities for independent use by clients.

Clinicians are likely to encounter software employing the CAI format, because it dominates the market. Competent clinicians will know how to choose appropriate tutorial or drill-and-practice software for client use, based on previously established communication goals. Clinicians should be able to change the default software settings to personalize activities with regard to factors such as stimulus type, number of trials, and type of feedback. The success of CAI must be measured not just in scores or percentages during a computer activity, but in observed improvement in communication.

WHAT DOES THE RESEARCH SAY ABOUT CAI AND YOUNG CHILDREN?

An early study of preschool children's use of computers gives insight into the importance of software design. Fazio and Rieth (1986) observed the free time choices of children in a preschool setting. They found that preschoolers with mild-to-moderate mental retardation chose to use the computer 70% of the time during free-choice periods, despite the presence of a wide variety of alternative activities. Peers who did not have mental retardation chose the computer 84% of the time. Both groups showed a marked preference for software considered learner-controlled rather than drill-and-practice in format. In other words, these preschoolers enjoyed being in control of the computer more than being "taught" by the computer.

This preliminary finding has since been supported by numerous studies of the use of computers with children. For example, Haugland (1992) found that preschool children who participated in a 24-week trial with classroom computer activities and used "developmental software" made significant gains in areas such as nonverbal skills, structural knowledge, and long-term memory. On the other hand, children who used "nondevelopmental software" during the same 24-week trial had significant gains in only one area—attention. The children who used nondevelopmental software also showed a significant decrease in creativity as measured by the researcher.

What is "developmental software"? Desirable characteristics of software chosen for use by and with young children include learner control over the activity, content and tasks that are age-appropriate, and instructional design that is consistent with the learning style of most young children. In other words, the software should offer children the opportunity to use it in an exploratory manner. Ideally, children should set their own learning pace and have unlimited opportunities for trial and error. Children's motivation to use the software should be intrinsic and based on their interest in finding out more about the possibilities inherent in the activity (see Haugland & Wright, 1997). A more detailed discussion outlining considerations for choosing software for use with young children is found in Topic 13.

Despite the evidence supporting the desirability of open-ended, exploratory, learner-controlled software, much of the software marketed for children with communicative disorders follows a distinctly different set of priorities more typical of CAI. This software is based on a stimulus-response-reinforcement learning paradigm in the classic CAI tradition. In such CAI, the learner completes a number of trials in which visual and auditory stimuli chosen by the software designer are used to elicit pre-determined responses. The computer provides feedback to indicate whether the response was correct once the user responds (usually by pressing a certain key or clicking in a certain place). Rarely are creativity or collaboration rewarded. The child may have to achieve a predetermined percent correct in order to proceed to another lesson because the software controls progression through the activities.

The effects of CAI on the language skills of children has yet to be thoroughly studied. Clements and his associates (Clements, 1987; Clements, Nastasi, & Swaminatha, 1993) observed that young children benefited from brief periods (10–15 minutes) of drill-and-practice with computer games that focused on specific skills. Their research assessed skills such as letter naming, sound–letter correspondence, and visual discrimination. In addition, children with a low level of prior knowledge in a skill area appeared to have greater difficulty using open-ended, exploratory software in an independent manner than children with greater initial knowledge (Clements et al., 1993). It is important to note that these studies did not focus on the needs or abilities of children with speech or language disorders. Also, they stressed children's independent (rather than adult-guided) use of computers. Unfortunately, most of the specialized drill-and-practice software designed to address goals such as vocabulary comprehension, concept development, and sentence formation, remains untested with special populations.

In an exploratory study of four children with language impairments ages 6.11 to 7.9, researchers documented the positive effect of intensive short-term use of CAI from Laureate Learning Systems (Gillam, Crofford, Gale, & Hoffman, 2001). In this study, two children had intensive exposure to *Fast ForWord* software, and two children had intensive exposure to a bundle of language intervention software from Laureate (approximately 140 minutes per day for 20 days over a 4-week period). According to the researchers, two children who received the Laureate software treatment and one who received *Fast ForWord* made clinically significant gains on mean length of utterance (MLU) in morphemes. One of the children receiving Laureate also had fewer grammatical errors after treatment. Although preliminary in nature, this is a hallmark study because it represents the first documentation of positive effects of independent use of CAI software in which crucial extraneous variables (e.g., clinician participation, subject selection) have been controlled, and in which behavior away from the computer (e.g., conversational language) was measured. Clinical trials of a larger scale remain to be done in order to explore questions such as which children are likely to benefit from such treatment and why.

Specialized drill-and-practice language software does not generally place high value on exploratory learning, flexibility, or creativity. For this reason and others, many clinicians give preference to other kinds of software for use with children in speech or language therapy. Alternatively, they investigate ways to use CAI software that increase its suitability.

Some CAI can be used as a group activity. For example, a clinician may want to use CAI such as *The Deciders Take on Concepts* (Thinking Publications, 2000) to reinforce basic concepts. In the example that follows, a pair of students is given the task of checking behind *all* (versus *some*) of the pieces of art in a museum scene. They must take turns controlling the mouse and finding the artwork. The "game" format of this drill-and-practice activity provides motivation, while the collaborative nature of the task arranged by the clinician requires using language to negotiate and explain (besides the concept reinforcement).

CASE EXAMPLE

Clinician:	*Okay Jenny and Kim, together you have to check behind all of the paintings to see if anything is hidden there.*
Computer display:	An art scene, in which an animated character is ready to help search.
Computer voice:	*Deciders, look behind* all *of the paintings now.*
Jenny:	*Here's one! Click there!* (Points to a painting in the scene)
Kim:	*Okay!* (Clicks on the painting)
Computer display:	Painting turns, revealing hidden musical notes.
Computer voice:	*Good work, Deciders. There may be more so check* all *the paintings.*
Jenny:	*Let me do one. We gotta do them* all.

CAI AND PHONOLOGIC AWARENESS

Phonologic awareness refers to a child's understanding of how sounds are combined to form syllables and words. For example, finding words that rhyme, clapping out the syllables of a word, or recognizing that a word begins with a certain sound are all activities that challenge and develop phonologic awareness. Research has consistently suggested a strong relationship between phonologic awareness and reading success. Computer activities can be an effective component in phonologic awareness instruction.

Torgesen and Barker (1995) evaluated the use of computer software to develop phonologic awareness skills in children with reading disabilities. The software activities provided instruction and practice in skills such as rhyme recognition, matching on initial consonants, matching on final consonants, blending words, and counting the number of sounds in words. The effect of instruction was measured with tasks designed to assess phonologic awareness as well as word identification and word analysis. The children who used the phonologic awareness software made greater gains than children who received traditional instruction or a control group who used math skills software.

With this research in mind, clinicians may want to work with parents and educators to facilitate phonologic awareness and emergent literacy in children with speech and language problems. Software such as *Simon Sounds it Out* (Don Johnston, Inc.) exemplifies CAI that presents phonics in a systematic way, focuses on sound–symbol relationships, and makes optimum use of digitized speech and animation to reinforce learning in a CAI format.

Software developers are responding to recent interest with new programs designed to help users of all ages acquire individual practice on phonemic awareness skills deemed most important for reading. Among the first of these to gain widespread attention and distribution is *Earobics* (Cognitive Concepts, Inc.). *Earobics* is CAI designed for individual use, although clinicians report using it with small groups of children as well (Masterson, 1999). *Earobics* consists of a series of games and puzzles that focus on rhyming, sound isolation and deletion, blending, and other phonemic awareness skills. Within the *Earobics* family of software, packages have been developed that are appropriate for various age levels (K–adult) and for home or professional use (see Figure 5.1). Professional versions allow for extensive individualization of activities so that focus on particular skills is possible in a therapy setting. Home versions are less flexible.

To date, the efficacy of *Earobics* software has been less studied than *Fast ForWord* (see discussion that follows) and more studied than most software available for use in speech or language therapy. Testimonials from parents, teachers, and clinicians on the Cognitive Concepts web site claim success with children and adults with a wide variety of learning problems and developmental disabilities. According to efficacy examples provided by Cognitive Concepts, in 1999 Bowden and Chalfonte-Evans did a controlled study of 18 children with Down syndrome using *Earobics*. Significant positive gains were found not only in phonemic awareness skills, but also in auditory word memory and receptive vocabulary, after 3 months (10–20 hours) of use.

CAI and Auditory Processing

Since its introduction, *Fast ForWord* (Scientific Learning, 1996) software has challenged the way many clinicians think about using computers with children. It began as a research tool in an investigation of the way children with language impairments hear and process spoken language (Merzenich, Jenkins, Miller, Schreiner, & Tallal, 1996; Tallal et al., 1996). Soon, *Fast ForWord* was released as a commercial product, accompanied by an extensive assessment and treatment protocol.

The developers of *Fast ForWord* theorize that language impairment in children results from an inability to process the rapidly changing auditory signals that make up speech. Using technology to manipulate the digitized speech in their software, the researchers

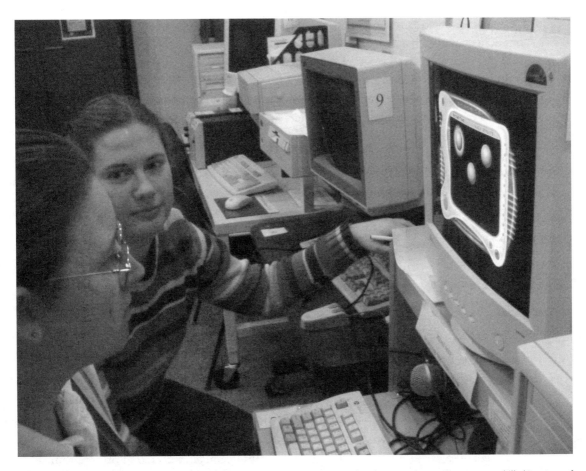

Figure 5.1. A clinician helps an adult use *Earobics* software (Cognitve Concepts) to improve phonemic awareness skills (Courtesy of Truman State university Speech and Hearing Clinic).

claim that they can make the speech signal easier to discriminate for persons who have this auditory processing deficit. In their treatment protocol, intensive exposure to their acoustically modified speech occurs through participation in computer-delivered drill and practice games (about 3 hours per day, 5 days per week, for 4 weeks in the first studies). The researchers claimed that improvement in language tasks results from improved auditory processing due to exposure to their acoustically modified speech and other auditory training tasks. In preliminary research trials, this intervention resulted in significant improvements on several standardized measures of language comprehension (Merzenich et al., 1996; Tallal et al., 1996). Since the original research, claims of dramatic positive impact on reading and other language skills have also been made on the corporate web site, in press releases, and in book chapters by the research team (Merzenich, Tallal, Peterson, Miller, & Jenkins, 1999; Tallal, 2000).

From the beginning, both the background research and the intervention program have received much media attention and sparked professional debate across several areas of expertise, including communication disorders, reading, and cognitive neuroscience (Brady, Scarborough, & Shankweiler, 1996; Rice, 1997). Experts have criticized the underlying research, including the basic theory of auditory processing deficit that it espouses (Bishop, Carlyon, Deeks, & Bishop, 1999; Thibodeau, Friel-Patti, & Britt, 2001).

Before and since the release of *Fast ForWord*, carefully designed research from many independent scientists has failed to corroborate the "rapid signal processing deficit" theory. It is important to consider the possibility that the dramatic improvements in test scores reported have occurred for reasons other than those claimed by the original developers.

Researchers have expressed many additional points of concern about the early *Fast ForWord* research published in peer-reviewed journals. These concerns include the nature and number of subjects selected for study and the measures used to assess change (standardized tests repeated at short intervals, scores reported in age equivalents rather than standard scores, and tests closely matching the software tasks in format). These concerns were directly addressed in the August 2001 issue of the *American Journal of Speech-Language Pathology*. A series of studies and articles from a total of 13 different authors contributed to this special forum. It is a mark of the impact of *Fast ForWord* and its proponents that they have drawn the attention of so many other language researchers. The studies considered the impact of *Fast ForWord* on language (Friel-Patti, DesBarres, & Thibodeau, 2001; Frome Loeb, Stoke, & Fey, 2001; Gillam, Crofford, Gale, & Hoffman, 2001), the influence of intervention setting (school, clinic, home) (Frome Loeb, Stoke, & Fey, 2001), impact on auditory processing (Marler, Champlin, & Gillam, 2001; Thibodeau, Friel-Patti, & Britt, 2001), and comparison to other computer-assisted instruction (Gillam, Crofford, Gale, & Hoffman, 2001). In a summary article, the authors stated,

> The collective results of our studies suggest that improvements in language abilities after [*Fast ForWord*] FFW training did not result from changes in temporal processing. It is possible that similar improvements in language may be obtained from a variety of interventions that are presented on an intensive schedule, that focus the child's auditory and visual attention, that present multiple trials, that vary task complexity as a function of response accuracy, and that reward progress. The validity of this hypothesis needs to be tested by large-scale randomized clinical trials. Only then can the efficacy of FFW be discussed with some confidence. (Gillam, Frome Loeb, & Friel-Patti, 2001, p. 73)

In addition to short-term efficacy, the long-term benefits of an intervention such as *Fast ForWord* are of interest to parents, teachers, and clinicians. According to reading specialists who completed a longitudinal study of *Fast ForWord*,

> The FFW group showed significant gains in phonemic awareness and in the spoken language areas of speaking and syntax immediately after treatment. However, gains made in spoken language were not maintained over two years, and progress in phonemic awareness and reading mirrored gains made over two years by a longitudinal control group that did not participate in FFW. Thus, benefits of participation in FFW for reading and spoken language were minimal. (Macaruso & Hook, 2001, pp. 7–8)

Clinicians and scientists have pointed out that the level of intervention intensity required in the *Fast ForWord* treatment protocol is unusual—in fact, few if any approaches to language therapy have been tested in this way. Claims that *Fast ForWord*'s results surpass traditional intervention, therefore, are premature. Nevertheless, many clinicians will testify to its efficacy, and it remains at this time one of the most notable examples of CAI ever designed and sold for clinical use.

SUMMARY

Much of the software marketed for children with communicative disorders incorporates the set of design features typical of CAI. This software is based on a stimulus-response-reinforcement learning paradigm in the classic CAI tradition. Although CAI software especially designed for use by children with communication disorders has been widely available since the early 1980s, little research documenting its efficacy has been published to date. This is a matter of concern because this software is primarily envisioned for independent use by children.

Researchers across several related fields have begun to investigate the claims made by one widely marketed CAI package called *Fast ForWord* (Scientific Learning). Some immediate positive gains were observed in some children in these preliminary studies, although long-term benefits were not substantiated. Researchers suggest that factors that may be important in accounting for and comparing the benefits of CAI packages may include intensity of the treatment schedule, appeal to auditory and visual attention, provision of multiple trials, varying task complexity, and reinforcement.

Values such as creativity, exploration, and flexible outcomes are rarely incorporated into CAI software. On the contrary, CAI is noted for specific objectives that focus on a particular receptive language task (similar to those found on a standardized language subtest). Some clinicians, therefore, will find CAI too limiting in their practice with young children. Other clinicians compensate for the limitations of CAI by using it in small groups, where interaction among participants is required.

REVIEW FOR TOPIC 5

1. Describe the learning paradigm that characterizes CAI.
2. What are the characteristics of software that is considered "developmental"?
3. Which language skills in young children does research suggest might be improved through the use of CAI?
4. Summarize the research regarding the efficacy of *Fast ForWord* to date.
5. How can a clinician facilitate oral interaction among children and also make use of CAI in therapy?

QUESTIONS FOR DISCUSSION

1. In your opinion, what standards should be used to determine whether or not a computer-based activity or intervention program is "effective"?
2. Visit the web sites for one or two of the software programs mentioned in this Topic. Discuss the claims made on the web sites and how a clinician could evaluate them before making software purchases. Are the web sites primarily aimed at professionals or parents?

RESOURCES FOR FURTHER STUDY

Cochran, P.S., & Masterson, J.M. (1995). NOT using a computer in language assessment / intervention: In defense of the reluctant clinician. *Language, Speech, and Hearing Services in Schools. 26*(3), 213–222.

Gillam, R.B., Frome Loeb, D., & Friel-Patti, S. (2001). Looking back: A summary of five exploratory studies of *Fast ForWord. American Journal of Speech-Language Pathology, 10*, 269–273.

Torgesen, J.K., & Barker, R.A. (1995). Computers as aids in the prevention and remediation of reading disabilities. *Learning Disability Quarterly, 18*, 76–87.

Using Computer-Assisted Instruction (CAI) with Adults

Clinical Computing Competency #1: The clinician will demonstrate the ability to choose, configure, and evaluate appropriate computer-assisted instruction (CAI) activities for independent use by clients.

Clinicians recommending the use of CAI by adolescents and adult clients should be aware of programs that directly address goals related to language and literacy, life skills, or education. Successful independent use of a computer by a client may require the clinician to change the default options of software such as speed of presentation, number of trials, type and content of stimuli, or feedback variables. The effect of CAI should be carefully assessed against specific communication and life skills goals.

There are many effective ways to use computers with adult clients who are working on improving speech or language skills. This topic offers suggestions to clinicians who want to use a computer as an instructor for an adult client. Recall from Topic 4: Introduction to Using a Computer as an Instructor, that there are several important questions to be considered before determining that CAI is the best option. CAI is usually designed so that the computer controls the sequence of instructional events and interaction is characterized by two-way communication between the computer and the individual user only. Therefore, CAI is primarily used in situations where interaction with a real conversational partner—such as a clinician or peer—is not crucial to the clinical objective. Alternatives that do include the participation of a conversational partner are described in Topic 12: Using a Computer as a Context for Conversation with Adolescents and Adults.

CHOOSE APPROPRIATE AND SPECIFIC COMMUNICATION OBJECTIVES

As with any other therapy activity, success depends on whether appropriate objectives are addressed by a CAI activity. Because one of the strengths of CAI software is record keeping, goals that involve specific right and wrong responses and that are validly measured in terms of percentage correct are the most appropriate choices. For example:

1. The client will unscramble and correctly spell words at his reading level with 85% accuracy or better.

2. The client will use capital letters and punctuate simple sentences with 80% accuracy or better.

3. The client will identify word opposites from among three choices in a silent reading task (no auditory cues) with 80% accuracy or better.

Several experimental studies have considered the independent use of computers by adults who have aphasia or traumatic brain injury (see, e.g., Katz, 1986; Katz & Wertz, 1997; Lynch, 1993; Mills, 1986). The computer has functioned successfully as an instructor when target behaviors involve improving literacy skills such as reading comprehension, spelling, or sight-word recognition.

Recall that during CAI, the computer is generally in control of the activity. Tasks have been designed to be completed independently by a learner, usually in a stimulus-response-reinforcement format. Goals intended for clients who will be making *independent* use of a computer should be written accordingly. The following goals for independent computer use illustrate this:

1. The client will independently complete a 10-minute spelling activity on the computer.

2. The client will complete a 15-minute reading comprehension activity on the computer, print the results, and file them in his folder with no more than two verbal cues.

The multi-disciplinary intervention plans for some adolescents and adults are designed to help them gain an increased sense of control and responsibility for their own rehabilitation. In such cases, independent use of computer applications capable of serving in the role of instructor may be particularly effective. In all situations, however, clients using computers should have access to competent people in case something goes wrong or becomes frustrating.

PREVIEW AND PERSONALIZE THE COMPUTER ACTIVITY

In most other types of computer-based therapy activities, the clinician will be present, tailoring the activity to the needs of the client as the activity progresses. During CAI, however, clinician control is minimal. Input from the clinician regarding content, difficulty level, number of trials, reinforcement, or success criteria usually comes prior to the activity, during software setup. It is crucial that clinicians take time to become familiar with all of the options available in CAI software, so that maximum personalization can occur. In addition, familiarization with the software ensures that the correct match between clinical goals and software selection has been made.

Rehabilitation centers and other clinical settings may have facilities for adults to use computers independently between sessions with therapists. Aides or volunteers may monitor computer lab facilities. When such computer use is part of a rehabilitation plan and

Table 6.1.   Educational software that provides practice with academic content or skills

Software title	Example activity
Earobics for Adolescents and Adults (Cognitive Concepts)	Phonemic awareness, word games
Aphasia 4: Reading Comprehension (Parrot) *AphasiaTutor* (Bungalow)	Reading comprehension
Picture Categories (Parrot)	Matching picture to written word
MoneyCoach (Parrot)	Number concepts and basic math

is intended to improve communication skills, clinicians should be involved. Clinicians should preview and customize software and directly supervise clients who are trying new software for the first time.

Clinicians, and others who serve as assistants, must guard against instances in which the computer misjudges the client's response. When this happens, the client receives misleading feedback.

CASE EXAMPLE: Client Using CAI Receives Confusing Feedback

Computer displays text and says aloud: *How many eggs are in a dozen?*

Client types: l2 [lower case "L" and number 2]

Computer display and voice: *No, there are 12 eggs in a dozen.*

Client has puzzled look on her face.

In this example, the client knew the correct answer but typed a combination of letters and digits that the computer did not recognize as correct. This shows why even clients using appropriate software to address appropriate goals should have access to competent personal assistance at all times.

CREATE GENUINE OPPORTUNITIES FOR CARRYOVER

All skills that are practiced at the computer using CAI should also be practiced in more realistic contexts. For example, if it is important for a client to learn to spell on the computer, there must also be frequent opportunities to use this skill in tasks that have authentic purpose in the client's life. Such tasks might include making a grocery list or writing a phone message. Computer-based activities for adults that involve conversation and interaction with others are discussed in Topic 12.

CONSIDER A VARIETY OF CAI SOFTWARE FOR USE WITH ADULT CLIENTS

Tables 6.1 and 6.2 list examples of CAI software that could be used to address either educational/vocational goals or specialized language goals.

Table 6.2. Specialized language software for language therapy

Software title	Example activity
My Town (Laureate)	CAI: match community vocabulary pictures/words
Functional Vocabulary Plus (Parrot)	CAI: choose best description of a picture
Sorting by Category (Parrot)	CAI: read and sort words into categories
Nouns and Sounds (Parrot)	CAI: match pictures to sounds/speech
Opposites and Similarities (Parrot)	CAI: find word pairs

SUMMARY

The effective use of CAI with adolescents and adults begins with the selection of appropriate goals. This kind of computer activity, when conducted independently, rarely provides opportunity for oral communication. CAI, therefore, is usually more appropriate for goals targeting receptive language or literacy. Clinicians can increase the likelihood that CAI will be effective by choosing appropriate goals, previewing and personalizing the computer program, and creating opportunities for carryover of new skills away from the computer. Clinicians should consider a variety of software that focuses on academic/educational content as well as CAI software that has been especially designed for practicing for persons with speech and language disorders.

REVIEW FOR TOPIC 6

1. List three things clinicians should do to increase the efficacy of CAI with adolescents and adults.
2. What are some of the parameters of a CAI activity that a clinician can often control through choosing the correct software setup options?
3. Why is it important for clinicians to be familiar with all CAI software used by their clients for language therapy purposes?
4. Why is it important for clients to have access to a person who can answer questions at all times during their use of CAI?

QUESTIONS FOR DISCUSSION

1. Some rehabilitation clients may need to learn to function more independently. In your opinion, how might computer-based activities be helpful to such a client?
2. Research has shown that using CAI targeted at literacy skills can benefit even persons with chronic aphasia. How could a clinician assess the carryover of such an intervention?

RESOURCES FOR FURTHER STUDY

Katz, R.C., & Hallowell, B. (1999). Technological applications in the treatment of acquired neurogenic communication and swallowing disorders in adults. *Seminars in Speech and Language, 20,* 251–269.

Katz, R.C., & Wertz, R.T. (1997). The efficacy of computer-provided reading treatment for chronic adult aphasics. *Journal of Speech and Hearing Research, 40,* 493–507.

Lynch, W. (1993). Update on a computer-based language prosthesis for aphasia therapy. *Journal of Head Trauma Rehabilitation, 8,* 107–109.

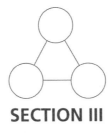

Using a Computer as a Context for Conversation

Introduction to Using a Computer as a Context for Conversation

Clinical Computing Competency #2: The clinician will demonstrate the ability to use computer-based materials to form a shared context for communication with clients.

Acquiring this clinical computing competency requires skills in choosing appropriate software, integrating it effectively into therapy, and ensuring that the computer activity directly addresses the goals chosen for the client. During the computer activity, the clinician remains responsible for tailoring conversation with the client so that genuine opportunities to practice communication goals are provided. The computer activity provides a shared context for three-way interaction among the clinician, the client, and the computer.

The notion of using a computer-based activity as a context for conversation with a client will seem intuitive to some clinicians, but may be difficult for others to envision. It is quite a departure from the vision of computer as a "teaching machine," or the CAI model described in Section II. Successful clinical uses of computers depend on a strong foundation of good clinical practice. Before jumping right into computer activities, this topic sets the stage by providing essential background information about the notion of "context" in language therapy. Then, strategies are outlined for integrating computers into this pragmatically appropriate approach to language therapy. Following up on this overview, later topics in Section III present more focused suggestions and activities for using the computer as a context with children, adolescents, or adults.

WHAT DOES "CONTEXT FOR CONVERSATION" MEAN?

In their seminal article "Therapy as social interaction: Analyzing the contexts for language remediation," Catherine Snow and her colleagues outlined the importance of acknowledging and designing the *context* of therapy activities (Snow, Midkiff-Borunda, Small, &

Proctor, 1984). According to Snow et al. (1984), clinicians should strive to establish a language therapy approach that places high value on the features of normal social interaction. This requires establishing a shared context in which conversational partners discuss a topic of mutual interest. Within this context, communicatively useful language should be emphasized and meaning should be continually negotiated.

Context is an ever-present influence when people are communicating, and competent speakers are continuously negotiating with each other about what is meant.

CASE EXAMPLE

Two people arrive home after work and are making a dinner plan:

Speaker 1:   Want to go out for pizza?

Speaker 2:   Uh, not really.

Speaker 1:   Okay, we could order in. (Thinking that Speaker 2 wants to stay home)

Speaker 2:   I had pizza for lunch. Let us go to the China Palace, want to? (Clarifies that going out is okay, but doesn't want pizza for dinner)

Speaker 1:   Deal.

Such negotiation requires understanding subtle cues from the other person and continuing the interaction until consensus is reached; not just consensus about where to have dinner, but shared understanding of what "Uh, not really" meant in this interaction.

Regardless of whether competent speakers consciously take context into account during such negotiation, their language reflects automatic contextual adaptations. For example, to communicate more efficiently, a speaker may refer to an object in the environment with a pronoun (it, his, that) rather than a specific noun (baby, dog, cookie, sandwich). This way of coding shared information signals to the conversational partner that the object in question is obvious—maybe even clearly visible.

CASE EXAMPLE

Speaker 1:   Do you want one?

Speaker 2:   Yeah, I'll take peanut butter.

Even in an interaction this brief, much "shared" information has been coded. We interpret these words based on what has been said as well as what has not been said. For example, we know that the object under discussion is either visible in the environment or has been previously discussed. Otherwise, Speaker 2 would say something like "One WHAT?" There must be multiple objects to choose from, because Speaker 1 used the word "one" instead of "it." We know there are multiple kinds of objects, because in Speaker 2's reply, the variety is specified (peanut butter); therefore there must be other kinds to choose from. From this interaction, we could hypothesize about a context: possibly the speakers are sharing a plate of sandwiches or buying cookies at the bakery. Regardless of the setting, however, the presence of certain objects, potential actions, and shared information, creates a context that influences the syntactic, semantic, and phonologic behavior of these speakers. The amounts and kinds of information that the speakers needed to convey were influenced by their environment and by their shared experience.

This is always true and so important that it warrants repeating: *The amounts and kinds of information that speakers need to convey are influenced by their environment and by their shared experience.* Communication does not take place in a vacuum. Clinicians can manipulate the therapy environment such that they provide contextual support for target language behaviors. This may increase the client's chance of learning target language behaviors successfully.

Alternatively, clinicians can think of therapy tasks as "practice" rather than as real communication that depends on context. A sports analogy helps illustrate the difference. In the latter case, clinicians attempt to have clients "practice" language the way a coach might have someone "practice" a tennis serve. If the player has seen a tennis match, then "practice" out of the context of a real match is understood. Such decontextualized practice is tolerated and even pursued by the tennis player who understands the value of a good serve. However, how does someone who has never seen a real game of tennis learn to play just by practicing serving the ball?

For children and adults who do not possess adequate cognitive and language abilities, decontextualized practice is often confusing. Interactions with such clients should be treated like "real" communication, because they *are* real communication. Clients, especially those with impaired language abilities, cannot be expected to suspend what they know about real communication for the sake of "practicing" in therapy. For example, in typical social interaction, people do not ask each other questions to which the answers are obvious unless they are being deliberately funny or sarcastic. This happens all too often, however, in the atypical environment of some therapy rooms.

CASE EXAMPLE

Clinician: What's this? [Holds her own pen up]

Child: [looks puzzled, grabs at a toy]

Does this child know the word *pen*? Maybe, maybe not. But asking a pragmatically inappropriate question is not the best way to find out. The clinician wants the child to "practice" labeling an object. From the child's point of view, however, there is no need to label an object that is known and visible to this strangely behaving adult. There is no information to convey, no purpose for this language in this context.

CREATING AN EFFECTIVE CONTEXT FOR CONVERSATION

Remember the three criteria associated with effective contexts for language therapy:

- Shared interest in the topic or task at hand
- Emphasis on communicatively useful language
- Opportunities for negotiating meaning with conversational partners

The clinician and client need shared experiences or shared goals; in other words, there must be something for the clinician and client to communicate about. Ideally, both are interested in the topic or goal because motivation will improve performance. In addition, the clinician should target communication behaviors (e.g., vocalizations, signs, words) that are communicatively useful for the client. A speech therapy session with a 5-year-old that focuses on the words *vest, vase, violin,* and *veil* may fail the "communicatively useful" test. Why would the clinician pick these infrequently occurring words? Most likely because it is easy to find pictures of them, not because these are the "v" words most 5-year-olds need to say intelligibly in everyday conversation. Words or concepts that are merely easy to illustrate are not necessarily powerful or frequently used in daily communication.

The third criterion to keep in mind is opportunity for negotiating meaning. There should be choices, options, or flexibility built into the activity to maximize opportunities for real communication. Nearly any kind of popular therapy activity can be implemented in a way that takes these criteria into account. Conant, Budhoff, and Hecht (1983) provided a rich collection of traditional language therapy games, all re-designed to include real communication at their heart. Examples include hiding games, picture-object matching games, lotto, and barrier games.

In addition, many computer-based activities lend themselves particularly well to providing an effective context for communication. However, the prevalence of the traditional computer-assisted instruction (CAI) model for software development has caused social interaction and the issue of context to be largely ignored in computer applications designed for use in language therapy. For the most part, clinicians must look elsewhere for software applications that will create a shared context for communication.

CONSIDER USING GENERIC SOFTWARE TO CREATE A SHARED CONTEXT

Many software applications intended for general education or entertainment make ideal candidates for using the computer as a context for communication. A product so popular that it became the model for a whole new genre of software, *Print Shop* (Broderbund) is a perfect example, equally appropriate for children and adults. Using *Print Shop*, a client and clinician could plan and produce any number of useful projects, including greeting cards, signs, posters, banners, and calendars.

CASE EXAMPLE

Using *Print Shop* as the context of conversation during language therapy, the client is seated in front of the computer, with the clinician slightly to one side. The client is an adult working on requesting clarification and using adequate vocal loudness.

Clinician: We could make a get-well card for Ms. Ikerd or a sign for your room.

Regan: Make a card.

Clinician: Okay, let's make a card. You start. (Waits to see if client asks for help or clicks card option on screen)

Regan: (Mumbles)

Clinician: Sorry, I didn't hear you.

Regan: What now?

Clinician: That time I heard you. Click here to start the card. [Points to screen icon]

In this example, the client and clinician are beginning a computer activity that will serve as a shared context for conversation. They are both interested in this task, and the clinician is already providing opportunities for the client to practice skills that are communicatively useful. They will have to negotiate with each other along the way to choose the shape of the card, the borders or graphics, what text will be inside, and so forth.

Certainly they could make a get-well card without a computer. But with a computer, there are new things to explore, procedures to discover, and a final product that will be personalized but professional looking. Additional examples of software that are effective for these kinds of activities are found in later topics, as well as other criteria to consider when choosing software.

CHARACTERISTICS OF COMPUTER-AS-CONTEXT ACTIVITIES

The software that underlies computer-as-context activities should have the following characteristics:

- Ease of use: Ideally, the client and clinician will share and/or alternate control over the computer.

- Flexibility of outcome: The outcome may be a product, such as a drawing, a story, a successfully solved puzzle, or a game, that can be repeated with variations from session to session.

- Flexibility of linguistic content: The computer activity should allow the clinician to easily tailor the linguistic content to meet the exact interests and language ability of the client.

Such characteristics contrast sharply with those that have been identified as priorities for drill-and-practice and other CAI software. For example, CAI may be more positively reviewed if it has narrowly focused outcomes, a limited range of correct responses, prompt and specific feedback about correctness, and a pre-determined instructional sequence.

ROLE OF THE CLINICIAN

What is the role of the clinician during computer-as-context activities? Choosing specific communication goals, providing consequences, providing linguistic content, and assessing client performance are functions rightly assumed by the clinician, not the computer, during computer-as-context activities. In addition, the clinician participates as a full conversational partner in such activities. The goals and direction of the activity may be negotiated in advance with the client. More negotiating may occur as together the client and clinicians consider specific choices offered by the software. In contrast to the two-way interaction (client–computer) that characterizes CAI activities, computer-as-context activities are better described as three-way interaction (see Figure 7.1).

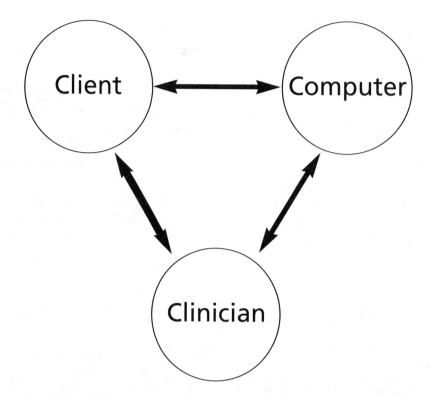

Figure 7.1. Computer-as-context activities are characterized by three-way interaction between the client, clinician, and computer.

In this three-way interaction, the clinician and client communicate with each other and share control over the computer activity. The computer provides feedback to both users, helping them accomplish the goal or complete the activity they have chosen.

DECIDING ON A COMPUTER-AS-CONTEXT ACTIVITY

In order to use the computer effectively as a context for therapy, each clinician must work through the following questions:

1. Is this software likely to be of interest to my client?

2. Using this software, can I tailor the interaction with my client to address our specific speech or language therapy goals?

3. Have I planned pre-computer activities that provide an adequate opportunity to observe whether the client is ready for the computer-based activity that I have in mind?

4. Have I previewed the software sufficiently to believe that this computer-based activity suits my client's cognitive, motor, and communication skills?

5. Will I need to adapt access to the computer to ensure that the client can participate in controlling the computer during our activity? (See Section VIII)

6. Have I thought through exactly what I could say and do during the computer activity to ensure that speech-language goals are addressed?

7. Have I thought through exactly what I could say and do during the computer activity to ensure that opportunities for negotiation will occur?

8. During this activity, will the client receive reinforcement or feedback from both me and the computer that will be useful for improving communication?

9. Have I planned post-computer activities that will help the client generalize to situations away from the computer?

10. If this computer-based activity goes as expected, what improvements in communication can I reasonably expect?

AVOIDING PITFALLS

Integrating a computer into speech and language therapy is just as challenging as learning any other new approach to therapy. Effectively using a computer as a context for conversation with a client requires practice. The questions listed above are designed to help clinicians have early success with computer-as-context activities. For example, Question 7 requires the clinician to think through the conversation that will take place at the computer. If this step is skipped, some clinicians may begin with the intention of using the computer as a context for conversation, but end up conducting a clinician-driven drill-and-practice style activity.

CASE EXAMPLE

A computer-as-context for conversation activity gone awry:

Clinician: Now we're going to make a card. Point to the card icon.

Stephen: (points to screen)

Clinician: Good! Do you need help?

Stephen: (nods head)

Clinician: Click here.

Stephen: (clicks on icon)

Clinician: That's right! Now say "I need help."

Stephen: I need help.

Clinician: Good! Click on that thing.

Stephen: (clicks on icon)

Clinician: Good! Pick the border you want.

Stephen: (chooses border from choices on screen)

Clinician: Okay, what is that?

Stephen: Leafs.

Clinician: Yes, that's a leaf border. Good!

What is wrong with the interaction in the previous example? The clinician is so busy being in control that no real communication has a chance to happen. The client can hardly get a word in, and none of the criteria of a shared context activity are present. Stephen may not have any interest in this task, the communication objectives for him (other than obedience) are not clear, and he has no opportunity to negotiate or use language to convey useful information.

Clinicians who are interested in learning how to design therapy that is in concert with the guidelines outlined here may benefit from video or audio taping sessions with new software. Or, they could explain to a colleague or supervisor what they are trying to do, and have them observe a few sessions to provide objective feedback. Pretty soon, the pitfalls will become more and more obvious, and creating a computer-based context for conversation more and more natural. With these basic principles in mind, specific strategies for working with children and adults can be developed.

CHOOSING CAI VERSUS USING THE COMPUTER AS A CONTEXT FOR THERAPY

From a client's point of view, there is a big difference between CAI and computer-as-context activities. In computer-as-context activities, open-ended possibilities are tailored to the client as the activity progresses. As the client and clinician negotiate, they make the computer serve their purposes. Having a computer do, say, or make what they want it to is an empowering experience for clients. This is quite different from the relatively passive role involved in drill-and-practice trials, over which a client has little control.

It may seem as if using the computer for CAI is easier for the clinician at first, because it offers pre-designed activities and pre-determined goals. In contrast, when using the computer to create a shared context for interaction between the client and clinician, the outcome may seem less certain and the whole thing may feel more complex to plan and implement. But the risk is worth taking. During the daily course of events, communication with human conversational partners always involves an element of uncertainty. But who would trade the freedom to communicate spontaneously, with the inevitable occasional misunderstandings, for a group of pre-determined messages that are absolutely clear? Similarly, the exact content and sequence can be known in advance during a CAI activity, which is not the case during open-ended activities. But when opportunities for genuine communication with human conversational partners are also placed on the scales, the balance usually tips heavily toward using more flexible software as a context for therapy.

SUMMARY

The rationale for paying attention to the role of context in language therapy is illustrated with examples that show how everyday interaction is influenced by contextual factors. During typical conversation, people are continuously adjusting their language to take context and shared information into account. Therapy that deliberately uses context to support and improve conversational language includes a task or topic of shared interest, emphasis on communicatively useful language, and opportunities to negotiate meaning between conversational partners. Much software designed for educational and entertainment use provides an excellent shared context for language therapy. Desirable software characteristics include: ease of use, flexibility of outcome, and flexibility of linguistic content.

The role of the clinician in computer-as-context activities is substantially different than when the computer is serving in the capacity of "teaching machine," as in CAI. In contrast to the two-way interaction that takes place in CAI, three-way interaction is characteristic of computer-as-context activities. The clinician is a crucial element in this interaction, bearing the responsibility for ensuring that throughout the activity, the linguistic content and communication opportunities presented to the client are appropriate. The clinician, not the computer, must evaluate the client's participation in the activity.

Clinicians are encouraged to plan carefully and evaluate their own success at creating a shared context that benefits the client. Self-evaluation or feedback from others can identify computer activities that need further fine-tuning to become effective contexts for client communication.

REVIEW FOR TOPIC 7

1. What are three important characteristics of therapy designed to acknowledge the rules of normal social interaction?
2. Give an example of how the amount and kind of information that speakers need to convey is influenced by their environment and shared experience. Include a sample dialog.
3. If pointing to a pen and asking "What's this?" is not the best way to find out whether the client knows the word *pen,* how could you find out in a more pragmatically appropriate way?
4. What is the role of the clinician in computer-as-context therapy activities? Draw a diagram that represents your understanding of this interaction.

QUESTIONS FOR DISCUSSION

1. Compare and contrast the role of the clinician during CAI versus computer-as-context activities.
2. Review the list of questions designed to help clinicians prepare computer-as-context activities. Have you ever tried a computer activity that failed? Discuss a possible cause based on this list of questions.
3. Describe a software program (real or invented) that could be used to meet the desirable characteristics of computer-as-context activities.

RESOURCES FOR FURTHER STUDY

Cochran, P.S., & Nelson, L.K. (1999). Technology applications in intervention for preschool-age children with language disorders. *Seminars in Speech and Language, 20*(3), 203–218.

Snow, C., Midkiff-Borunda, S., Small, A., & Proctor, A. (1984). Therapy as social interaction: Analyzing the contexts for language remediation. *Topics in Language Disorders, 4*(4), 72–85.

Using a Computer as a Context for Conversation with Young Children

Clinical Computing Competency #2: The clinician will demonstrate the ability to use computer-based materials to form a shared context for communication with clients.

In general, clinicians who have had experience using word processing or electronic communication have enough technical expertise to begin using computers for clinical purposes with young children. This competency, therefore, focuses on planning and implementing computer activities that are developmentally appropriate and guided by the clinician to address specific speech or language goals. The computer activities should inspire genuine conversation between the child and the clinician. Competency also requires integrating computer activities effectively into larger intervention plans so that carryover to other contexts is achieved.

For this chapter, the term *young children* refers to children who are ages 3–6 years or who are functioning within that range linguistically and/or cognitively. The software chosen for use with young children should be based on teaching methods that are consistent with their capabilities and motivation for learning. (See Topic 13 for guidelines pertaining to choosing software for young children.) Many people are surprised to find that even some 2-year-olds, with adult assistance, can attend to and control a computer activity effectively. Some children will not show interest in computer-based activities until age 3 or 4. Even young children with developmental delays, however, may surprise everyone and show high motivation to interact with and about a computer.

When planning computer-based activities for young children, it is especially important to think about how the computer activity relates to the "real world" experiences of children. Special attention should be paid to the transfer of concepts and symbols from the three-dimensional form children may know (e.g., a toy car) to a flat, untouchable, immovable representation such as a cartoon car on the computer screen. Computer activities can be ideal for helping children make the transition to this more symbolic form, but clinicians must plan accordingly. Pre-computer activities making use of "real" objects and post-computer activities that facilitate carryover to other contexts are crucial in this regard. It's also important to remember that children learn through play. Sometimes, a child needs extra time just to explore new software. During this time, the child may not talk much. During subsequent encounters with the activity, however, the child may be more verbal than usual, because now the child is ready to communicate about this new experience. This topic describes strategies that increase the likelihood that computer-as-context activities with young children will be successful.

CHOOSE AND IMPLEMENT APPROPRIATE COMMUNICATION OBJECTIVES

The identification of goals for a particular child or group should happen prior to the selection of instructional materials. Computers or other technologies are then considered as one of several possible approaches for working on those objectives. For young children, communication goals frequently focus on expressing basic wants and needs (requests), requesting and giving clarification (questions), following and giving directions (prepositions), increasing semantic diversity (vocabulary), increasing grammatical complexity (syntax and morphology), and increasing narrative skills (personal narratives and scripts). Emergent literacy skills are supported with attention to phonemic awareness (rhyming, sound–symbol activities) and print awareness activities (reading and writing). All of these communication goals can be addressed effectively with or without the help of computers. For some clinicians and some clients, however, use of computer-based activities to address these goals will be a motivating and effective choice.

A word of caution is in order. It is deceptively easy for new technologies to distract a clinician's attention from the most important communication objectives for clients. Among the many ways this can happen, two seem to be the most common. One is an error in planning, the other is an error in implementation. In the first instance, the clinician knows of a computer activity that the client will enjoy, so the client's goals may be adjusted accordingly. In the second case, during the course of a computer-based activity, the clinician may become distracted from the original intent. This happens when a compelling computer activity causes both the clinician and client to focus on the software's inherent purposes and procedures, even if they are not top priority for improving communication.

CASE EXAMPLE: A Well-Intentioned Computer-Based Language Activity Targeting *Under, Over,* and *Beside* Goes Astray

This activity could be implemented with any software that allows the user to rearrange items shown in the scene on the monitor. Rearranging is more powerful than just clicking on items, and more useful for working on spatial relationships. In the example that follows, the clinician and client are using the ABC Book activity from Broderbund's classic children's software *The Playroom*. In this program, users are presented with a background scene showing a farm, a city street, or a fantasy castle. Clicking on an alphabet letter at the top of the screen brings forth an item associated with that letter. Items coordinate with the background scene (C is for Cow in the farm scene, C is for Car in the city scene, C is for Crystal ball in the fantasy scene). After a letter is pressed, the item can be added to the scene by moving the mouse. At any time, more items can be added and existing items can be selected and moved or deleted. In the session presented in this case example, the client and clinician are using the farm scene. They take turns giving and following directions using the words *under*, *over*, and *beside*.

Clinician:	Yes! You put the frog beside the rock. Way to go. My turn. (takes mouse and looks expectantly at child)
Sheila:	(finger touches monitor on the rock)
Clinician:	Tell me where to put the frog. Put the frog . . .
Sheila:	on rock
Clinician:	(moves frog on the rock and looks to child for approval)
Sheila:	Uh-huh (nodding approval)
	(So far, so good—this activity is going well up to this point, and then it takes a turn away from the focus on spatial concepts.)
Clinician:	The frog is on the rock. Let's add a pig. Find the P for pig.
Sheila:	Presses the letter C.
Computer voice:	C! Cow! (cow appears on monitor)
Clinician:	Is that P?
Sheila:	(shakes head no)
Clinician:	Find the P.
Sheila:	(presses the letter B)
Computer voice:	B! Boy! (boy appears on monitor)
Clinician:	Here's the P. (points to letter P)

During the moment, this clinician may not realize what is happening to his lesson on spatial concepts. What began as a language activity quickly became an alphabet/typing lesson. It is fine to address multiple goals in a single activity, as long as the primary communication goal remains in focus and is not unintentionally pushed aside. This way of using a computer depends upon the clinician (not the software designer) to introduce and implement specific communication objectives. Therefore, clinicians may need to adapt the "rules" of the game or modify the steps of an activity to ensure that the individualized language objectives for a particular client are emphasized. This extra effort (and vigilance!) is worth it—because the clinician and client remain in control of what happens during such an open-ended activity.

PREVIEW AND PERSONALIZE THE COMPUTER ACTIVITY

Software that is developmentally appropriate for young children usually has options or preference settings that clinicians can use to make a computer-based speech or language activity optimally suited to a child or group. Such options might include whether speech or music is on or off, how or when feedback is available, and choices regarding task complexity. It is worth a few extra minutes of preparation to review these options and learn how to change the settings of software to optimize it for a session. Also, this gives the clinician the chance to review any special procedures/key combinations that are necessary in order to skip a demo, interrupt the activity, or save it midway through.

Software previewing provides the ideal opportunity for the clinician to think through the upcoming interactions with children and how the software will be used. Especially for clinicians who are new to using computers with young children, it is valuable to consider exactly what children will be expected to say and do, to ensure that opportunities to focus on target speech and language behaviors will occur. Who will control the mouse (or other input device)? Will participants take turns telling the other person what to do? What will provide the reason to talk during this activity?

Some children will require adapted access to the computer in order to participate in a shared activity. The range of alternatives to the regular keyboard and mouse are discussed in Section VIII. For example, many young children enjoy using a touch screen interface to control a computer, even if their motor abilities are intact (see Figure 8.1).

Software that accommodates the use of adapted access devices is widely available for young children, although much of it is developed and distributed by publishers who target the special education market. Examples of accessible software that could be used in computer-as-context activities are found in Table 8.1.

USE PRE-COMPUTER ACTIVITIES TO INTRODUCE IMPORTANT CONCEPTS OR CHECK ON PREREQUISITE COMPREHENSION

Consider a clinician who wants to help a child improve comprehension of spatial relationships in two-dimensional tasks. Many kindergarten activities, for example, require the child to draw a line under something, a circle around something else, or make a mark beside a picture on a page. To be successful, the child must understand the concepts of *under, around,* and *beside* within the flat two-dimensional framework of the worksheet. A computer-based activity can provide an ideal context within which to practice and discuss these concepts. However, the wise clinician will do a warm-up activity with three-dimensional objects to ensure that the child can handle the target concepts in this more immediate, more realistic context. A toy barn with animals and fences can be used to quickly check how the child is doing with *under, around,* and *beside* in three-dimensional space. If difficulties are present, the planned computer activity should be reconsidered. If the child does well, together they proceed to use a software program that allows them to move animals and objects around in a farm scene (see *The Playroom* case example).

These are the same considerations that any skillful clinician would have in mind, regardless of whether a computer activity was planned. The point is that effective computer-based activities rely just as much on clinician planning and execution as other kinds of therapy activities do.

CREATE A GENUINE CONVERSATIONAL CONTEXT

When a clinician thinks of language therapy as social interaction, the following question must be considered: "How will communication be an integral part of this activity?" It is helpful to recall the criteria outlined by Snow et al. (1984) and discussed in Topic 7. Ide-

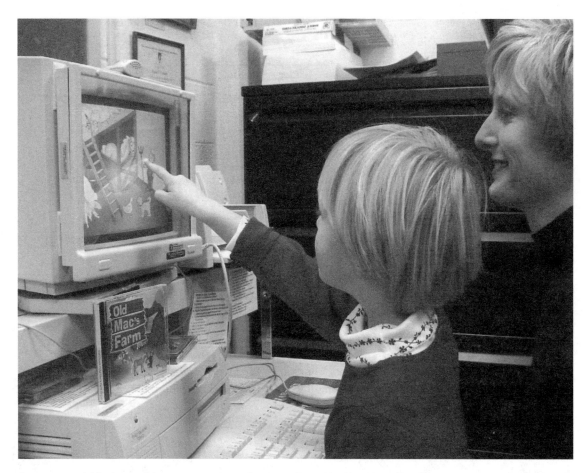

Figure 8.1. A child using a touch screen as an alternative to a traditional keyboard (Courtesy of Truman State University Speech and Hearing Clinic).

ally, the therapy context (environment, materials, activities, and previously shared knowledge) provides a topic of mutual interest, opportunities to experience communicatively useful language, and negotiation of meaning with conversational partners. The case example below illustrates how computer activities can help create such a context with young children.

CASE EXAMPLE: Using the Kitchen Scene from Edmark's *Imagination Express: Neighborhood* Multimedia CD-ROM to Establish a Shared Context

Specific language goal: The client will request and provide clarification when insufficient information is provided in nine of ten opportunities.

Clinician: Look, Shana! This kitchen is really messy. How could we clean it up?

Shana: I don't know.

Clinician: Well, we could move some things around or get rid of things that don't belong here. Which should we do first?

Shana: Get rid of stuff.

Clinician: What do you mean by "stuff?"

Table 8.1. Examples of software for young children that is compatible with adapted access (keyboard alternatives) and a computer-as-context approach to therapy

Software examples	Sample activities
Sesame Street Baby (Encore) (single switch)	Play Peek-a-boo, imitate Ernie, find hidden pictures
Spider in the Kitchen (Encore) (touch screen, single-switch scanning, Intellikeys overlays included)	Put things away in the kitchen, find the spider, make cereal or a sandwich
Old MacDonald's Farm Deluxe (SoftTouch) (switch, touch screen)	Sing about animals, match babies to mothers
Single Switch Software for Preschoolers (Simtech) (single switch)	Five programs that help children learn switch control through cause-effect, for example make a frog catch a fly

Shana: Like that sofa.

Clinician: Okay. That sofa doesn't belong here. I'll delete it (selects and deletes sofa). Your turn. You delete that ugly thing (moves mouse toward Shana's hand).

Shana: What?

Clinician: I'm glad you asked before you deleted! I mean that ugly car. It doesn't go here.

Shana: (deletes car)

Clinician: It's your turn to tell me something to move or something to delete. No pointing allowed.

Shana: Move the chair.

Clinician: Which chair?

Shana: The one by the fridge.

Clinician: (moves chair slightly and hesitates, looking at Shana)

Shana: Put it beside the table.

Clinician: Will do. I'll put the chair beside table. (moves chair on screen)

The clinician in this case example has previously prepared and saved a messy kitchen scene with appropriate objects and probably used this same file with several children for various goals. Today she made sure to take turns with Shana, both giving directions and controlling the computer. That way, she is certain that they have opportunities to negotiate (Which chair? What do you mean?) and use language that has genuine communicative value (the clinician is acting on the information provided by Shana, giving Shana a purpose for providing clear and complete directions).

USE POST-COMPUTER ACTIVITIES TO PROMOTE GENERALIZATION AND CARRYOVER OF NEW COMMUNICATION BEHAVIORS

No matter how successful the computer-based activity is at providing a context for practicing speech or language skills, it is crucial that children use these new skills in tasks away from the computer. Generalization and carryover to other contexts can be facilitated if it is planned right from the start. The clinician working with a child on spatial concepts could do another two-dimensional activity, such as moving reusable vinyl stickers on a farm scene or drawing a picture of a farm with crayons or markers.

Many open-ended software programs that are developmentally appropriate for young children have components that make carryover easier to implement. For example, sometimes the computer screen itself can be printed out in full color. Some software for young children includes support materials such as story starters, puzzles, or finger puppet patterns. Products of the therapy activity, such as a story or a picture, can be printed out and used for a post-computer activity. For example, a picture developed by the client and clinician could be printed, glued to stiffer paper, or laminated, then cut up into pieces to make a simple puzzle. The child can take this product home, and it can stimulate conversation with family members which further extends the opportunity to use new skills in various contexts.

CONSIDER DESIGNING A THEMATIC UNIT OR A SCRIPT-BASED THEME

Many young children with special needs receive services in the context of a preschool, nursery school, or child care. Professionals working in such settings often develop thematic units to organize various aspects of the curriculum. Ideally, such a unit uses a single theme to incorporate multiple aspects of a well-balanced early childhood program. Themes are a natural way for teams to collaborate in meeting the individual education needs of children who are receiving special services in schools. Themes can be as simple as "frogs" or "healthy snacks" and as complex as "the USA" or "zoo animals." Often themes are related to seasons, traditions, and recognition of different cultures. Activities that focus on fine and gross motor skills, socialization, creativity, emergent literacy, music, drama, and communication may be included. Thus a single thematic unit might include not only computer activities but also a special song or finger play, arts and crafts, storybooks, an action game, a special bulletin board or learning center, and a cooking activity. There are excellent examples of thematic units available on web sites for parents and professionals who work with young children.

Thematic units have benefits for both professionals and the children in their care. For teachers and clinicians, themes provide a structure that makes planning easier. Having a theme for a day, a week, or even longer allows children to explore new ideas and concepts through a variety of media and a range of familiar and novel experiences. One of these experiences could be a thematically related computer activity. Much of the software that is developmentally appropriate for use with young children would lend itself to incorporation in a thematic unit (see Table 8.2). A clinician could make use of the theme while still targeting specific speech or language goals for each child.

For preschoolers, "script-based" themes may be ideal for facilitating language development and other important aspects of child development such as social skills. Scripts are based on the routine events that children experience frequently with their families and friends. Such event sequences include getting ready for school or bed, shopping for gro-

Table 8.2. Examples of generic, developmentally appropriate software that clinicians could use for computer-as-context activities with young children

Software examples	Sample activities
Bob the Builder (THQ)	Knock down and build a bridge, build a tunnel
Jump Start Animal Adventures (Knowledge Adventure)	Explore various animal habitats, take animal photos, print stickers
Leaps and Bounds 3 (Tool Factory)	Noisy painting, make a body, monster band, water flowers
Dragon Tales Dragon Land Festival (Encore Software)	Plant seeds, create songs, make clouds
Barbie Software: Kelly Club (Mattel/Vivendi)	Dress Kelly, hunt for wild flowers, have a tea party, decorate a cake, plant seeds, look for hidden treasure
Teddy Games (Inclusive)	Build a room, make a garden, dress Teddy
Disney Bundle (Disney Interactive)	Solve puzzles, create stories, sing-a-long
Ollo in Sunny Valley Fair (Plaid Banana/Hulabee Entertainment)	Adventure game with songs, puzzles, games in 28 different scenes

ceries, going to the doctor, having a birthday party, or having a picnic. Scripts generally have a specific vocabulary and sequence associated with key objects and people involved in the event. Computers can easily enhance script-based therapy activities. For example, the client and clinician could use a computer to create an invitation to a birthday party. A more detailed discussion of how to use computers to help children acquire narrative skills is presented in Topic 9.

SUMMARY

There are many developmentally appropriate generic and specialized software programs designed for use by and with young children. Although many embody a CAI model of software design, many others include activities and options that are ideal for creating more flexible, open-ended computer activities. Such software can be used by clinicians to create a shared context for language therapy with children.

Successful computer-as-context activities are more likely to occur when clinicians 1) preview and personalize the software, 2) plan pre-computer activities that teach and assess the key skills necessary for the computer activity, 3) implement activities that are linguistically tailored to the child and provide opportunities to use communicatively useful language, and 4) provide post-computer activities that facilitate carryover of skills to other contexts. Sometimes the software itself makes off-computer projects easier to develop by providing printable materials like pictures, finger puppets, stickers, or posters. These materials can be taken home and discussed with family members to further reinforce generalization.

A successful strategy used in many preschool environments is the development of thematic units of instruction that include computer activities along with music, art projects, storybooks, cooking activities, or field trips.

REVIEW FOR TOPIC 8

1. What is the clinician's role in using the computer as a shared context for conversation with a young child?
2. Why are pre-computer and post-computer activities recommended when using a computer as the context for therapy with young children?
3. Describe a common pitfall encountered by clinicians when they first start to use a computer as a context for therapy with young children. How could this be avoided?

QUESTIONS FOR DISCUSSION

1. Suppose there was a software program about having a birthday party. The software contains various party scenes, characters, games, food, and presents. Users can choose sound effects (e.g., singing, balloons popping, laughing, music) and add text. A section of the software allows the user to design and print paper party supplies such as invitations and party hats. What are some of the ways this software could be used in language therapy with a young child?
2. Describe the pre-computer and post-computer activities you would use with the software described in Question 1.

RESOURCES FOR FURTHER STUDY

Clements, D.H., Nastasi, B.K., & Swaminatha, W. (1993). Young children and computers: Crossroads and directions from research. *Young Children, 48,* 56–64.

Cochran, P.S., & Nelson, L.K. (1999). Technology applications in intervention for preschool-age children with language disorders. *Seminars in Speech and Language, 20*(3), 203–218.

Fallon, M.A., & Sanders Wann, J.A. (1994). Incorporating computer technology into activity-based thematic units for young children with disabilities. *Infants and Young Children, 6,* 64–69.

Using a Computer as a Context for Conversation with School-Age Children

Clinical computing competency #2: The clinician will demonstrate the ability to use computer-based activities as a shared context for communication with clients.

This competency can be achieved through the open-ended, flexible computer activities used directly with school-age children in order to accomplish specific communication goals. Competent clinicians will know how to choose software that lends itself to creating a shared context for conversation and will integrate computer activities into a larger intervention plan. Clinicians should be aware that there are computer activities available that complement the classroom curriculum of school-age children.

Matching appropriate software to appropriate goals is the key to the success of all computer-based activities. Goals for computer-as-context activities with school-age children may be traditional in nature. Examples include articulation of a target sound, use of a target syntactic structure, or demonstration of a particular pragmatic skill. Three-way interaction between the clinician, the child, and the computer will focus on these goals through genuine communication opportunities. Computer activities provide a focal point and a purpose for this interaction.

School clinicians will find that computer-as-context therapy activities can serve several purposes simultaneously. They can address speech and language therapy goals, complement the overall school curricula, and reinforce an individual's academic IEP objectives. For example, computer-as-context activities can facilitate the development of both oral and written narrative skills as well as emergent and advanced literacy.

Recall from Topic 7 that certain features are associated with software suitable for computer-as-context activities. Ideally, the software should be 1) easy to use, so that the clinician and client can share control; 2) flexible in outcome, so that the clinician and client can choose or change what they are doing; and 3) flexible in linguistic content, so that the exact speech and language needs of the client can be addressed.

Topic 9 describes and discusses the use of such software with school-age children, emphasizing traditional speech and language goals other than literacy. Later topics in Section III focus on emergent and advanced literacy skills. Even with only a business-quality word processing program, much can be accomplished in therapy. Ideas for capitalizing on more specialized software are also illustrated. Computer-as-context software is flexible enough for clinicians and interesting enough for school-age children to be well-suited for inspiring conversations between them.

AWARENESS OF CURRICULAR GUIDELINES AND CLASSROOM COLLABORATION

Clinicians working with school-aged children frequently collaborate with other professionals to reinforce instructional and developmental objectives for their clients. Current trends in education have centered everyone's efforts on achieving standards established by state and local school administration. Table 9.1 presents examples of what schools expect children to achieve in language arts at various grade levels.

Administrators and teachers bear most of the responsibility for ensuring that standards of learning are met, however, related service providers, such as clinicians, should become familiar with the major instructional goals in place for the school-age children with whom they work. Successful professional collaboration depends on shared goals. Effective inclusion of children with communication disorders depends on successful professional collaboration. Computer-based activities can be an especially powerful way for clinicians to address a child's communication goals while reinforcing specific content learning.

BASIC WORD PROCESSING ACTIVITIES FOR THERAPY WITH SCHOOL-AGE CHILDREN

Many of the features that make word processing software invaluable for administrative tasks are also useful during therapy activities. All word processing software allows a user to enter text that can easily be amended, saved on disk, or printed. Word processing software facilitates manipulation of small or large amounts of text that goes beyond just perfecting the text's appearance. Search and replace functions, for example, automatically search the entire text for words or symbols specified by the user and may replace them if necessary (e.g., all instances of "Paul" could be replaced with "Carl" in a matter of seconds). Almost any sort of mistake is easily corrected by inserting, deleting, or moving text. Early in the instructional use of computers, Rosegrant (1985) contended that this forgiving quality of word processing lowers the risks for learners with language impairments when they attempt writing tasks. "Young writers appreciate the lack of finality to text they put on the screen. Errors caused by inexperience or motor difficulties can be corrected without recopying every word . . . Children are willing to experiment with word choice and sentence structures since words/lines can be quickly removed" (Rosegrant, 1985, p. 114).

Table 9.1. Examples of state curriculum guidelines for language arts

Academic area	Level	Sample state guideline (not presented in their entirety)
English—Oral language	Grade 1	The student will continue to demonstrate growth in the use of oral language. • Tell and retell stories and events in logical order • Be able to express ideas orally in complete sentences • Increase oral descriptive vocabulary • Begin to ask for clarification and explanation of words and ideas • Give and follow simple two-step oral directions
English—Reading	Grade 1	The student will read and comprehend a variety of fiction and nonfiction selections. • Relate previous experiences to what is read • Make predictions about content • Ask and answer questions about what is read • Identify characters and setting • Retell stories and events, using beginning, middle, and end • Identify the theme or main ideas • Write about what is read
English—Writing	Grade 2	The student will write stories, letters, and simple explanations. • Generate ideas before writing • Organize writing to include a beginning, middle, and end • Revise writing for clarity • Use available technology

Source: Commonwealth of Virginia Standards of Learning (www.pen.k12.va.us/go/Sols).

The activities in Table 9.2 can be accomplished with any word processing software and a printer. If time or printer availability is a problem, printouts can be made after a session or with the help of an aide or parent volunteer. These activities have several features in common. They involve the child in conversation with the clinician and interaction with the computer; they require the child to convey a message to an audience; they require a clinician to tailor the linguistic interaction to the needs of the child so that communication objectives are addressed during the activity; and they constitute a context for language therapy. Although these activities indirectly reinforce and encourage literacy skills, they are not primarily designed to teach either reading or writing. Rather, these activities could be used as a context for addressing a wide variety of traditional speech or language goals.

ORGANIZING A SESSION AROUND A WORD PROCESSING ACTIVITY

If clinicians plan therapy activities which require students to write more than a few words, they should be aware of the approach to writing that their clients experience in the classroom (see Nelson, Bahr, & Van Meter, 2004, for extensive examples and information about using computers to assist children with writing in a lab or classroom setting). It is important to be consistent, even if the clinician does not plan to provide explicit writing instruction. For example, among the various approaches to teaching writing, one that is widely favored is called the "process" approach. This approach views writing as a process involving four phases: pre-writing, writing, revision, and publication.

Table 9.2. Creating a shared context for conversation with school-age children using generic word processing activities

Word processing activity	Possible variations
Making a sign	Make a sign for the speech room, for a child's room at home, to announce a special event or achievement: Knock Before Entering! or Today is Yvette's Birthday! or No Chewing Gum Beyond This Point, No Speech Today, Jamie Completed Speech Homework 10 Times!
Making labels	Label possessions, special objects, warnings, and directions: Speech Store Box, Hot/Cold, Tiffany's Speech Book, Ms. Hartfield's Tape.
Making a card	Send well wishes to a sick classmate, thank the school cook or custodian or bus driver, send holiday greetings. If your word processor does not have a greeting card template, print the greeting in one half of the page, fold and let children decorate with stickers or crayons.
Writing a letter	Say hello to a teacher on leave or a sick classmate; write to a grandparent or well-known author, athlete, musician, or TV star.
Captioning pictures	Write captions for photos taken at a school event, or pictures drawn by students: The Winners of the Recycling Contest, The Fourth Grade Opens School Store, Jay's Favorite Things to Do at Recess, Our new custodian, Ms. Sinha.

These phases of the process approach to writing can parallel the previously outlined steps for integrating computer activities into therapy. Thus *pre-writing* (any activity that helps to get the writer's ideas going) could be accomplished in a *pre-computer activity*. Writing and revision are comparable to the computer activity itself, and publication is comparable to post-computer activities, which promote generalization.

Activities that employ a computer to establish a shared context for conversation can be designed with individuals or small groups in mind. Small groups are the typical configuration in most school settings (see Figure 9.1). The pre-computer activity serves to review previous instruction and to assure the clinician that the children have the knowledge and skills necessary for the computer activity. A pre-writing/pre-computer activity for making a sign with a word processor might include talking about signs the children recall in the school or community, looking at some actual signs, and talking about why people put up signs. Clinicians can provide models and opportunities for children working on WH-question formation to ask each other, "Where did you see that sign?" Alternatively, regular (printed, posted, taped, tacked) or irregular (saw, read, found, made) past tense verbs can be brought into the discussion if appropriate. Note that the goals for the children have previously been established. The clinician, not the computer, remains responsible for goal attainment in activities such as making a sign.

Once the computer activity begins, to maintain focus on oral language rather than keyboarding, younger children "dictate" the text while the clinician types. Or, children who have developed some keyboarding skills take turns talking and typing. Possibly the group will come up with several alternative texts for the sign; the clinician types them all in rather than trying to force the group to reach consensus at an early stage. When one or more complete versions are ready, drafts are printed. Revisions are discussed, and the group votes on a preference, or decides to produce more than one version of the finished product. Using this structure for a therapy session (pre-computer, computer, post-computer activities) the clinician has reinforced the approach to writing which many classroom teachers are trying to instill (pre-writing, writing, revision, and publication).

Once the signs are printed, they can be decorated with colored markers, stickers, or stamps during a post-computer activity. While the children are working, the clinician con-

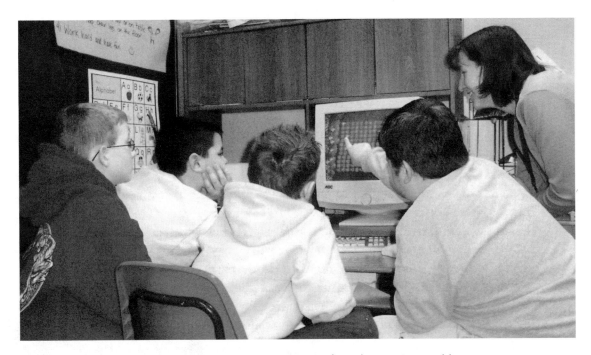

Figure 9.1. A clinician mediates the conversation during a group session focused on a computer activity.

tinues to tailor the linguistic interaction to the individual communication goals for each child. This time, the conversation might be geared to rehearsing an explanation, "Could you tell your mom how we made this sign?" The discussion could also be used to introduce a more abstract event, "What do you think Mr. Hendler will say when he gets these signs for his door?" Well-conceived post-computer activities encourage the use of emerging language skills outside the therapy room. This can be accomplished by having children take their computer projects to show and explain to someone else, "Before we put up this sign, let's show it to Ms. Kline, okay? What should we tell her about it?"

A fertile context for therapy is especially likely to develop if activities like those in Table 9.2 are part of a continuing project that involves a series of related activities. In an ongoing context for therapy such as an extended project, some key vocabulary, procedures, and concepts stay constant. When such information is familiar to all conversational partners, then the client and clinician can focus on other specific language skills in need of improvement. The clients and clinician have the opportunity to use language to plan, implement, discuss, and recall such activities. Making a sign or writing a letter could be components of an anti-litter campaign, a reading week project, a puppet show, a school athletic event, or a fund raising project. (See Topic 11 for more examples of extended projects.)

WHY USE A COMPUTER?

Clearly, these activities could all be done without a computer. So, why should clinicians consider using computers for such activities? First, many children like using computers. In studies comparing closely matched computer-based and traditional table-top speech therapy activities, most children expressed a preference for the computer-based version (Ott-Rose & Cochran, 1992; Shriberg, Kwiatkowski, & Snyder, 1989).

Second, a computer can help maintain the attention of a small group working together on a single product. When writing appears on the computer monitor, in contrast to a piece of paper under the writer's hand, it is easier for several people to watch, participate in the authoring, and discuss the content. Remember that the activity has another agenda, namely practicing specific speech or language skills. The primary goal is not making a sign—the primary goal is talking about making a sign, in such a way that children have opportunities to hear and use language that they need. Children respond to the genuine demands of this communication context by trying to make their preferences known and their messages clear enough for peers and the clinician to understand. Scaffolded activities of this sort often involve as much or more oral language than written language.

Third, word processing makes it painless to manipulate lots of different words. During an activity such as making a card or labels, the participants usually explore alternate wording and layouts. Such major changes mean starting over on a handwritten document, but a word processor easily accommodates revision. Even multiple versions can be readily developed for experimentation, because words can be switched around or substituted so easily.

MAKING CURRICULAR CONNECTIONS

Even with a modest budget and limited experimentation, clinicians can greatly expand their use of the computer as a context for conversation with software that combines basic word processing capabilities and multimedia features like graphics, animation, or sound. Software with these features is readily available, relatively inexpensive, and usually easy to learn.

Since personal computers became widely available, there has been children's software that encourages the user to write and illustrate a story. Often the illustration fills part of the computer display, leaving space for text to accompany the picture. Display "pages" can be linked together to make a longer story. Stories can be saved and printed out. Outstanding examples of such software include the *Imagination Express Series* of CD-ROMs from Riverdeep/Edmark. This series of multimedia CD-ROMs presents a variety of settings and themes upon which users can build their own stories or reports, including: *Imagination Express: Neighborhood, Imagination Express: Castle, Imagination Express: Ocean, Imagination Express: Pyramid,* and *Imagination Express: Rainforest.*

Imagination Express and similar software appeals to children of a wide age and ability range (grades K–8). With the help of an adult, younger children can manipulate a library of graphics to produce a picture and stop right there. The picture can be used as the beginning of an oral personal narrative ("One time when my mom took me to the park . . ."). An especially motivating feature in the *Imagination Express* series is the ability to record speech or other sounds and then link the sound to an object or character on the screen.

In *Imagination Express* and similar software, the selection of graphics includes backgrounds, people, objects, and animals. The libraries of graphic stickers are interesting to children and seem to quickly inspire creativity. Not only can the software be used to address many different goals but also the same activity might serve different purposes for different children. For example, if a clinician encouraged a child to select a shark and place it beside a ship on a story page from *Imagination Express: Ocean*, two stimulus words for /sh/ production would be available for practice. Alternatively, the shark beside the ship assists another child with practicing two-dimensional representations of spatial concepts such as *beside*. For a third client, the graphics already in place might serve as the impetus to make up a story.

The clinician can use such flexible software to provide opportunities for practicing skills like sequencing information, developing elements of an episode, negotiating with peers, or giving and requesting clarification. The pragmatic language case example that follows demonstrates three desirable characteristics in action.

1. Use of the computer activity to provide a context for conversation between students and the clinician

2. Use of flexible software that allows the clinician to tailor this activity to exactly meet the needs and abilities of these students

3. Use of software with curricular content that complements classroom goals

CASE EXAMPLE: Using *Imagination Express: Ocean* as a Context for Language Therapy

Objectives: 1) When presented with incomplete or confusing directions, the child will request clarification. 2) When presented with the clinician's puzzled facial expression and/or a request, the child will provide clarification including more information (not just repetition of previous utterance).

Preparation: An underwater scene showing rocks and seaweed, a diver, several fish, a shark, a treasure chest, and an octopus has been created by the clinician, printed out, and placed in an envelope. Then characters and objects in the scene were rearranged and the file was saved prior to the session (3–5 minutes, total prep time). The basic scene used for this activity was created by other students working on a different objective.

Clinician: Today we are going to practice giving directions. It is important to be able to tell people what they need to do. We'll take turns. First, one person will look at the picture in this envelope. That person gives the directions and the other person will do what they say on the computer, until the scene matches the picture. Who wants to be first?

Katie: I want to do the computer.

Clinician: Okay, Katie (pushing mouse toward Katie). Dakota, here's the picture we're supposed to make on the computer (giving envelope to Dakota). Don't let us see it! Tell us what we should move first.

Dakota: Geesh!

Clinician: (looks expectantly at Dakota)

Dakota: Put that guy over on the other side.

Katie: (looks confused) Huh?

Dakota: That swimming guy—put him over by that chest. (Katie moves diver)

Clinician: The diver goes beside the treasure chest?

Dakota: Yeah, the diver goes beside the treasure and up a little.

Katie: Okay, how's that?

Note that both students in this example are communicating with a purpose. Along the way, they are getting experience with vocabulary and relationships that are being presented in their regular classroom through a science unit about oceans. Neither the students nor the clinician are asking questions to which the answers are already known by everyone in the group (non-communicative interaction). On the contrary, Dakota has new information to convey to Katie as clearly as possible, and Katie is attempting to act on the information provided by Dakota. So, both students are engaged in genuine communication about concepts they need for classroom success.

ENHANCING NARRATIVE SKILLS

Software for classroom or home use can often be incorporated into a series of therapy sessions or a long-term project. *Imagination Express (Neighborhood, Castle, Ocean, Pyramid,* or *Rainforest)* exemplifies this kind of software. In group language therapy, the students might begin by exploring the extra resources included in the software, such as information about fish and other ocean life. Speech output is available for supporting reading text aloud to students who have weak or emerging reading skills.

There are various ways to facilitate narrative skills using software like the *Imagination Express* series. One approach would begin when students have a general familiarity with the content of the software. A plan for a story or report is then negotiated between group members. The planning stage is crucial, because important opportunities for practicing oral communication inevitably occur. They might plan the main points in storyboard style on pieces of paper, or outline them in a word processor. Or, they could organize their information using graphical organizing software such as *Kidspiration* (Inspiration Software, Inc.) or describe their ideas on a tape recorder for future reference. Then the group works on the computer in teams to develop illustrations and the exact narrative text. Again, working in teams ensures that opportunities for conversation, misunderstanding, negotiation, and clarification will arise. Some group members add recordings of their own voices narrating each page or speaking for characters. Depending upon the specific speech and language goals for the group, the story is shared with younger students, printed out into booklets to take home, or turned into a bulletin board display.

Although the computer provides a shared focus in the previous examples, the clinician provides the communicative purpose, models, and feedback that ensure effective speech or language activities. Clinicians can use story-making software to help children improve their narrative skills at all levels. Naremore, Densmore, and Harman (2001) suggested a hierarchy of narrative skills that builds upon a child's familiarity with routine events (script knowledge). They provided clinicians with assessment and intervention suggestions for three levels of narrative development

Table 9.3.   Software and activities for encouraging oral and written narrative skills

Sample Language Objectives (Narrative)	Software Examples	Activities
Telling personal event narratives: Personal event narratives are organized around a high point, which is the reason for telling someone what happened. Children can tell well-formed personal narratives by age 6 (McCabe & Rollins, 1994).	*Just Grandma and Me, Imagination Express: Neighborhood, The Cat in the Hat,* Digital camera and generic word processor, slideshow, or movie software	Software is used to model and practice telling what happened from a personal perspective ("When the clown came to my school . . ." "Saturday I went to visit my Grandma . . ." "When mom and I went to the mall yesterday . . ." "This year at my birthday party . . ." "When Dorothy and I went to the park last night . . .").
Episodic story re-telling: Episodes consist of three elements: an *initiating event* or problem, an *attempt* or response, and a *consequence*. Children who have had exposure to good books for young children are able to re-tell episodic stories in kindergarten (Naremore, et al., 2001).	*Thinking Out Loud, Tiger Tales, P.B. Bear's Birthday Party*	Software is used for listening to and viewing an engaging story, describing episodes in the story, and retelling single and multi-episode, multi-scene stories. Some software permits re-arrangement of story pieces and recording of children's voices in key scenes.
Creating original episodic stories: Understanding and using underlying story structure develops over time. By fifth grade, children can independently tell coherent, goal-based, original stories (Naremore, et al., 2001).	*Sunbuddy Writer, Stanley's Sticker Stories, Imagination Express Series*	Software is used to plan original stories, develop illustrations of key episodes, and write text to accompany illustrations. Finished stories are viewed on the computer (with animations and sound) or printed out in book pages.

- Personal event narratives
- Story retelling
- Creating episodic stories

Work on narrative development can be extended and enhanced with appropriate computer tools and a computer-as-context clinical approach. Table 9.3 presents software examples and activities for each level.

Included in Table 9.3 is the possibility that the clinician and clients will use generic software tools as a shared context for therapy. For example, a digital camera could be used to record key school or classroom events (e.g., "Our Trip to the Zoo") or stages in a long-term project (e.g., "How We Planted and Tended Our Class Garden"). Using the pictures as a starting point, a book could be developed that matched the language and literacy skills of any group of students. Section IV discusses the many ways in which computers can be used to generate therapy materials, including multimedia memory books and journals.

WHAT A COMPETENT CLINICIAN NEEDS TO KNOW

Clinicians who are working toward competency at creating a shared context with a computer and school-age clients should be well-informed about the general goals of the curriculum as well as other IEP objectives that are in place for each child. If computers are being frequently and appropriately used in classrooms, appropriate software may already be available for accomplishing this competency. It may take some scouting and consultation with classroom teachers or technology coordinators to find it. Even regular word processing can be used to enhance an extended project and to serve as the context for therapy interactions. Clinicians who have more advanced computer skills themselves may want to explore the possibilities of including digital photography and other multimedia in their projects with children.

It is important to note, however, that the competency discussed in this topic requires minimal technical knowledge–the emphasis is on creating a context for conversation with a computer activity at the core. Experienced clinicians who happen to be computer novices will probably make faster progress on this competency than computer whizzes who are novice clinicians. What will make the difference is identifying appropriate goals and thinking through what each person in the therapy session will actually do and say, to ensure that the goals are actually addressed.

SUMMARY

A variety of available software programs are appropriate for creating a context for therapy with school-age children. Even with only a word processor, however, clinicians can integrate computer-based activities into therapy sessions, which address specific and individualized communication goals and complement curricular objectives.

Clinicians are encouraged to explore multimedia toolkits for story making that integrate word processing with graphics and sound. Such software is attractive to school-age children and helps clinicians plan activities that focus on oral language and facilitate the development of academic skills.

REVIEW FOR TOPIC 9

1. Describe three purposes that can be achieved when using computer-as-context therapy activities.
2. Give an example of software and a computer-as-context activity you could use to accomplish one of these purposes.
3. What are some advantages to using the computer to make projects that could also be done with traditional paper, pens, and crayons?
4. What are the four steps involved in the "process approach" to writing? Discuss how pre-computer, computer, and post-computer activities are parallel to the steps in the "process approach" and give an example activity for each.
5. Review a software program listed in this topic or one that is similar (open-ended, flexible). Give examples of speech or language goals that could be addressed as well as pre- and post-computer activities that you would like to try.

QUESTIONS FOR DISCUSSION

1. Describe a school-age client and choose a likely speech or language goal. Decide what software could be employed as a context for conversation including this goal, and write a

sample dialogue showing how the clinician will make sure that your speech or language goal is addressed.

2. Reconsider the example above in which the clinician and students are using *Imagination Express: Ocean* to practice giving directions and requesting/giving clarification. Discuss the difference between this approach to using the computer and using CAI software to teach direction words (beside, between, above/below, and so forth).

RESOURCES FOR FURTHER STUDY

Cochran, P.S., & Bull, G.L. (1991). Integrating word processing into language intervention. *Topics in Language Disorders, 11*(2), 31–48.

Gardner, J.E., Wissick, C.A., Schweder, W., & Canter, L.S. (2003). Enhancing interdisciplinary instruction in general and special education: Thematic units and technology. *Remedial and Special Education, 24*(3),161–172.

Justice, L.M., & Kaderavek, J. (2002). Using shared storybook reading to promote emergent literacy. *TEACHING Exceptional Children, 34*(4), 8–13.

Naremore, R.C., Densmore, A.E., & Harman, D.R. (2001). *Assessment and treatment of school-age language disorders: A resource manual.* San Diego: Singular.

Nelson, N.W., Bahr, C.M., & Van Meter, A.M. (2004). *The writing lab approach to language instruction and intervention.* Baltimore, MD: Paul H. Brookes Publishing Co.

Wood, L.A., & Masterson, J.J. (1999). The use of technology to facilitate language skills in school-age children. *Seminars in Speech and Language, 20*(3), 219–232.

Using a Computer as a Context to Facilitate Literacy

Clinical computing competency #2: The clinician will demonstrate the ability to use computer-based activities as a shared context for communication with clients

Clinicians can achieve this competency by choosing and using appropriate open-ended software to help children acquire emergent literacy skills. Competent clinicians will know how to envision and implement computer-based activities that provide communication opportunities for all participants. Such activities can be used to create a context that teaches and reinforces phonemic awareness and the functions of literacy.

Research into the relationship between language development and later academic success has focused on the complexities of early and emergent literacy. A large body of research confirms the relationship between specific language skills, such as phonological awareness, and acquisition of literacy (for summaries, see Catts, 1993; Koppenhaver, Coleman, Kalman, & Yoder, 1991; Stahl & Murray, 1994). As professionals become increasingly skilled at assessing and teaching the language skills that underlie academic success, they look for effective new materials and methods. Complementing more traditional interventions, open-ended computer activities can facilitate both oral language development and emergent literacy skills. Computers can also be used to help children acquire the language skills that underlie advanced literacy, as discussed in Topic 11.

THE LANGUAGE DEVELOPMENT CONTINUUM: LISTENING, TALKING, READING, AND WRITING

A current perspective on the clinical applications of computers requires a contemporary perspective on language development. The transition from oral language to literacy used to be described in terms of prerequisites and readiness skills. Mistakenly, clinicians and teachers viewed language development as a hierarchy through which children passed on their way to literacy (see Figure 10.1).

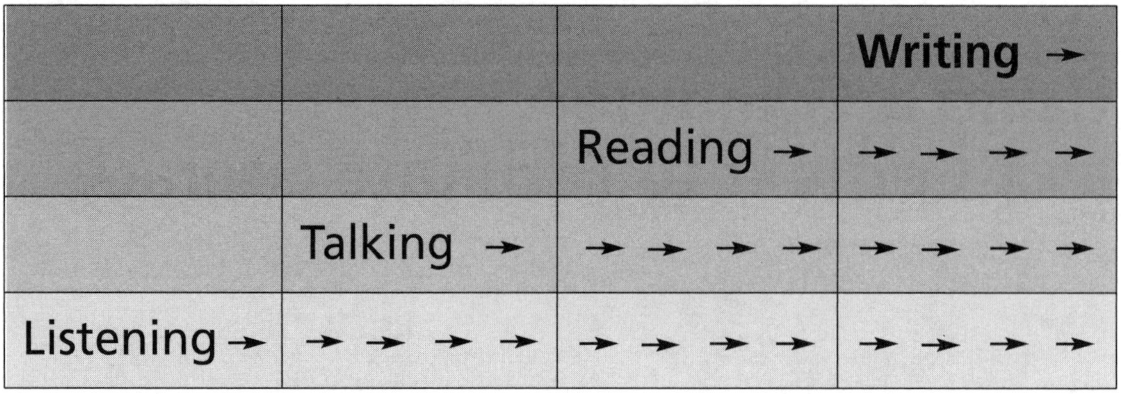

			Writing →
		Reading →	→ → → →
	Talking →	→ → → →	→ → → →
Listening →	→ → → →	→ → → →	→ → → →

Figure 10.1. Outdated view of language skills as a hierarchy of levels.

At each level in the hierarchical view, there were "prerequisite" skills on which goals for instruction were based. For many children with speech, language, and hearing impairments, failure to succeed at the lower levels of the hierarchy resulted in low expectations for achieving literacy and instruction that was modified accordingly (Koppenhaver et al., 1991). According to some researchers, children with physical and cognitive impairments had substantially less exposure to print at home and less (instead of more!) instruction in reading and writing than typical peers (Pierce & McWilliams, 1993). The resulting vicious cycle (low expectations–less exposure and instruction–low achievement–low expectations, and so forth) may have contributed to low literacy levels in children and adults with moderate to severe delay and disorders in communication skills.

An updated perspective holds that language development should be thought of as a continuum, rather than as a hierarchy (see Figure 10.2). "Developing speaking abilities enhances children's listening abilities, which improves their writing abilities and facilitates their reading development" (Koppenhaver et al., 1991, p. 39).

In this view, developing language is acquiring competency with symbols of all types–sounds, words, gestures, pictures, and graphemes. Koppenhaver et al. (1991) summarized the findings of emergent literacy research involving typically developing children. The following conclusions derive from their review:

1. Learning to read and write is a process that begins at birth.

2. Reading, writing, talking, and listening are interrelated in development.

3. Learning the functions of literacy is as important as knowing the forms.

4. Children achieve literacy (as other language skills) through active participation in their environment.

An important implication for clinicians lies within these conclusions. When clinicians deliberately consider literacy in their work with children, they are reinforcing all aspects of language development. What is the rationale for clinicians using computers to facilitate literacy? Just like many other areas of communication and academics, computers can be interesting and motivating tools that also promote the acquisition of literacy skills.

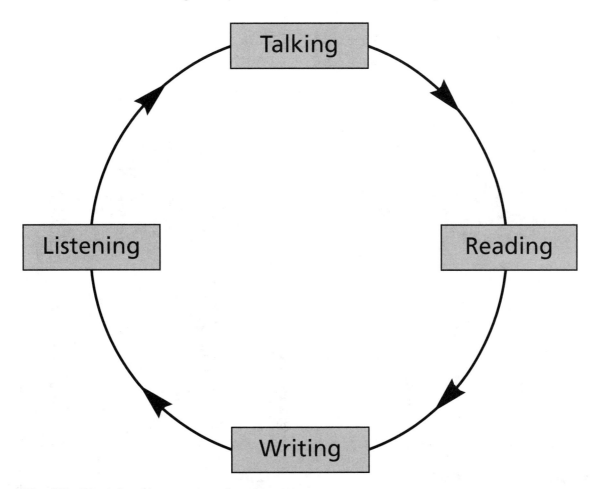

Figure 10.2.   Current view of language as a continuum.

PHONOLOGICAL AWARENESS:
USING THE COMPUTER AS A CONTEXT FOR DISCOVERY

Children with language impairments are at risk for difficulties with phonological aware-ness, and are likely to need more instruction and practice than a typical classroom provides (Blachman, Ball, Black, & Tangel, 1994; Catts, 1993; Kamhi & Catts, 1986; Naremore et al., 2001). Naremore et al. (2001) identified four levels of phonological awareness that may warrant clinical attention: syllabification; rhyming; attention to indi-vidual phonemes (beginning sounds, ending sounds, then blending sounds); and ability to add, delete, or move phonemes and regenerate the resulting word.

Clinicians are encouraged to consult resources such as curricular guidelines when choosing assessment and intervention goals specific to phonological awareness. For ex-ample, the Commonwealth of Virginia Standards of Learning suggest that kindergartners should orally identify words that rhyme; sort words orally according to shared begin-ning, ending, or medial sounds; blend sounds orally to make words or syllables; and divide syllables orally into sounds. Motivating computer-as-context activities can be planned once appropriate goals are established. Software exemplars that could be used to address such goals with individuals or small groups are found in Table 10.1.

Table 10.1. Software examples for creating a shared context and working on phonemic awareness

Sample language objectives (phonemic awareness)	Software exemplars	Software description	Computer activities
Learning nursery rhymes and rhyming songs	*Five Little Monkeys Jumping on a Bed*, *Old MacDonald's Farm Deluxe*, *Fall Fun* (SoftTouch)	These simple computer games and song activities emphasize uncluttered graphics and adapted access.	Individual children or small groups can choose when the computer presents the next scene or line of a rhyming song (e.g., "Five fat turkeys are we; we live in a giant tree . . ."). When children become familiar with the songs and rhymes, they can predict the next line and then see and hear whether they were correct.
Auditory identification of words that rhyme (in a meaningful context)	*The Cat in the Hat*, *Green Eggs and Ham*, *Dr. Seuss ABC's*	These electronic storybooks presented well-known children's books in a format that includes high-quality speech, music, and animations.	Together, children and clinician watch and listen as the computer reads a page and each word is highlighted. A single story page might be the focus of the entire session. The clinician and children take turns clicking on individual words and finding other words that rhyme on the page. "Let's find a word that rhymes with Sam. Sam." When auditory identification of words that rhyme is mastered, children can be asked to make up words that rhyme. "Can you think of a word that rhymes with ham?" Other language skills (verb usage, spatial relationships, negotiating) can be simultaneously addressed during this activity.
Auditory identification of beginning, ending sounds in words.	*A Whale of a Tale: Leap into Language 1* (Innova Multimedia) *Learning to Read with Phonics: 1st and 2nd Grade* (Riverdeep/ The Learning Company)	Games focussed on sounds, rhymes, and other aspects of language.	PreK – 2 activities, including rhymes, songs, stories, animations of language concepts. Some of the activities in these packages are more like CAI in design, but clinician could tailor small group interaction to create a shared context and turn-taking.
Matching beginning sounds to alphabet and keyboard	*Literacy: Phonemic Awareness* (Locutour/Learning Fundamentals) *Simon Sounds it Out* (Don Johnston)	This software is designed for use in speech therapy and to facilitate phonemic awareness.	In the Read My Lips module of *Literacy: Phonemic Awareness*, the computer plays a close-up video of a person saying a sound, and describing the sound. Users can record their own productions and compare them to the model. This activity could be a fun and beneficial way to explore, discuss, and practice the idea of how sounds are associated with letters and begin words. *Simon Sounds it Out* is switch-accessible and has scanning options, allowing children who need adapted access to participate in phonemic awareness and phonics activities.
Matching sounds to individual letters, syllables, and words	*Dr.Peet's Talkwriter Windows*, *Dr.Peet's Talkwriter Mac* (Interest-Driven Learning, Inc.) *Intellitalk* (Intellitools) *Write:Outloud* (Don Johnston)	Talking word processors that allow users to type and hear one letter/sound at a time, or whole words.	Sound–letter relationships can be explored with this flexible tool, without the pressure or distraction of a competition or game environment.

Addressing phonemic awareness through individual computer activities was previously mentioned in Topic 5: Using Computer-Assisted Instruction (CAI) with Children. In that topic, the focus was on drill-and-practice with computer-controlled goals, activities, and performance measures. In this topic, the emphasis is on using flexible computer activities as a context for discovering, discussing, and exploring the phonological aspects of language. The difference is not merely a matter of software selection (e.g., choose X software versus Y software). The distinction also comes in the clinician's intent—is this computer activity intended to be something the child does independently to practice skills that do not require interaction with another person, or is this computer activity intended to address communication skills, in which case a human conversational partner is essential. Planning and implementing these distinctly different activities require different clinical computing competencies of clinicians.

WHAT IS A TALKING WORD PROCESSOR?

A talking word processing program makes it possible to hear whatever a writer writes. Sometimes this software is called a word processor with speech output. Early talking word processors required special hardware to be added to computers to provide speech output. Now most computers come equipped with speech output capability, but usually special word processing software is required to take full advantage of sound/speech capabilities. This is especially true for users who have special needs. Examples of software designed particularly for users with special needs or emergent skills include *Clicker for Windows and Mac* (Crick Software, Ltd.), *Dr. Peet's Talkwriter* for Windows or Mac (Interest-Driven Learning, Inc.), *Write: Outloud* (Don Johnston, Inc.), *PixReader* (Slater Software), *IntelliTalk* (IntelliTools), *Kurzweil 3000* (Kurzweil Education Systems), *Aurora 3 for Windows* (Aurora Systems), *WriteAway2000* (Information Services, Inc.), and *WYNN 3.0* (Freedom Scientific).

Most talking word processing software can be configured to allow the user to hear each letter as it is typed, each word as it is typed, a whole line of text, or a whole page. An increased sense of audience may result as the writer has the opportunity to consider the writing from a listener's point of view. Empirical studies and anecdotal reports suggest that such auditory feedback has a positive impact on writers who are young or who have language impairments (Blischak, 1995; Collis, 1988, 1989; King & Hux, 1995; Rosegrant, 1984). Despite the positive research findings and the availability of well-designed, reasonably priced software choices, many teachers and clinicians remain unaware of the benefits of talking word processing. It is a powerful addition to a repertoire of clinical computing tools.

Talking word processors began as utilities for writers with visual impairments. Refined over the years, these programs hold potential for many special populations, including children and adults with developmental or acquired language disabilities and speakers of English as a second language. In some settings, talking word processing may serve as a component of an augmentative and alternative communication (AAC) system. For example, a child with severe communication impairment could deliver an oral book report by writing it with the talking word processor and having the computer "read" it aloud to the class.

It is desirable for talking word processing programs to include a feature that allows the user to change the pronunciation of a selected word. This is an important capability, because speech synthesizers may mispronounce personal names and other words that are exceptions to regular spelling rules. Rather than having to choose between the correct spelling and the correct pronunciation, the user can add a more acceptable pronunciation for the computer to use whenever the problem word is encountered. For example, suppose the speech synthesizer mispronounced the name "Michelle" with a hard /ch/ as "Mitchel." This is easily fixed by selecting the word "Michelle" and typing in a preferred pronunciation, such as "Mishell." The computer adds the word "Michelle" to its dictionary of exceptions so that this correction need be made by the user only once. From then on, when the word appears correctly spelled on the screen, it is pronounced according to the alternative in the exceptions dictionary.

Talking word processing programs may provide additional user support features such as spell-checking, word prediction, background/text color alternatives, or spoken punctuation. More comprehensive reading and writing tools, such as *WYNN* and *Kurzweil 3000*, include speech output as just one of many features designed to facilitate successful access to and production of text materials. Matching software features to individual needs is particularly important when choosing a program for the long-term use of a certain child or adult. Hunt-Berg, Rankin, and Beukelman (1994) and Sturm, Rankin, Beukelman, and Schutz-Meuhling (1997) provided detailed discussion of such considerations, along with matrices of features included in various software. For general clinical and classroom purposes and the activities described in the following section, any talking word processing software will work well.

USING TALKING WORD PROCESSING TO EXPLORE SOUND–SYMBOL RELATIONSHIPS

It is one thing to read about how a talking word processor works and an entirely different thing to actually use one. Imagine the difference between riding a bicycle and reading about bicycles—there is no comparison. Talking word processing is fun. Adults as well as children enjoy hearing what the speech synthesizer does with their words, and trying out new combinations of letters just to see and hear what happens. Together, they can discover dozens of ways to explore sound–symbol relationships.

Anecdotal reports suggest that preschoolers often respond to talking word processing in similar ways (Rosegrant, 1984). One example often described is a youngster who types the same letter repeatedly, just to hear the computer say it. If a child asks an adult to name a particular letter, most readily comply at least once or twice. A patient teacher or parent might repeat the name of a letter four or five times in a row upon request. But how many adults would patiently repeat the name of the same letter 25 or 30 or 40 times in a row? This is how many times some children want to hear the names of the letters they type; the computer says them as cheerfully the 40th time as the first. (Note that headphones can be attached to the computer whenever speech output is likely to disturb other people.)

Explorations can extend to sound combinations. A common occurrence in beginning spelling is for children to invent combinations of sounds/letters in order to approximate words they wish to use. If a talking word processor is available they hear what these combinations sound like. Adding this multi-sensory feedback to the beginning writing process is interesting and motivating for most learners.

In a study of children in a rural Head Start program, the motivating effects of speech output were examined (Windham, 2000). The purpose of the study was to compare how children used a word processing program when speech output was activated and when it was not. Eighteen children ages 4–6 participated. Both quantitative and qualitative data were collected over a 6-week period during which repeated observations took place. Children worked individually and in pairs at the computer with an informed adult. Results suggested that children demonstrated more behavior considered "exploratory" when speech output was activated. In this condition, children were also more likely to offer help to each other, more likely to talk about what was happening on the computer, more likely to express pleasure or excitement, and more likely to attend to what they typed on the screen than when the computer was silent.

EMPHASIZING THE FUNCTIONS OF LITERACY

Researchers tell us that children must learn that reading and writing are useful and fun (the functions), not just how to do them (the forms). Some clinicians have difficulty envisioning oral language activities that could make use of a talking word processor. Other clinicians may hesitate to try a talking word processor because they feel inadequately prepared to teach "writing." However, experience suggests that actually using a tool like this with children will lead most clinicians to see many possibilities. Three general purpose activities follow. These activities take advantage of the speech output capabilities of talking word processing and help children learn about the important functions of literacy through personal experience. They also could be used to facilitate a wide range of other speech and language goals.

Daily News

"Morning news" is the name that Rosegrant (1985) gave the oral language activity with which many preschools start the day. Sitting on mats in a circle around the teacher, children take turns reporting some "news" about themselves or their family. When talking word processing software is available, the news can be revisited throughout the day. A clinician or aide can type as each child talks during circle time (see Figure 10.3). When the news for the day is complete, children listen to their own sentences by placing the cursor on their name and pressing a "say it" key. They hear their own or someone else's news as many times as they desire, without depending on an adult to read it to them over and over again. The news can be printed out and sent home for parents to reinforce and discuss with their child.

You've Got a Message

A clinician can use a talking word processing program to prepare a message for an individual child ahead of time. Even non-readers can get "mail" if they can find their names on the screen and put the cursor beside the right name. When the "say it" key is pressed, the computer reads the line of text following the child's name (see Figure 10.4).

Daily News

Juan: *My mom said I can bring my Pokemon for show and tell.*

LaToya: *My dog was lost but now he came home!*

Alex: *I'm going to Walmart to get Halloween stuff. My grandma is going to take me. I like Walmart.*

Sheila: *I want to be a bumble bee for Halloween.*

Figure 10.3. Sample Daily News activity implemented with talking word processor.

Word Swap: It's a Good Thing

Older children enjoy experimenting with language when incongruities, puzzles, or exaggerations are involved. A talking word processor can be used to create amusing texts that focus on either syntactic or semantic aspects of language. For example, as the context for a lesson about descriptive words, the clinician could prepare a short story which includes several general adjectives like "good, neat, okay, fine, great" (see Figure 10.5). This activity could be done with any talking word processor, but is a perfect example of how to use one that has a frozen text option, such as *IntelliTalk II* (IntelliTools). Everything but the descriptive words could be frozen text. Ahead of time, the clinician highlights the undesirable descriptive words (the not-so-"good" ones) by changing their text to a different color. This gives the students an additional cue regarding which words are going to be changed during the activity, but the remainder of the passage does not get accidentally deleted or rearranged.

During the language therapy session, the group could listen to the story and discuss how it could be improved. They could experiment by replacing the words "good" and "okay" with more explicit adjectives. Thus, Amy could be a talented musician playing cool music. This activity could lead to another in which synonyms are discussed—how many words that mean "good" can they think of?

WHY THE DIFFERENCE BETWEEN SYNTHESIZED AND DIGITIZED SPEECH IS IMPORTANT

Talking word processing software converts text into computer-generated speech. This synthesized speech is based on the pronunciation rules of a particular language. The primary advantage of text-to-speech synthesizers is that they can and will try to pronounce anything a user types—in this sense, the "vocabulary" is infinite. Synthesized speech is often used in

Before therapy the clinician creates a message:

Sheila, Happy Birthday!

Missy, I noticed that you were NOT yelling on the playground yesterday—congratulations on using your good voice!

James, your /s/ sounds were super in the school pageant—superb performance!

During therapy, children read messages that start with their own names, and can plan group or individual messages for classmates who will see them later that day:

Fontaine and John, pizza is on the school menu today!

Carl, see you later on the bus, from Fontaine.

Janet, I like your new Barbie lunch box , love from Connie Sue.

Figure 10.4.   Examples of personal messages children listen to using talking word processing.

AAC devices where the user wants unlimited vocabulary capability. Typical listeners find even the best synthesized speech slightly less intelligible than regular human speech (Hustad, Kent, & Beukelman, 1998; Klatt & Klatt, 1990; Logan, Greene, & Pisoni, 1989; Scherz & Beer, 1995; Venkatagiri, 1996) It also sounds a bit artificial or robotic because getting stress, intonation, and timing features right is so difficult (and dependent on context).

Synthesized speech should not be confused with digitized speech, which is often found in educational and entertainment software. When a computer records a person talking, stores that file, then plays it back, the result is digitized speech. It is common to have professional actors record the narration for electronic books, games, and CAI. A range of factors can affect digitized speech quality, but generally it is perceived to be intelligible and often indistinguishable from live human speech. High-quality digitized speech files require large storage capacity. So, digitized speech and music first became routine features in educational and entertainment software with the popularity of CD-ROM drives (see more about digitized speech in Sections IV and V). Because a human speaker must pre-record every word, digitized speech is best used in situations where a finite, known vocabulary is required. For this reason, it is not used in talking word processing programs.

In the minds of many, the issues surrounding digitized speech, synthesized speech, and speech recognition overlap. Speech recognition technology involves digitizing the dictation of a speaker and converting it into text displayed on the computer screen (in many ways, the opposite of the process involved in synthesized speech). The clinical use of speech recognition technology is covered in Topic 39.

> ## A Good Musician
>
> Once upon a time there was a good musician named Amy. She thought playing music was a pretty good way to make a living. Whenever she played, the audience would yell, "Amy is a good musician!" During the big concert, Amy wanted to play a song that her fans would say was okay, or maybe even good.

Figure 10.5. Example of a "good" paragraph that could be improved with more specific and descriptive adjectives.

WHAT THE COMPETENT CLINICIAN NEEDS TO KNOW

CAI software as well as the software listed in Table 10.1 could be used to address phonological awareness or emergent literacy goals. However, using non-CAI software or a tool such as a talking word processor requires a different set of clinical skills than does choosing an appropriate CAI program. It helps enormously to be familiar with the software. Talking word processors are easy to use, but clinicians need a little time to explore, just as their clients will. In the long run, such familiarization yields results in therapy ideas and time savings.

Exploring with the software also makes an excellent "shared context" for conversation with a client, "What happens if we change the voice? What will happen if I click here? How will it say my name?" There is plenty to do and plenty to talk about, with individuals or small groups of clients. The clinical challenge comes in planning and managing this interaction in a way that is therapeutically or educationally beneficial. That everyone will probably enjoy the activity is a given; that everyone will learn or practice important communication behaviors is less certain unless the clinician is skilled in planning and implementing session objectives.

A talking word processor provides a context for exploring the sounds and symbols of language, the way a sandbox encourages people to weigh and measure sand. Crucial learning takes place, although it may look and feel like play. It may not be simple learning of the rote-recall type. Therefore, clinicians and teachers should look beyond X% correct criteria for estimating the ways in which learners using talking word processing are progressing. Such additional documentation might include, for example, time-on-task, preference for task over other choices, motivation to complete task, cooperation with others, use of content-related questions, and printouts of activity results (typing) showing which letters/sounds were of particular interest.

SUMMARY

Open-ended computer activities (non-CAI) can facilitate both oral language development and emergent literacy skills. Contemporary perspectives on acquisition of literacy view it as a component of language development that occurs in parallel with oral language development. A range of flexible software types such as electronic books and talking word processors can be used effectively to help children acquire emergent literacy skills such as rhyming, sound isolation at the beginning and ending of words, alphabet familiarity, and sound–symbol relationships. It is important for teachers and clinicians to emphasize both the forms and the functions of literacy.

Research suggests that the use of talking word processors has many benefits for beginning readers and writers. Talking word processors make use of synthesized rather than digitized speech, because an unlimited, unpredictable vocabulary is desired. Suggestions for individual and group activities using talking word processors as a context for therapy include Daily News, You've Got a Message, and Word Swap. Clinicians are encouraged to explore the use of such flexible software to create a conversational context for communication with clients. The learning that occurs in such contexts can be measured in multiple ways.

REVIEW FOR TOPIC 10

1. What is meant by the "forms" versus the "functions" of literacy?
2. Why do talking word processors use synthesized speech instead of digitized speech?
3. What is the difference in intent between selecting a CAI software program to practice specific computer-determined phonemic awareness skills and addressing phonemic awareness using a talking word processor?
4. Explain why using a talking word processor might be more likely to encourage emergent literacy than using a traditional word processing program without speech output.

QUESTIONS FOR DISCUSSION

1. Tell about an example from your family or friends, which illustrates that very young children are learning to recognize all kinds of symbols, visual and auditory (e.g., the baby who recognizes the right cereal box in the grocery store).
2. Find an example of electronic storybook software to try, or look for a demo on the Internet. What aspects of literacy are reinforced by this software? What additional speech or language goals could be addressed while talking about this software with a client?
3. Consider the statement that compared a talking word processor to a sandbox. How does this analogy work?
4. Discuss the ways in which the examples in this topic could also be applied to adolescents and adults who need to work on literacy skills. Which clinical populations might especially benefit from the auditory feedback provided by a talking word processor?

RESOURCES FOR FURTHER STUDY

Cochran, P.S., & Bull, G.L. (1991). Integrating word processing into language intervention. *Topics in Language Disorders, 11*(2), 31–48.

Hustad, K.C., Kent, R.D., & Beukelman, D.R. (1998). DECtalk and Macintalk speech synthesizers: Intelligibility differences for three listener groups. *Journal of Speech, Language, and Hearing Research, 41*, 744–752.

Laine, C., & Sitko, M. (2001). Using computer assisted writing in inclusive settings. *Closing the gap: Computer technology in special education and rehabilitation, 20*(1), 1, 12, 31.

Nelson, N.W., Bahr, C.M., & Van Meter, A.M. (2004). *The writing lab approach to language instruction and intervention.* Baltimore: Paul H. Brookes Publishing Co.

Wood, L.A., & Masterson, J.J. (1999). The use of technology to facilitate language skills in school-age children. *Seminars in Speech and Language, 20*(3), 219–232.

Using a Computer as a Context to Facilitate Advanced Language and Literacy Skills

Clinical Computing Competency #2: The clinician will demonstrate the ability to use computer-based activities as a shared context for communication with clients.

This competency can be achieved by clinicians who design flexible computer activities for helping clients practice the language skills that underlie advanced literacy, such as finding the main idea in pictures, words, sentences, and paragraphs. Other language skills that are necessary for success in reading comprehension and effective writing include identifying given versus inferred information and using language to negotiate and persuade. Competent clinicians will know how to use computer-based activities to teach and reinforce all of these important language skills through extended projects.

A review of national and state curricular guidelines will assure clinicians and teachers that good communication skills are crucial not just for early academic success, but also for continued advancement in school. Emergent literacy success depends heavily on phonological awareness and learning decoding strategies. According to Moats, "Eighty percent of the variance in reading comprehension at the first-grade level is accounted for by how well students sound out words and recognize words out of context" (2000, p. 9). Moats argued that the relationship between decoding and comprehension changes as children move into the middle grades. "Comprehension strategies and knowledge of word meanings become more of a factor in reading success as students move into more advanced stages" (p. 9).

Mature readers and writers depend upon language abilities that are subtle, complex, and comprehensive. This topic presents computer-as-context therapy ideas that emphasize the language skills that school children need for the more challenging academic tasks encountered in upper elementary school and beyond. The emphasis in this topic is on using language during computer activities:

Table 11.1. Examples of state curriculum guidelines for advanced language and literacy

Academic area	Level	Sample state guideline (not presented in its entirety)
English—Oral language	Grade 4	The student will use effective oral communication skills in a variety of settings. • Present accurate directions to individuals and small groups. • Contribute to group discussions. • Seek the ideas and opinions of others. • Begin to use evidence to support opinions. The student will make and listen to oral presentations and reports. • Use subject-related information and vocabulary. • Listen to and record information. • Organize information for clarity.
English—Reading	Grade 4	The student will demonstrate comprehension of a variety of literary forms. • Use text organizers such as type, headings, and graphics to predict and categorize information. • Formulate questions that might be answered in the selection. • Make inferences using information from texts. • Paraphrase content of selection, identifying important ideas and providing details for each important idea. • Write about what is read.
English—Writing	Grade 4	The student will write effective narratives and explanations. • Focus on one aspect of a topic. • Develop a plan for writing. • Organize writing to convey a central idea. • Write several related paragraphs on the same topic. • Edit final copies for grammar, capitalization, punctuation, and spelling. • Use available technology.

Source: The Commonwealth of Virginia Standards of Learning (www.pen.k12.va.us/go/Sols).

- To identify and convey the "main idea"

- To infer new information from given information

- To negotiate with and persuade other members of a group

Clinicians working with adolescents and adults who have language and literacy skills impairments will find these therapy ideas and strategies useful as well.

AWARENESS OF CURRICULAR GUIDELINES AND CLASSROOM COLLABORATION

Close collaboration among school personnel helps inclusion efforts to succeed, which helps children obtain maximum benefit from their educational opportunities. Educationally relevant IEP goals for communication and appropriate computer-based activities for therapy are easier to develop with reference to overall curricular priorities. Table 11.1 presents sample standards of learning from Virginia, but similar guidelines can be found across many states and within the recommendations of content-related educational associations.

As indicated in Table 11.1, fourth graders are expected to listen to presentations and record (write) information. This is the beginning of note taking. Presumably, children are to pick out the most important or central information and write that down (or otherwise record it, if assistive technology is in use). Fourth graders are also required to convey a central idea in writing and understand how headings and layout of text convey information.

Standards provide benchmarks to use in gauging students' progress but they do not prescribe instructional approaches or suggest strategies to address students' basic deficits in language. Some children may require intensive work on the concept of "main idea" before achieving a curricular benchmark calling for the application of this idea to a new situation. The same may be true for guidelines that require children to make inferences based on reading. The skills described in many curricular guidelines depend heavily on language abilities that some children may not yet possess. Clinicians can help by developing educationally relevant IEP objectives for children who are working on improving language skills under their guidance. Computer-as-context activities can be used to implement such objectives.

FINDING THE MAIN IDEA

The ability to look at a variety of stimuli and verbally summarize their commonalities is an important cognitive and linguistic skill. People depend on such categorization all the time in everyday tasks and events. Category labels like "dairy, produce, and meats" help people get groceries. Most adults take this "main idea" arrangement for granted until they cannot find something. For example, where should a person look for a recipe item like cream of tartar? Is it in dairy? Spices? Condiments? What *is* cream of tartar anyhow?

Anyone looking for an unfamiliar grocery item may momentarily feel puzzlement or frustration. Likewise, children whose summarization or categorization skills are inadequate may routinely experience puzzlement and frustration. When weak language skills

Table 11.2. Computer-as-context activities for identifying the main idea

Sample language objectives (Main Idea)	Software exemplars	Software description	Computer activities
Find the main idea in a group of pictures. Work on transition from describing the main idea in a group of pictures to labeling the main idea of a list of words.	*Kidspiration*	Called a "visual learning organizer," this software is a tool for creating concept maps with pictures, text, or both. Writing mode provides automatic outline based on visual concept map.	An illustrated "concept map" can be developed about almost any topic. An extensive symbol library is available, or images from the web are easily incorporated. Maps can be developed in advance for individual or group use, or children choose illustrations from the clip art library that match a main idea.
Find the main idea in a list of words. Make transition from pictures to words.	*Usborne's Animated First Thousand Words*	A collection of "scenes" filled with related objects and activities, like an electronic picture dictionary. In explore mode, user clicks on pictures and hears label; in game mode, user is given a list of items to find within a scene English or Spanish.	Play with or without text labels. Before using the computer, discuss the theme or main idea for the day (e.g., kitchen, classroom, restaurant, farm, beach, city street). What words to children think of when they hear the main idea? Ask what they expect to find if you go on a pretend trip to see a _(theme)_. At the computer with an adult, children take turns finding objects and talking about why that object is in that scene. Why does it "go with" these other things? Afterwards, reverse the process – say words or show pictures and ask, "where would you find ____?"
Find the main idea in a list of words. Find the main idea in a list of sentences.	*Intellitalk II*	Talking word processor with "frozen text" option. In frozen text mode, user listens to words read aloud but can't accidently delete or change the words.	Lists of single words or sentences of appropriate difficulty can be created and saved in advance. Word groups can be related to previous activities done with pictures and symbols. Good for beginning readers. Pairs or small groups can hear the words as many times as needed while discussing the "main idea" or choosing from a list of possibilities. Fill-in-the-blank activities are possible with frozen text.
Find the main idea in paragraphs where it is explicitly stated.	*Imagination Express: Castle, Ocean,* or *Rainforest*	This software series provides multimedia toolkits that each focus on a different theme. Each package provides background files similar to a brief encyclopedia, scene backgrounds, music, and libraries of characters and objects. Text and speech can be added to story pages created by the user. Resource files have a read-aloud option.	Pre-prepared scenes can be used to elicit "main idea" labels for pictures, or children can view a scene and choose a paragraph that best expresses the main idea of the scene, or scenes can be used to cue the main idea in a paragraph and children can discuss how to figure out the main idea. Children could create a scene that illustrates the main idea in a paragraph of text. With an adult, children can practice identifying the main idea in text-only paragraphs found in the background information files (e.g., the life of servants in a castle, or a bird in the rainforest).
Find the main idea in paragraphs where it is only implied.	*Start-to-Finish Books* (Don Johnston)	This high-interest, low vocabulary reading series provides stories and expository text in three forms: electronic book, paperback book, and audiocassette (grades 2/3 or 4/5).	These electronic books include selections from literature, sports, historical characters, mysteries, and science. Although language-level controlled, mature looking in format and illustrations.

are applied to the abstract task of reading, the processing load further increases. "What *is* this chapter in my social studies book about, anyhow?" The ability to find and describe the main idea in a body of text is considered a crucial reading comprehension skill. Underlying language ability in categorizing and summarizing must be present to support reading comprehension.

Informal and formal testing can be used to assess children's abilities with "main idea" tasks using oral and written language. Naremore et al. (2001) provided an informal assessment instrument based on the work of Baumann (1986). Their tasks are designed for use with children in third to seventh grade. They allow the clinician to observe a child identifying the main idea in a group of pictures, single words, phrases, sentences, and paragraphs. The computer-as-context therapy ideas presented in Table 11.2 follow the same task sequence.

MAIN IDEA TASKS AND GRAPHIC ORGANIZERS

Children develop main idea skills gradually during school years (Naremore, et al., 2001). Clinician's expectations for clients should be adjusted to match their individual language abilities. The examples that follow show how a clinician could use a graphic organizer to help children visualize and use category labels that tell the main idea. Graphic organizers are a type of software that helps users outline or otherwise arrange pieces of information to make them easier to understand or remember. Family trees, system flow-charts, and business management hierarchies, for example, are more easily conveyed in a format that combines text and graphical elements such as boxes, arrows, and other symbols. Many users find graphic organizers helpful for additional purposes, including thinking through and representing relationships that may or may not exist between items, facts, or people. Among the most widely used and highly rated graphic organizers for general use is *Inspiration* (Inspiration, Inc.).

Many teachers and clinicians use visual organization strategies as teaching tools. Terms that are often used for visual organization strategies include *webbing*, *idea mapping*, or *concept mapping*. For example, an idea map could be used to help students keep track of ideas during a prewriting brainstorming session. Traditionally, individual students would draw an idea map on a chalkboard, an easel pad, or on sheets of paper. Educators who wanted an easier way to color-code, duplicate, illustrate, and revise the maps and webs they were making with students quickly adopted software tools such as *Inspiration*. With a click, a graphical concept map made with *Inspiration* can be converted into a text outline, so students can use the method of organization that best meets their needs. *Inspiration* is now marketed for educational purposes and is recommended for students in grades 4 and higher. Special materials are available from Inspiration, Inc., to help teachers and clinicians make optimal use of *Inspiration* in classrooms.

A special version of *Inspiration*, called *Kidspiration* (Inspiration, Inc., 2000), was designed for students needing an even stronger pictorial component and a simpler user interface. Marketed for students in grades K–3, clinicians use it with a much wider age range of children (and adults) with special needs. *Kidspiration* includes a library of 1,200 images, so children's ideas can be readily represented with pictures. The images are categorized by themes such as foods and health, animals and plants, geography, people, and others. Importing graphics from other sources, such as clip art libraries or the Internet is supported by *Kidspiration* so that custom symbol libraries can be developed. Individual images and whole concept webs can be copied and pasted into word processing files, if desired. *Kidspiration* is the sort of open-ended, flexible software tool that a creative clinician could use in a thousand different ways.

CASE EXAMPLE: Using *Kidspiration* to Practice Identifying and Labeling the Main Idea in Pictures

Language objective: The student will correctly label the main ideas illustrated by a group of pictures in eight of ten trials.

Preparation: Choose an easy theme or main idea (things that are red, animals, food [see Figure 11.1]). In a group with an adult, children choose illustrations from the clip art library that match the main idea. Talk about why these things go together (see Figure 11.2).

Talk about whether these things could be divided into more groups to work on the next time. For example, sports could be divided into group and individual sports, musical instruments could be divided into wind and stringed, or wild animals could be divided according to how they move, as in Figure 11.3.

Clinicians may choose to use *ThemeWeaver* or *Kidspiration* to develop some examples (saved files) that have items that clearly do not belong, so children can "fix" them (see Figure 11.4). When main idea or concepts are well established, clients can make their own "funny" concept maps with mistakes, too. It is difficult for children to generalize skills from a single workbook page or an isolated classroom exercise to the "real world" of academic texts and other information media. Computer-as-context activities provide scaffolded (gradually more complex and less supported) opportunities to apply new skills in novel situations.

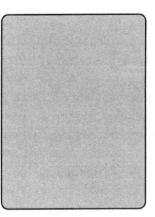

Figure 11.1. Starting a picture concept map with animals as the main idea. The software is *Kidspiration* (Inspiration Software, 2000).

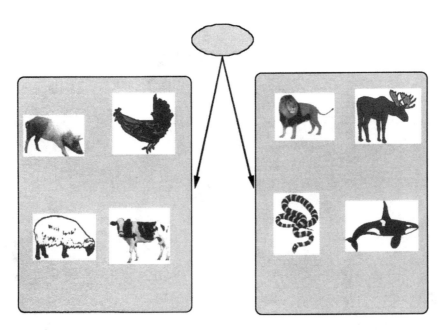

Figure 11.2. Choosing farm animals or wild animals from the clipart library. The software is *Kidspiration* (Inspiration Software, 2000).

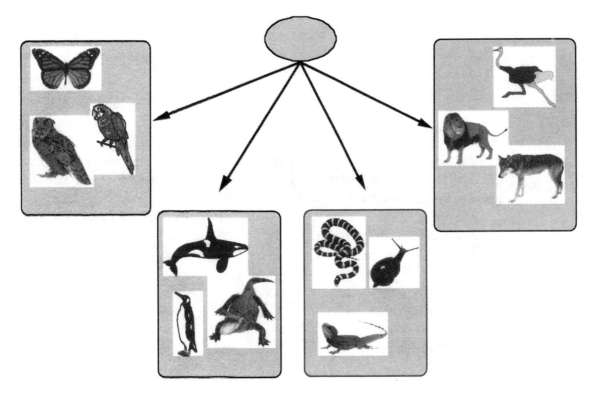

Figure 11.3. Choosing wild animals from the clipart library according to how they move. Category labels for flying, swimming, crawling, and running are missing, waiting for children to decide which label is appropriate. The software is *Kidspiration* (Inspiration Software, 2000).

Figure 11.4. Simple idea map for things that are round, including a mistake for children to find and correct. The software is *Kidspiration* (Inspiration Software, 2000).

FINDING GIVEN VERSUS INFERRED MEANINGS

Reading comprehension success at the fourth-grade level and beyond depends heavily on "reading between the lines." Good readers continuously apply their knowledge of the world and experiences as they read. Without realizing it, they frequently and correctly infer information that is not explicitly stated. This ability is sometimes called "constructive comprehension" or "inferencing." Read the following brief narrative and then respond to the questions that follow it.

Lee opened the door and got into the car. The drive was short, but it was hard to find a place to park downtown. When Lee arrived at the theater, the movie had already started.

Indicate whether the following sentences are based on explicit or implied information:

	Explicit	Implied
Lee knows how to drive a car.	[ ]	[ ]
Lee went to a movie theater.	[ ]	[ ]
The movie was downtown.	[ ]	[ ]
Lee went to the movie alone.	[ ]	[ ]
Lee was late.	[ ]	[ ]

Most readers use a multitude of subtle linguistic and contextual cues to arrive at these kinds of conclusions. For example, we know that Lee went to the movie alone. How? Because it would violate normal pragmatic and syntactic behavior to say "Lee arrived at the theater" if, in fact, Lee picked up a friend on the way and "they" went to the movie together. Mature language skills allow people to draw conclusions based on given information, assuming that other information would have been given if those conclusions were untrue. Therefore, we infer that Lee knows how to drive, that the movie was downtown, and that Lee was indeed late. These pieces of information are not explicitly given, but are implied in the story and assumed by typical readers.

Children with language impairments may have difficulty making inferences based on the information that they hear or read. According to Naremore et al., the relevant research suggests that the constructive comprehension ability of children with language impairment "is like that of normally developing children who are 2 to 3 years younger" (2001, p. 125). The precise cause of this gap is not known but could be due to several related factors. Clinicians need to be aware of this relationship between language impairment and the potential for reading comprehension deficits. Identifying given versus inferred information and using language to make inferences should be included in the assessment of school age children. Naremore et al. (2001) provided an informal assessment tool to help clinicians determine whether improving ability to make inferences is an appropriate goal for a child with language impairment.

Computer-based activities involving a clinician and individuals or groups of children can create a context within which to introduce and practice making inferences. Table 11.3 presents examples of software and activities that can be used for this purpose.

Naremore et al. (2001) recommended that clinicians use materials that are directly related to classroom activities for working on given versus implied information. If skills are taught in the same context and with the same materials in which they will be required, the need for carryover is minimized. It is important to remember the role of motivation in learning, however. It may be much more motivating to practice making inferences in a challenging computer game than to complete a more traditional classroom assignment. Some children may feel like they are always doing the same thing if materials are not varied enough. Computers can be used to add variety, while keeping relevant goals foremost. Although classroom connections should be considered, clinicians should explore and use materials that intrigue and reward children for whom regular classroom activities are difficult. Some classrooms will have software that can be used by the clinician to address advanced language goals, too. The ideal is to find the right balance between regular classroom materials and motivating alternatives.

MAKING INFERENCES ABOUT THE OREGON TRAIL

Consider, for example, the well-known classic in educational computing, *The Oregon Trail* (Riverdeep/The Learning Company). This simulation of pioneer life has undergone several updates since the original version distributed by MECC in the early 1980s. More than two decades of learners have enjoyed the adventure of traveling west from Missouri to Oregon in covered wagons. *The Oregon Trail* is interesting and challenging for users of almost any age. Because it is widely available in schools and widely used by social studies teachers, it provides a good example of content-related software that clinicians could use to help students practice inferencing skills.

Table 11.3. Computer-as-context activities for learning to make inferences

Sample language objectives (Inferencing)	Software exemplars	Software description	Computer activities
• Identify given information vs. implied information. • Practice answering "how do you know that?"	Thinkin' Things Series: Collection 1, 2, or 3, Sky Island Mysteries, Fripple Town, Hoyle Puzzle Games	These programs include a variety of puzzles, stories, and adventure games that deliberately encourage problem-solving and logic.	Together, clinicians and children take turns discussing and trying choices and using logic to accomplish the goal of the game.
• Practice answering "How do you know that?" • Contrast questions that require given vs. inferred information. • Answer questions using inferred information.	Where in the USA is Carmen Sandiego? Where in the World is Carmen Sandiego?	In the award-winning Carmen Sandiego series, users chase and catch elusive criminals, if their knowledge and attention to detail and detective skills are good enough.	Solve a mystery by gathering information, linking clues to existing knowledge, recognizing important details, and synthesizing what is learned to narrow choices. Use what is known and deduced to crack the case. Each program focuses on a content area such as U.S. geography, world geography, space, or history.
• Identify and answer questions that involve making an inference.	Oregon Trail, Hot Dog Stand, Ice Cream Truck, SimTown, Road Adventure USA, GeoSafari USA Search	These programs present age-appropriate simulations of historical events or everyday activities.	Simulate a "real-life" experience by taking off on an adventure, opening a business, or running a town. Retrieve and collect information and data, use tools to solve problems. Users make decisions based on what they know, what they learn, and the consequences of mistakes they make.
• Identify and answer questions that call for making an inference.	Reader's Quest I, II	Interactive, multimedia workshops provide direct reading instruction.	Read a passage and use an electronic highlighter "pen" and other program tools to identify clue words and details that signal information needed to support inferences or deductions. Use background knowledge and information from text to draw logical conclusions.

Table 11.4.   Activity guide illustrating how to teach inferencing using *Oregon Trail* simulation software (Riverdeep/The Learning Company)

Getting Ready to Go on the Oregon Trail
Say or write the names of all 12 months of the year, in order. Look at a calendar if you need to. (Get explicit information.)
What does "early" mean when you are talking about months of the year? (Make an inference.)
Name some months you think are "early" months of the year. (Make an inference.)
What does "late" mean when you are talking about months of the year?
Name some months you think are "late" months. (Make an inference.)
Look at the following list of months (possible departure dates): Which is the earliest? (Explicit information.)
March   April   May   June   July   August
Which of these months is the latest? (Explicit information.)
If you want to avoid traveling too early or too late in the year, which of these months should you choose?
Does the program tell you exactly when to leave? (Explicit information.)
Then, how do you know which months are best? (Explain an inference.)

At the beginning of the trail, users must make several important choices. For example, they must choose which month to start their journey. They are warned that if they leave for Oregon too early, the weather may be too cold and there won't be grass for the oxen and that if they leave too late, the winter storms may come before they arrive. Clinicians can help students think through their early decisions through a guided conversation such as the one outlined in Table 11.4.

Clinicians must preview software to be used with children working on inferencing, to identify examples of explicit information and opportunities for making inferences. Reviewing a computer-based activity after-the-fact can provide additional opportunities to help clients think about the activity, the choices they made, and how they might choose differently in the future. For example, consider the conversation guide or worksheet activity for *Oregon Trail* (Table 11.5).

EXTENDED PROJECT IDEAS FOR ADVANCED LANGUAGE AND LITERACY

The activities described in Table 11.6 could be used to address a wide variety of oral language and literacy objectives with individuals or groups, depending on how they are implemented. Most of the extended projects described here could also be enhanced through the use of the Internet. For example, children planning a recycling project or a fund-raiser for a good cause, could find background information for the project on related web sites. Or, it may be that students in other schools are working on similar projects, and have put the story of their experience on the web to share.

Effective use of the Internet requires all of the language skills that have been emphasized in this topic. For example, choosing search terms is an exercise in labeling the "main idea." The Internet can be both a source of inspiration and frustration for most people. Clinicians and teachers should consider exactly what they expect students to do and learn when incorporating the Internet into a session, and try web site addresses in advance to make sure the content is appropriate. Some students will need additional help organizing their use of the web and staying on task despite the inevitable distractions present. A worksheet with prompts or key words or a pre-determined set of focused questions may ensure that children with language or learning difficulties have a productive web experience. If more support is required, clinicians and teachers may want to investigate software that can screen or highlight certain parts of web pages with color filters, provide speech output for web page text, and other helpful features. *Aurora 3 for Windows, Kurzweil 3000, Read & Write v.6: textHELP*, and *WYNN* are examples of writing/study software with such features.

In a school setting, extended projects simplify the day-to-day planning of therapy sessions for older children. When the clinician and the students know what is happening and what the shared goals are, there is a greater sense of continuity. Less time is spent orienting everyone to new goals and materials every session. Shared goals and subsequent experiences are behind "creating a shared context." (Recall the discussion in Topic 7.) Children respond with greater effort when something or someone actually depends on their effective communication. Having a shared context makes it more natural to work on conversation skills such as negotiating, as seen in the example that follows:

CASE EXAMPLE

Clinician: What do you think we should do next? Why? Michelle, make a deal with Shane. One of you should go ask Ms. Garrett if we can borrow her yardstick and one of you should stay here and help me make a sign.

When children are using the computer to accomplish part of the project, genuine opportunities for negotiation are likely to arise. For example, a pair of children may be

Table 11.5   Discussion questions to be answered after the *Oregon Trail* activity

What Happened on Your Trip?
How many people survived the trip? (Explicit information.)
If some people died, what killed them? (Explicit information.)
Is there anything you could have done differently to help them survive the trip? (Inference.)
Did you talk to anyone along the way? (Explicit information.)
Did you learn anything that helped you make a good decision? (Explicit information.)
Why is it a good idea to talk to people along the trail? (Inference.)
Did you hunt for food on your trip? (Explicit information.)
Did you ever kill more animals than you could carry back to the wagon? (Explicit information.)
Did you lose food due to spoilage? (Explicit information.)
Is there anything you will do differently when you hunt on your next trip? Why? (Inference.)
Did you consult the travel guide during your trip? (Explicit information.)
Give an example of something you learned by reading the guide. (Explicit information.)
Why does reading the guide help people win the game and get to Oregon? (Inference.)
Did you ever run out of food or ammunition? (Explicit information.)
Did supplies or wagon parts run short during the trip? (Explicit information.)
Is there anything you will do differently the next time when you buy supplies? (Inference.)

using the computer to make a sign for the upcoming bake sale. If they are using a "sign-making wizard" or template, they will need to agree on a background or border design, choose clip art showing baked goods, decide exactly what the sign should say and what font to use (see Section IV for more about wizards, templates, and using the computer to generate materials). These are real decisions required in a real communicative context, occurring under the watchful eye of the clinician. The clinician can jump in to model a good question or help a child who is having trouble getting a chance to talk in a busy group. Children in a group can be encouraged and supported as they learn to use language to express their opinions or persuade others to their points of view, as seen in the following example.

CASE EXAMPLE

Clinician: Sarah and Heather, you two should get together and discuss why posters would be a good way to advertise the bake sale. Type a list of three reasons on the computer. Lori, Aaron, and Mark, you discuss why P.A. announcements would be a good way and make a list of reasons. Then both groups can present their ideas and we'll all vote on what to do, okay?

Extended projects do, however, involve coordination with other people. The clinician must do some of this coordination and collaboration in advance, but some can be part of the responsibilities (and communication practice) of the students. What if the principal's approval is required for posters that are hung on school property? The group planning publicity has already developed a list of reasons why posters are a good way to advertise the upcoming bake sale. The list is already typed into the computer. Therefore, it forms the start of a letter from the group to the principal, asking for permission to post bake sale signs. The group could negotiate who wants to write the letter, who will take it to the principal's office, and who will make a sample bake sale sign to go with the letter. Then the letter team chooses who will type first and who will talk first. A third student is responsible for spell checking and printing the final copy. Clinicians and teachers are often tempted to assign such responsibilities, which may be a better strategy in some cases. But recall that curricular guidelines for older students are likely to include goals such as using oral language to express an opinion or giving directions to a group (review Table 11.1). Giving students the task of dividing up responsibilities provides an excellent, genuine opportunity for using advanced conversation skills.

WHAT THE COMPETENT CLINICIAN NEEDS TO KNOW

To achieve this clinical computing competency, clinicians should be familiar with curricular guidelines, typical language development in school-age children, and computer applications that are age and content appropriate. Clinicians should understand how general language abilities—such as grasping the central theme in a collection of pictures or words, inferring information that was not given, and using language to convince or persuade—are important to acquiring mature literacy skills.

Table 11.6. Sample language objectives, pre/post-computer activities, computer activities, and possible extended projects for school-age children

Sample language objectives	Computer activities	Pre/Post computer activities	Extended project ideas
• Giving directions • Taking another's point of view • Sequencing events • Personal narrative • Tailoring written language to an audience	• Choose a recipe from an Internet web site or type one in from a cookbook (keep citation) • Use a word processor or talking word processor to add notes that explain special terms, or rewrite the recipe for younger children to use	• Prepare a dish according to the recipe • Tell others how it was done • Take photograph of finished dish	• Collect recipes into a notebook with appropriate credits • "Publish" the recipe book for parent, teacher, or class, with web citations • Make bulletin board display with photographs
• Summarizing information • Taking another's point of view • Verb tenses • Personal narrative	• Compose daily entry in "speech journal" (5 minutes at end of each session) using word processor • Make a concept map of what happens when a person "goes to speech"	• Discuss the therapy session (what was the "main idea" today?) • Plan what to write • Discuss goals and how to celebrate accomplishing them	• After a week or two, make a success report for mom, dad, teacher
• Initiating a topic • Using correct question syntax • Making inferences • Maintaining a topic • Changing a topic • Closing conversation • Tailoring written language to an audience	• Draft an interview plan or make an interview concept map • Write a "dialogue" of the interview (what will you say?) (focus on content, not punctuation) • Based on the dialog write a biography or story	• Watch videotape of an interview on TV, read or watch a celebrity interview on the Internet • Interview someone familiar (cook, bus driver, music teacher) • Role-play being the interviewer and/or interviewee	• Make a "This is Your Life" display • Start a school newsletter (paper or on the school web site, get permission before putting personal photos or information about someone on a public web site)
• Carryover of any new syntactic or phonologic skill • Sequencing events • Predicting what will happen • Identifying the main idea • Explaining what did happen • Making inferences • Tailoring written language to an audience	• Make a project concept map and draft the project plan • Write a letter asking for permission to have contest/event • Make signs and invitations • Write a letter inviting a newspaper or yearbook photographer to the event • Take digital photographs for making an event book later • After the event, write an announcement of the results to be read over school PA system	• Plan the event • Discuss what will be needed • Discuss what participants must do • Discuss what makes "news"	• Hold a contest (bubble blowing, poster making, ball throwing, recycling) • Raise funds for a worthy cause (hold a bake sale, car wash, rummage sale, or dog wash) • After the event, make a bulletin board or memory book celebrating the highlights—take turns reading the book to younger students.

From Cochran, P.S., & Bull, G.L. (1991). Integrating word processing into language intervention. *Topics in Language Disorders, 11*(2), 31–48; adapted by permission.

Clinicians should consider planning an extended project or joining a school-wide initiative. Computer activities are often easy and rewarding to include as a component of an activity that goes beyond the scope of a single session. Computer activities integrated into tasks that students view as important and relevant to them provide a context for genuine communication between participants.

SUMMARY

Advanced literacy and conversation goals are often complementary, and computer activities can address both. Some of the language skills underlying mature reading and writing include comprehending and conveying the "main idea," making inferences based on given and implied information, and using language to negotiate and persuade. Several types of software are available for use in activities that address these goals. Examples include educational games, problem-solving software, simulations, visual learning organizers, and story-making programs. This software has the characteristics desirable for creating a shared context (e.g., flexible outcomes, easy control, flexible language) as well as clear curricular content. Extended projects permit students to use computer activities to work on both conversational goals and literacy skills in a motivating and realistic context.

REVIEW FOR TOPIC 11

1. Choose one of the following and list at least five subcategories or "main ideas" that come to mind for each: animals, vehicles, clothing, food, rooms in a house, books, restaurants, and sports.
2. How could an organizer (like *Kidspiration*) be used to help children learn to find the main idea in a group of pictures? Words? Sentences?
3. Search an available clipart library and consider what "main ideas" are represented. How could you develop a therapy activity based on these materials?
4. What is the difference between information that is stated explicitly and information that is inferred?
5. Visit story web sites designed for children, or look at some familiar children's books. Identify three examples of information that must be inferred by a user, because it is not directly stated in the text.
6. Find computer simulation software (for children or adults), and try it out. As you go, think about what information is directly given and what is implied by the situation. How do you use inferences to improve your performance in the simulation?

QUESTIONS FOR DISCUSSION

1. Review the extended projects described in Table 11.6. Develop an addition to the table, including information for each column: the extended project idea, sample language objectives, computer activities, and pre/post computer activities.
2. How could computer activities in therapy help support the goals of using language for negotiating and persuading?

RESOURCES FOR FURTHER STUDY

Anderson-Inman, L., & Ditson, L. (1999). Concept-based concept mapping: A tool for negotiating meaning. *Learning and Leading With Technology, 26*(8), 6–13.

Council for Exceptional Children (2000). *Developing educationally relevant IEP's: A technical assistance document for speech-language pathologists.* Reston, VA: Author.

Moats, L.C. (2000). *Speech to print: Language essentials for teachers.* Baltimore: Paul H. Brookes Publishing Co.

Naremore, R.C., Densmore, A.E., & Harman, D.R. (2001). *Assessment and treatment of school-age language disorders: A resource manual.* San Diego, CA: Singular.

Nelson, N.W., Bahr, C.M., & Van Meter, A.M. (2004). *The writing lab approach to language instruction and intervention.* Baltimore: Paul H. Brookes Publishing Co.

Using a Computer as a Context for Conversation with Adolescents and Adults

Clinical computing competency #2: The clinician will demonstrate ability to use computer-based materials to form a shared context for communication with clients.

With adolescent and adult clients, a wide variety of speech and language goals can be addressed with activities that create a shared context for conversation. Competent clinicians will identify appropriate software for this purpose, based on client goals. Clinicians must know how to provide language models and communication opportunities as they use the computer together with clients to accomplish a shared purpose.

Most software applications especially intended for the use of adolescents or adults with language impairment have a CAI design. Similarly, most of the published research pertaining to computers and adult language clients has focused on CAI, usually with narrowly defined reading and spelling skills as the objective (see Topic 6). Published studies of clinical computing with children have included few children older than 10. Thus, a review of the literature to date provides an inadequate picture of the potential use of computers with both adolescents and adults.

Clinical observation and experience suggests that using open-ended, flexible computer activities with adolescents and adults can provide similar advantages and benefits as with younger children. The addition of auditory feedback to word processing, for example, may help an older client sustain attention to a writing task, monitor spelling and typos, and increase willingness to revise or check written work. King and Hux (1995) described the use of a talking word processor in writing intervention with an adult with mild aphasia. They reported an immediate decrease in overall error rate and an overall improvement in writing quality. Similar results were found in an experimental master's thesis study of two adolescents using talking word processing (Siemsen, 1993). Even relatively brief exposure to word processing with speech output resulted in improved writing and spelling in an adolescent with moderate developmental disability and an adolescent with severe language-learning disability. Talking word processors represent just one software tool that can be used to create a shared context in therapy with adolescents and adults.

This way of using a computer in intervention relies heavily on the clinician (see Topic 7). The clinician must manage the activity and the conversation in such a way that it truly becomes a therapeutic interaction. Participating in such an activity is just one of the ways adolescent and adult clients may use computers effectively to improve communication skills. For the clinician, success with such activities depends less on advanced technical skills than on good planning and thoughtful implementation.

CHOOSE APPROPRIATE AND SPECIFIC COMMUNICATION OBJECTIVES

The identification of speech and language goals for a particular client or group should happen prior to the selection of instructional materials. Computers or other technologies are then considered as one of several possible approaches for working on those objectives. For adults and adolescents, communication goals should be directly related to daily living, their educational/vocational goals, or recreational activities. Ideally, such goals are also geared toward increasing their communication success with their most frequent or most important conversational partners.

Consider one extended example in which recreational vocabulary and concepts are emphasized. Software that simulates participating in a sport is widely available, inexpensive, and easy to run on almost any kind of computer. Sports that users can "play" through such software include baseball, golf, car racing, and bowling to name a few. It may be that the client likes to participate in the real sport and needs to brush up on key expressions to make communication with friends more natural, or it may be that the client is practicing using language in the context of this computer activity as an end in itself. In either case, the first step is to consider how talking about a computer-based game with a clinician can address the goals established for the client. Following are some examples.

Potential Goals to Be Addressed While Using "Bowling" Simulation Software with Adolescents or Adults

- Anticipating future events and sequencing: *What should we do next?*

- Topic maintenance: *What do you like best about bowling?*

- Direction concepts: *Move a little to the left or right, pick up the ball, throw the ball toward the 7 pin, let go when you are near the line.*

- Number/Quantity concepts: *How many pins are left? How many did you knock down? What is the score?*

- Vocabulary: Specific bowling vocabulary: *pins, ball, lane, frame, strike, spare, bowling shoes*; or for ESL clients: bowling as an aspect of U.S. culture.

- Articulation or voice: This activity may provide a context that distracts or excites the client, providing an opportunity to test self-monitoring and carryover.

- Self-initiating, persisting, and completing a task: *Is it your turn?*

PREVIEW AND PERSONALIZE THE COMPUTER ACTIVITY

Software usually has options or preference settings that clinicians can change to make a computer-based speech or language activity optimally suited to the individual or group. For example, in bowling simulation software, on-screen score keeping and background music could be enabled or disabled, depending on client needs.

It is important for clinicians to preview software that they intend to use in order to create a shared context for conversation. This will prevent unanticipated delays or set-up problems and ensure that the software has appropriate content for the client's skills and needs. Most important, during the preview the clinician can be thinking about how best to engage the client in communication during the computer activity.

The Internet is an attractive context for therapy with adolescent and adult clients. Often, free shareware versions of popular games and simulations are available for downloading onto personal computers. More and more clients are likely to have Internet access in their homes, and some computer-based activities might be practiced with family members and friends as conversational partners. Clinicians should recommend software or web sites that are likely to be successful during these "homework" sessions and coach conversational partners about how to encourage the client's new skills. This can be an excellent way to encourage carryover from therapy to other settings.

CREATE A GENUINE CONVERSATIONAL CONTEXT

The first time a new program is used, it will be necessary to think through in advance how the goals for the client will be addressed during the computer activity. If the goal is for the client to demonstrate not only comprehension but also expressive use of direction words, for instance, the clinician must provide an opportunity for the client to give directions. This seems obvious, but one of the pitfalls of using computers as a context for conversation in therapy is getting distracted from the original therapy goal in favor of a game objective or rule. In the case of bowling, one person could bowl (control the mouse) while the other person gives directions (see Figure 12.1). The clinician could model giving directions while the client "bowls," then the client could tell the clinician what to do (e.g., *Move over a little*). An even better idea would be to have the client explain to a family member how to play, or to have a pair of clients helping each other with the game.

CASE EXAMPLE: Adult Shows Bowling Simulation Software to Spouse at the End of a Session

Spouse: *How do I let go of the ball?*

Client: *Let up button. Wait . . . near the line.*

Spouse: *I see. Wow!*

In this case, the client has genuine, new information to tell his spouse, which becomes a highly motivating context for conversation between them.

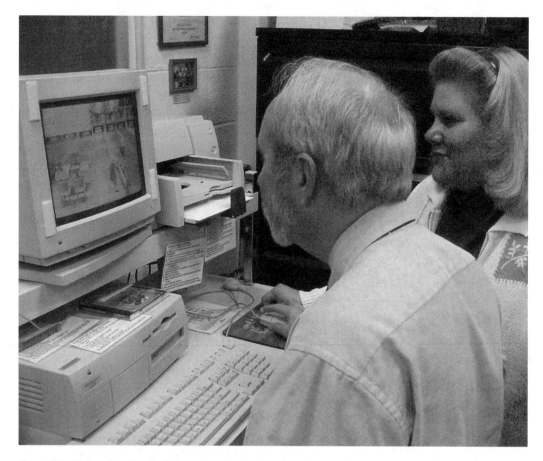

Figure 12.1. Using a bowling simulation program to create a shared context for conversation with an adult client (Courtesy of Truman State University Speech and Hearing Clinic).

CASE EXAMPLE: Adolescent Shows
Peer How to Make More Profit Selling Hot Dogs

Goal: The client will use oral language to offer and support an opinion or course of action in an appropriate manner.

   Software: *The Hot Dog Stand* (Sunburst) is a simulation in which the user is put in charge of a concession stand at a major sports arena. To succeed, it is necessary to consult attendance records for the upcoming sports event, check the weather forecast, order supplies, and set the prices of items for sale. The more thoughtfully these tasks are done, the greater the profit. Experience also helps, as the user learns what kind of events draw large crowds who are willing to pay higher prices.

   Client: We gotta charge more.

     Peer: Whaddya mean?

   Client: More for hot dogs. We can make more money.

     Peer: You mean, we gotta raise the price of the hot dogs this time?

   Client: Yeah.

Clinician: How do you know the customers will pay more?

   Client: They did last time!

Even though the examples above involve simulated bowling and entrepreneurship, the communication between participants is real. Participants ask questions because they need information from each other, not just for "practice." Such interaction provides an authentic context for developing communication skills, which motivates clients and promotes carryover.

SOFTWARE EXAMPLES FOR COMPUTER-AS-CONTEXT THERAPY ACTIVITIES WITH ADOLESCENTS AND ADULTS

For creating a conversational context with an adolescent or adult client, clinicians should consider software dealing with life skills, software that provides recreational entertainment, and software that enhances educational or vocational abilities. The software programs listed in Tables 12.1–12.3 are grouped according to the purpose each could have in the life of the client. In the tables that follow, software titles designated with an asterisk do not refer to a single specific program but rather a type of software. Game software is widely available in office supply and discount department stores, through public domain software distributors, and via the Internet.

The selection of software that has life skills as a major theme depends on the overall functioning level of the client. "Life skills" generally refers to the activities of daily living that include grooming, eating, transportation, shopping, emergency procedures, and interactions with family and caregivers. A young adult client with mild cognitive and language impairment from a TBI will need to be challenged in an entirely different way than an older client with severe aphasia. As usual, software choice is best guided by the previous selection of appropriate therapy goals.

Being able to participate in recreational activities with family and friends can be a major factor in successful acquisition or rehabilitation of social skills. Clinicians should consider including concepts and conversations related to entertainment in their therapy plans, because this is an important part of a well-rounded life. In therapy, practicing vocabulary and concepts and conversation scripts related to recreational activities is often enjoyable and productive. Outside of therapy, such activities provide rich opportunities for carryover in communication and expression of feelings.

Table 12.1.   Software that could provide practice with language related to basic life skills during computer-as-context activities with a clinicians and/or peers

Software	Example activity
Print Shop	Make greeting cards for family and friends
Quicken	Balance checkbook, make a budget
Bake & Taste	Choose recipes and follow directions in simplified cooking simulation
Community Exploration	Identify locations, activities, and objects around town
Trip planning software* or web sites	Read a map, calculate mileage, use time concepts
Shop 'Til You Drop (adapted access options available) (SoftTouch)	User goes shopping and can choose which outfits to purchase; another activity is a video arcade game about money (designed specifically for preteens and teens with moderate and severe disabilities)

Table 12.2.   Software that could provide practice with language and concepts encountered in recreational activities

Software	Example activity
Sports simulations*	Golf, baseball, racing, bowling, hockey, football, basketball, soccer, flying airplanes
Card games*	Solitaire, bridge, poker
Board games*	Checkers, chess, many others
TV games*	Popular television game shows are available on disk and on the Internet
Arcade games*	Pinball, darts, and so forth
Action/adventure games*	Creating simulated families, cities, civilizations
Quiz/puzzle games*	Trivia, crossword puzzles
Teen Tunes Plus (adapted access options available) (SoftTouch)	Large interesting graphics, a variety of musical interludes, and animations are combined with music in this software specifically designed for preteens and teens with severe cognitive delays and/or physical disabilities, and older clients learning to use a switch.

Some adolescent and adult clients are in a position to benefit from computer-based educational and vocational activities. For example, using the computer to look up information or to enter text could be a crucial vocational skill. Goals of this sort can be simultaneously reinforced when the clinician uses computer-based activities to work on communication skills as well.

SUMMARY

Although there is minimal published research regarding the use of computers as a context for conversation in therapy with adolescents and adults, many possibilities exist. The clinician must tailor three-way interaction between the client, the computer, and the clinician to meet appropriate communication needs and goals. In general, communication goals with older clients should focus on daily living, recreation, or education/vocational skills. Open-ended, flexible computer applications in all three categories are widely available.

REVIEW FOR TOPIC 12

1. What three aspects of life should be targeted by communication goals for adult and adolescent clients?
2. What does successful use of a computer to establish a shared context for conversation with an adult or adolescent client depend more on, technical expertise or good planning? Why?
3. Why is it important for the clinician to preview the software?
4. What does it mean to "create a genuine conversational context"?

QUESTIONS FOR DISCUSSION

1. Suppose there was a golf simulation available to you and your client. What are some language goals that could be addressed as you use this program together?

Table 12.3. Software that could provide practice with language for academic goals or job skills during computer-as-context activities

Software	Example activity
Write: Outloud (Don Johnston)	Talking word processing
Co:Writer 4000 (Don Johnston)	Talking word processor with word prediction
The Hot Dog Stand (Sunburst)	Simulation stressing applied math, making inferences and predictions based on weather reports, previous experience.
Inspiration (Inspiration)	Graphical organizer/visual map tool
Imagination Express Series: Rainforest, Pyramids, or Ocean modules (Riverdeep/Edmark)	Multimedia story-making toolkit with science and social studies content
The Oregon Trail (Riverdeep/The Learning Company)	Pioneer simulation providing practice with budget, planning, making inferences
GeoSafari (Educational Insights)	Interactive talking map focused on U.S. geography; rivers, states, & capitals; famous historical trails

2. A colleague has a positive attitude about using computer-based activities in therapy, but expresses concern that her clients do not talk enough during them. She concludes that computer-based activities are good for comprehension goals, but not for conversation or expressive language goals. What is your opinion?

RESOURCES FOR FURTHER STUDY

Nippold, M.A., Schwarz, I.E., & Lewis, M. (1992). Analyzing the potential benefit of microcomputer use for teaching figurative language. *American Journal of Speech-Language Pathology*, *1*(2), 36–43.

Wood, L.A., Rankin, J.L., & Beukelman, D.R. (1997). Word prompt programs: Current uses and future possibilities. *American Journal of Speech-Language Pathology, 6*(3), 57–65.

Selecting Software for Use in Speech and Language Intervention

Clinical computing competency #9: The clinician will demonstrate awareness of resources that provide continuing education, research results, technical support, and information about availability, funding, efficacy, and efficiency of new clinical computing products as well as assistive technology devices and services.

Software selection is one of the most important decisions that clinicians make in the process of using computers for assessment and intervention. Competent clinicians understand what to look for to ensure that choices are age and developmentally appropriate. They consider the role of the computer in therapy (e.g., instruction, context for conversation) and then they ensure that software chosen for use with and by a particular client has the essential features to fulfill that role.

Software review checklists of the 1980s and early 1990s (e.g., Rushakoff, 1984) were disproportionately concerned with technical adequacy (Will this software run on your computer? Is it compatible with your printer? Does it crash frequently?). In contrast, the criteria discussed in this topic draw attention to the content and design of the software and role it will play in intervention. This is not to say that other more practical factors in software selection should be dismissed. Prospective purchasers should make sure that their hardware meets the minimum configuration requirements of the software and that the software can be returned for refund or exchange within a reasonable period if it does not operate correctly or meet their expectations. More about the logistics of finding and purchasing software is included in Topic 14.

When a clinician chooses particular software for a session with an individual client, he considers what they worked on together during previous sessions, the interests and communication needs of the client, the client's cognitive, motor, vision, and language abilities, and especially the client's current intervention goals. Many client-focused con-

The author thanks Lauren Nelson, University of Northern Iowa; Glen Bull, University of Virginia; and Christine Appert, University of Virginia Children's Medical Center, for their contributions to the content of this topic.

siderations and the questions clinicians should address when deciding which role the computer will play in a particular session or activity, have been discussed in previous topics. In this topic, a broader perspective on software evaluation is presented. Software selection features will be discussed such as developmental appropriateness, the role of research in software development and marketing, the issue of open source software, and suggested criteria to be applied to selection or purchase of software for use as an instructor or as a context for conversation.

GENERIC VERSUS SPECIALLY DESIGNED SOFTWARE

Computer activities for clients with speech and language impairments employ either software deliberately intended for this target population or generic software intended for a wider audience of children or adults. Generic software is available from more sources, offers a larger selection of programs, and usually is less expensive than specially designed software. Examples of generic software that are widely used in clinical settings include *Print Shop* (Riverdeep/Broderbund), *KidPix* (Riverdeep/Broderbund), *Usborne's Animated First Thousand Words* (Usborne), and *The Oregon Trail* (Riverdeep/MECC/Broderbund).

For the sake of this discussion, most educational software, such as *Oregon Trail*, is considered generic in the sense that it is not remedial or clinical in original purpose. What some people would consider educational software is often designed and marketed with a large home-consumer audience in mind. The *JumpStart* series from Knowledge Adventure (*JumpStart Kindergarten, 1st grade, 2nd grade*, etc.) can be found in almost every office supply and discount department store where software is sold, along with other clinically useful but less academic-sounding titles based on popular television shows (Jeopardy, American Idol, Blues Clues), sports (golf, baseball, car racing), and toys (Barbie, Tonka, Fisher-Price).

Examples of specially designed clinical software include *Earobics* (Cognitive Concepts), *Nouns and Sounds* (Parrot), and *My Town* (Laureate Learning). Such software, in contrast to generic software, rarely appears in bargain bins and typically is ordered through specialized distributors. Software intended for clients with communicative disorders usually focuses on a specific skill area in greater depth, offers more opportunities for skill practice, and often includes more flexibility in adjusting program features such as sound, speed, visual effects, and alternatives to traditional mouse and keyboard control. Clinicians who make frequent use of computers in intervention activities are likely to maintain a software collection that includes both specialized and generic software titles.

IDENTIFYING DEVELOPMENTALLY APPROPRIATE SOFTWARE

Many professionals in early childhood education have qualms about young children's use of computers. Often this concern changes to excitement once they actually watch a young child using a computer (a picture is worth more than 1,000 words in this case). The problem often originates from the perception that somehow using computers is an isolated, anti-social, and artificial activity. Studies have shown, however, that children often enjoy using a computer with a peer, benefit from talking about computer activities, and sometimes prefer using a computer over other free-time materials (Clements, 1987; Fazio & Rieth, 1986). There is no reason to assume that computers are keeping young children from experiencing other exciting learning materials such as blocks and Play Doh. However, software selection is an important factor determining the benefits that children derive from computer activities.

Haugland and colleagues (Haugland & Shade, 1988; Haugland & Wright, 1997) developed a scale for evaluating children's software. These criteria, described with some amendments in Table 13.1, can be used to identify software that might be used independently (i.e., without full-time adult guidance and assistance) by typically developing preschool children. Haugland and Wright (1997) used these criteria to evaluate approximately 150 software programs for developmental appropriateness and then assessed the effects of children's exposure to high and low-scoring software. Some of their results were presented in Topic 5: Using Computer-Assisted Instruction (CAI) with Children.

Clinicians may want to consider the features in Table 13.1 when purchasing software for use with young children (other important criteria are discussed later in this topic). If nothing else, such scales remind clinicians and teachers to check for certain characteristics they may value. However, no single checklist or rating scale is likely to account for all of the software features that clinicians will want to consider. A case in point is a design flaw that has been a barrier that many clinicians have observed but rarely documented. In much generic software designed for young children, unfortunately, there is a mismatch between the developmental level of the content or instructional goal, and the cognitive and motor demands of the computer activity. For example, software based on the theme of popular toys and television shows for preschoolers may require sustained attention to task, advanced mouse navigation ability, or literacy skills well beyond those typically mastered by children who are still interested in preschool characters and content. The only way to discover such mis-matches is with the help of excellent software reviews or personal software explorations.

An important consideration in choosing software for young children is the nature of the learning experience. As noted previously, many early childhood educators and researchers have recommended that software for young children should encourage exploration in an open-ended learning environment (Judge, 2001). Clinicians should note, however, that much of the software designed especially for use with children who have communication disorders is based on a drill-and-practice approach to learning and uses a stimulus-response-reinforcement learning paradigm (i.e., CAI). In contrast, generic software includes many titles that allow young children to explore and learn at their own pace. As discussed further below, such software often has more of the features that are desirable in activities that make use of a computer as a context for conversation.

Early childhood specialists are not the only ones with concerns about the notion of developmentally appropriate software. Just as important is the idea of finding and choosing software for adolescent and adult clients that is well-suited to their specific therapy goals, but also to their cognitive abilities, motor and vision status, interests, and age (Gardner, Taber-Brown, & Wissick, 1992). Software may have appropriate content, but may have the look and feel of juvenile software that makes it inappropriate or offensive for use with older clients. To avoid this situation, occasionally software developers produce a parallel version of their software that is designed for adults or adolescents. An excellent exam-

Table 13.1. Evaluation criteria for determining the developmental appropriateness of software for young children

Evaluation criteria	Explanation
Age appropriate	To be age appropriate, the software should be based on teaching methods that are consistent with young children's capabilities and motivation for learning. Software objectives should address concepts and skills that relate to the needs and interests of young children.
Child in control	The software offers children the opportunity to use it in an open-ended exploratory manner. Children (and conversational partners) set their own learning pace and have unlimited opportunities for trial and error.
Clear instructions*	Because most preschool children are not able to read instructions, the software should provide clear auditory instructions and/or demonstrations. Instructions should be presented in simple, direct statements accompanied by appropriate graphics to facilitate understanding.
Expanding complexity*	Software should be easy enough for the youngest children in its intended audience to use it with minimal initial adult guidance (about 20-30 minutes). As children become proficient they should be able to access more complex aspects of the software.
Independence*	Children should be able to control at least some aspects of the software independently after a brief period of instruction (less important during adult-facilitated activities).
Non-violence	The software should not require children to use violent objects, interact with violent characters, or perform violent actions. In addition, the software should foster positive social values (e.g., cooperation, sharing, and friendship).
Process orientation	The software is based on a discovery approach to learning and fosters exploratory behavior. Children's motivation to use the software is intrinsic and is based on their interest in finding out more about the possibilities inherent in the activities.
Real-world model*	The visual representations of objects and events are realistic and objects behave as they would in the real world. The relative sizes of objects are accurately depicted. Note: Sometimes explicit violation of "reality" is delightful for children, such as the Little Critter in *Just Grandma and Me* (Riverdeep/Broderbund) and Dr. Seuss characters.
Technical features	Examples of desirable features include ease of installation, a clearly written manual, quick access to activities, rapid response to the child's input, appropriate use of colorful graphics, realistic animations and sound effects, easy exiting and re-entry, and reliable printing.
Transformations	Children are provided with opportunities to change objects and situations. Children should be able to revise their creations and explore realistic physical changes (e.g., plant growth, color blending, and objects in motion).
Anti-bias deduction	Although this category does not contribute to the positive point score in the Haugland et al. system, a 1/2-point deduction was assessed for negative bias attributes. Positive attributes are multiple languages, objects and situations that are familiar across cultures, mixed gender and role equity, and depicting people of different cultures, abilities, age groups, and family styles.

From Cochran, P.S., & Nelson, L.K. (1999). Technology applications in intervention for preschool-age children with language disorders. *Seminars in Speech and Language, 20*(3), 203–218; adapted by permission.

* These criteria are less important when an adult is assisting the child, as in computer-as-context activities.

ple of this is the auditory processing/phonological awareness software *Earobics 1 for Adolescents and Adults* (Cognitive Concepts). It provides similar skill practice as the version for children (*Earobics Step 1*), but with age-appropriate screen design and reinforcement for older users.

Clinicians who work with clients of wide ability and age ranges may gravitate toward software that is flexible enough for appropriate use with many of them. Word-of-mouth and personal exploration is the best way to find such software. Examples of generic software with this extreme clinical flexibility include *PrintShop* (Riverdeep/Broderbund) and *Kidspiration/Inspiration* (Inspiration). Examples of specialized software with comparably broad applications include *Write:Outloud* (Don Johnston), the *Articulation I, II, III* series (LocuTour), and the *Speech Viewer* (IBM/Psychological Corporation).

Keyboard alternatives, such as a touch screen, may help a young child or an adult with cognitive or motoric limitations share in the control of a program that is otherwise a developmentally appropriate choice for therapy. Some software is more compatible with adapted access options than others, so this can be an important selection feature. Adapted access technology is discussed in detail in Section VIII.

RESEARCH-BASED CLINICAL SOFTWARE AND THE PUBLISHERS' DILEMMA

Clinicians often assume that specialized intervention software (rather than generic software) has been developed based on research. The assumption is that clinical experts design such software and that the software has undergone trials with clients, the results of which support its use with particular populations. For the most part, this is a fantasy in current clinical and educational software markets. "Market" is the key word here. Because they have to make money, publishers develop and distribute software according to what they think will sell. They listen closely to what clinicians tell them they like and dislike about available products. (This is one reason why it is so important to return software that does not meet expectations.) Software publishers who specialize in products for special populations often support efforts to document the efficacy of their products and may generously contribute to related professional organizations, scholarship funds, and so forth. They are good citizens, but their products are most often based on market research and the ideas of individual clinicians and experts. Rarely is clinical efficacy research involved before, during, or after the final product is distributed.

This situation is one of the reasons that *Fast ForWord* (Scientific Learning) was so eagerly embraced at first. Its authors were well-known researchers who were claiming documented positive effects based on clinical trials (see Topic 5 for a more detailed discussion and critique of *Fast ForWord*). The development of commercial software products based on formal clinical research has occurred through the years, but it remains a rarity. Many such products, unfortunately, are no longer commercially available due to rapid technology changes (e.g., the excellent *PepTalk* phonology therapy series developed by Shriberg, Kwiatkowski, and Snyder and published by Communication Skill Builders for Apple II computers).

So, why doesn't research drive the development of new intervention software more often? There are many reasons, including

- It takes too much time (years can go by in software development and testing)

- It's too expensive (efficacy research is always resource-intensive)

- Even if the software is great, the investment may not show a return (because technology will change)

In defense of the specialized market publisher, then, it seems like the only way to publish research-based software for a profit would be if the software was developed and tested by scholars using grant funding, and then delivered to the publisher for distribution as a finished product. This puts publishers (and clinicians) in the passive role of waiting and hoping that such software will appear. Meanwhile, they may choose to take the best ideas they can find and develop them, even in the absence of any "data."

A notable exception to this line of reasoning is found in high-end hardware and software combinations such as those developed for speech and voice analysis and dysphagia therapy. Part of the reason that these systems are so expensive is that the risk as well as investment in research and development are high. Generally, clinical experts and researchers do drive the development and modification of such products, in close cooperation with the manufacturer/distributor. Because such systems often take on the role of medical equipment and research instrumentation, part of the cost of development lies in ensuring that the system does what is promised in a reliable fashion. Products without such reliability and validity information are likely to be less expensive and less frequently used in medical and research settings.

THE CLINICIAN'S DILEMMA

The lack of research-based intervention software may be unsettling news for the clinician who only wants to invest in software that has been proven (or who has supervisors who think this is a realistic expectation). It may be of small comfort, but the fact is that many of the techniques and most of the materials that clinicians routinely use have not been rigorously evaluated through empirical research. They may work well, but no one has documented that they work in a formal manner. Much intervention software, so far, is no exception.

Even when a technique or method has the benefit of objective evidence behind it, there is no guarantee that it will work with any particular client. Clinicians are accustomed to trying various methods with clients and pursuing those that work best for individuals. This is exactly how competent clinicians use clinical and generic software, evaluating the reactions and progress of the client to ensure a good match. They use software reviews, recommendations from peers, on-line resources and demonstration discs to help them screen potential additions to their software libraries and increase the chances of a worthwhile investment.

A POTENTIAL SOLUTION:
THE NOTION OF OPEN-SOURCE SOFTWARE

The open source software movement is one of the most significant technological advances that occurred in the past decade (Bull, Bell, Garofalo, & Sigmon, 2002). When the underlying code of a software program can technically and legally be modified by the user, it is labeled "open source" software. One of the best-known examples of open source software is the operating system Linux. In 1992 a programmer in Finland, Linus Torvalds, created an open source version of the widely used mainframe operating system, Unix. This open source version of Unix became known as "Linux." Torvalds demonstrated that it was possible for programmers around the world to improve and update the software by collaborating over the Internet. Open source software is gaining an increasing percentage of the business and industry software market, and the international open source community continues to grow.

A key component to making open source work as a method of sharing, improving, and distributing software is the way the results are copyrighted. A special form of copyright called a General Public License (GPL) is used to ensure that open source products are changed and shared appropriately. With a GPL, the author conveys the right to modify and distribute the program to others, provided that certain conditions are met. For example, derivative works must be made available to others in turn, through a GPL (Bull et al., 2002). It is important to note that a GPL does not prevent the sale of open source software for a profit, providing that the software also remains available at no cost through a public forum such as the Internet. "Accordingly, open source products such as Linux can be downloaded from the Internet without charge, but can also be acquired as commercial products from firms such as Red Hat, Inc., and IBM" (Bull et al., 2000, pp. 13–14). Some users are willing to pay for the convenience and peace of mind that a distributor provides through technical support and regular updates of open source software. (Additional software licensing information and issues are presented in Topic 14.)

What does the open source movement have to do with software for speech and language therapy? Throughout this book, excellent clinical software is mentioned that is no longer commercially available. It has been pointed out that software developers and publishers face high development costs that prohibit, in most cases, research-based software development or modification. Bull et al. (2002) made the case that similar difficulties impede educational software development, and could potentially be addressed through an open source approach. Thus, if the code for tried-and-true clinical and educational software was made available under a GPL, perhaps volunteer programmers around the world would undertake the task of updating it for new technologies (e.g., new operating systems), translating it for use by speakers of other languages, or improving it in response to clinical research findings. Software publishers could benefit by saving the research and development costs, but still offer distribution and technical support services to customers for a price.

Actual implementation of this idea may be more complex than it sounds, but the notion of open source clinical software is extremely attractive. No longer would clinicians have to either abandon a favorite software program or maintain an outdated computer in order to provide clients with some of the best computer-based therapy activities that have been developed. Our collective wisdom and knowledge about the strengths and weaknesses of particular computer-based activities and approaches would not be at the mercy of the next innovation.

JUDGING SOFTWARE ACCORDING TO ITS PURPOSE AND PROSPECTIVE CLINICAL OR EDUCATIONAL USE

One of the problems with early software evaluation checklists was the assumption that all kinds of instructional and clinical software should be measured with the same yardstick. This approach was strongly influenced by early educational software evaluation.

With "teaching machines" in mind, these rubrics tended to be overly focused on features desirable in tutorial and drill-and-practice software, to the exclusion of simulations, games, and learner-based tools (Bull & Cochran, 1991). Now it is more apparent that the features that are most important for software intended to be used independently by a client or student (i.e., CAI) would be different than those sought in software the clinician intends to use as a topic, or context, for conversation.

Table 13.2 provides criteria that clinicians and others could use to help identify software that incorporates what have traditionally been the most desirable features of CAI. That is, if a clinician has clients for whom using the computer as an instructor is an appropriate and recommended option, she could use this list to help her screen software for potential purchase and use.

Some of the criteria in Table 13.2 may need a brief explanation. The sixth criteria listed in Table 13.2 refers to frequent interaction between the client and the software. It is desirable for most software to be what software reviewers call "highly interactive." This is achieved by requiring users to participate/respond at frequent intervals. No one, especially not a user with special needs, likes to sit in front of a computer screen with nothing to do for long periods while the computer "teaches" (tells a story, gives directions, explains a concept).

Near the end of the list in Table 13.2 and again in Table 13.4, the role of "bells and whistles" like music, sound effects, and animation is mentioned. The multimedia features that computers bring to learning materials are powerful; they hold the attention of learners, they improve the demonstration and illustration of complex ideas, and they make learning more fun. Ideally, features like animation, sound, speech, music, and movie clips are incorporated into the software in a way that is integral to conveying information and involving the user. If so, they enhance the learning process. In contrast, when such features are present for no apparent reason, they merely distract the learner. Early in educational CAI history, researchers discovered that when dramatic consequences occurred as the result of a user error, children using CAI software would deliberately answer incorrectly just to see the animated monster and hear the buzzer. Such ill-considered use of multimedia features is counter-productive.

Table 13.2. Evaluation criteria for computer-as-instructor (CAI) software (clinical and educational)

Goals or learner outcomes are clear and specific.

Directions for using the program are clear and concise.

The program's language, content, and theme are developmentally appropriate for target users.

Options are available for individualizing the program for particular users.

Target clients are able to use the program independently.

The program frequently requires a client response and evaluates client learning/progress.

Record keeping is simple and reliable.

Response options/accessibility features are present.

Feedback to the client is informational (hints and explanations) rather than merely judgmental (right or wrong).

It is easy to enter, exit, and resume program activities.

The program makes deliberate and non-trivial use of multimedia features such as sound and animation.

The support documentation includes all essential information.

Table 13.3. Evaluation criteria for learner-based tools

Flexibility in choice of goals is available to users.

Feedback to users is informative rather than judgmental.

The software encourages prediction and successive approximation.

Explicit access to curricular content is facilitated.

Learning occurs within a context that is meaningful for the user.

The focus is on the process, not just the product of the activity.

The software facilitates three-way interaction between the clinician/teacher, client/student, and computer.

Users can create new applications or activities not necessarily envisioned by the creator of the tool.

Novices can use the software creatively almost immediately.

Experts can develop sophisticated applications of the tool.

From Bull, G., Bull, G., Cochran, P., & Bell, R. (2002). Learner-based tools revisited. *Learning & Leading with Technology, 30*(1), 10–17; adapted by permission.

The final criteria for both CAI and computer-as-context software pertain to documentation. Either on-line or hard copy support documentation should be available with all software. Such documentation should include system requirements, installation information, an overview of available activities, examples of record keeping or reports that the software generates, directions for options that can be configured to meet individual needs, and a source for additional information or questions. For educational or clinical software, examples of how the software can be used should be included.

Highlighting very different instructional values compared to CAI, Table 13.3 presents criteria that describe a category of software called "learner-based tools." The case for establishing this instructional software category (as distinct from others such as simulations, drill-and-practice, productivity tools, games, or tutorials) has been made elsewhere (Bull, Bull, Cochran, & Bell, 2002; Bull & Cochran, 1991; Russell, 1986). The list of characteristics of learner-based tools is presented here for the purpose of 1) contrast to CAI, and 2) transition to a discussion of the features clinicians will value in software they use to create a context for conversation in therapy.

There have been relatively few examples of learner-based tools over the years that have met each of the criteria described in Table 13.3. The most notable examples are *Logo, HyperCard,* and *HyperStudio,* which have nearly disappeared in educational and clinical settings compared to former periods of high popularity. The criteria are useful to consider, however, because many software programs share some of them, even if not all of them. So, software falls along a learner-based continuum, according to the number of learner-based features that it has. Examples of currently popular programs that have a high number of the features of learner-based tools include *Kidspiration/Inspiration* (Inspiration), *Write:Outloud* (Don Johnston), *IntelliPics Studio* (IntelliTools), and the *Imagination Express* series (Riverdeep/Edmark).

Clients and clinicians use learner-based tools to accomplish tasks they choose themselves, rather than activities completely pre-determined and controlled by a software designer. For clinical purposes, this is the most important distinction between learner-based tools and CAI. The same key distinction holds in identifying software most likely to succeed in creating a context for conversation in therapy. Clients and clinicians use computer-as-context software to accomplish a shared goal, through which many oppor-

Table 13.4. Evaluation criteria for computer-as-context software

A shared topic or theme or task of mutual interest is present in the software.

The program promotes flexible outcomes and diverse possible goals.

The program's language, content, and theme are developmentally appropriate for target users.

It is easy to share control of the software with a partner or peer.

The theme, tasks, and content are non-violent and non-biased (gender & ethnicity-balanced).

Feedback is designed to assist the user rather than judge the user's performance.

The program makes deliberate and non-trivial use of multimedia features such as sound and animation.

The support documentation includes all essential information.

tunities to model and practice particular communication skills occur. Flexibility, more than accountability, is required for success. Features that clinicians should look for in choosing computer-as-context software are presented in Table 13.4. This list reflects the influence of software evaluation efforts that have gone before, and that have been outlined above.

Clinicians who use the criteria in Table 13.4 will quickly learn that software they find effective in creating a shared context may not meet all of the criteria. This list is a beginning. It provides clinicians who may be more familiar with CAI and the features valued in CAI with an alternative starting point in the evaluation of potential software choices. Clinicians who may have been hesitant to choose or use software that did not have strong performance tracking features, for example, can see that when software is being used for an alternative purpose in therapy, other priorities are justified. (Recall that when using the computer as a context for therapy, the clinician is responsible for evaluating and documenting client performance, not the computer.)

Software that meets many of the criteria for use in computer-as-context activities can be acquired through almost any software source. That is, clinicians will find this software available on line, in specialized clinical materials catalogues, as well as in the bargain bin at their favorite discount store. The process of finding and purchasing software and installing and using it in accordance with copyright regulations is discussed in the next topic.

SUMMARY

Generic (general purpose or educational) and clinical (specialized for clinical purposes) software evaluation checklists from the 1980s and 1990s tended to focus on technical stability, documentation, accountability, and logistics (does this software work with your printer?). When instructional design issues were addressed, they were heavily weighted toward features most desirable in tutorials and drill-and-practice software (CAI). In addition to criteria for assessing CAI software, three alternative sets of software characteristics are presented in this topic that focus on the role the computer will play in intervention or instruction. They include features to look for in software that is likely to make a successful context for conversation in therapy, such as flexible outcomes and goals, content of mutual interest to the client and clinician, and feedback that is designed to help rather than judge the user.

The barriers to developing research-based software include time, resources, and rapid changes in technology, which prevent publishers from recouping investments in research and development. The open source software movement is introduced as a potential alternative to traditional software publishing, in order to facilitate research-based software modifications and prevent the loss of effective software products due to frequent technology updates.

Traditionally, clinicians are accustomed to trying various therapy methods and materials with clients and pursuing those that work best for individuals. Competent clinicians use the same strategy to identify the best clinical and generic software, evaluating the reactions and progress of the client to ensure a good match.

REVIEW FOR TOPIC 13

1. Review the criteria for determining the developmental appropriateness of software for young children in Table 13.1. Select the three items that you consider the most important considerations and discuss the reasons for your priorities.
2. Explain three reasons why there is a lack of research-based clinical software.
3. In clinical practice, there is no guarantee that a technique, method, or software product will work with an individual. Discuss how a competent clinician should evaluate and use clinical and generic software for a particular client.
4. Why is a general purpose license (GPL) a key component to making the concept of open source software work?
5. Explain how the open source concept could have a significant impact on the development and use of educational and clinical software.
6. Discuss why flexibility, more than accountability, is an essential ingredient for success in computer-as-context software.

QUESTIONS FOR DISCUSSION

1. Either look at an actual software program for young children or recall a favorite with which you are very familiar. How would this program score using the criteria suggested in Tables 13.1? Table 13.2? Table 13.3? Table 13.4?
2. Describe three key features that should be considered in selecting computer-as-context software. How do these features compare to criteria for learner-based tools and CAI software?
3. Sometimes not-so-perfect software can nevertheless be used effectively to meet the needs and goals of a particular client. How should clinicians balance these priorities?

RESOURCES FOR FURTHER STUDY

Buckleitner, W. (1999). The state of children's software evaluation—yesterday, today, and in the 21st century. *Information Technology in Childhood Education Annual* (pp. 211–220). Charlottesville, VA: Association for the Advancement of Computing in Education.

Bull, G., Bell, R., Garofalo, J., & Sigmon, T. (2002). The case for open source educational software. *Learning & Leading with Technology, 30*(2), 10–17.

Bull, G., Bull, G., Cochran, P., & Bell, R. (Sept 2002). Learner-based tools revisited. *Learning & Leading with Technology, 30*(1), 10–17.

Clements, D.H., Nastasi, B.K., & Swaminatha, W. (1993, January). Young children and computers: Crossroads and directions from research. *Young Children, 48,* 56–64.

Gardner, J.E., Taber-Brown, F., & Wissick, C. (1992). Selecting age-appropriate software for adolescents and adults with developmental disabilities. *Teaching Exceptional Children, 24*(3), 60–63.

Haugland, S.W., & Wright, J.L. (1997). *Young children and technology: A world of discovery.* Boston, MA: Allyn and Bacon.

Judge, S.L. (2001). Integrating computer technology within early childhood classrooms. *Young Exceptional Children, 5*(1), 20–26.

Understanding Software Licensing

Clinical computing competency #8: The clinician will demonstrate familiarity with legal and ethical considerations that apply to assistive technology and the use of computers in the management of communication disorders and will adhere to appropriate standards.

Clinicians who are responsible for using, recommending, ordering, or installing clinical software should be informed about software licensing. Competent clinicians will be aware of the technical and legal distinctions between copy-protected, copyrighted, licensed, shareware, and public domain software.

FINDING CLINICAL SOFTWARE

Many people approach the purchase of hardware or software with the same trepidation as they have when buying a car, and for some of the same reasons. Venturing into the computer hardware and software market can be intimidating for reasons such as fear of the unknown, fear of not getting good value, and lack of familiarity with brand names. Some clinicians lack information about the quality and reputation of brand names and familiarity with the process of software and hardware purchase. Others have too much familiarity with tales of woe and intrigue from the grapevine about the tribulations of computer/software shopping.

In a work setting, some of these considerations are simplified by internal purchase procedures and some are made even worse. Topic 13 presented information about the characteristics to be sought in software for particular clinical purposes, especially using the computer as a context for therapy. In contrast, the present topic is designed to allay some of the concerns and confusions of newcomers to the software market. Clinicians will benefit from knowing how to find software, how to purchase and register software, and how a user's rights differ with regard to licensed software versus shareware versus public domain software.

"How do I find good software?" is at the top of the most frequently asked questions at workshops about clinical computing. Fortunately, the process of identifying and previewing software is becoming easier every day thanks to the availability of Internet resources. Clinicians typically rely heavily on word-of-mouth recommendations from peers as well as catalog descriptions to guide therapy materials purchasing decisions (Ballanger, 1997). Many times a personal recommendation from a colleague is the best possible way to find good software. However, over-reliance on catalogs can backfire. Especially when a significant amount of money is at stake, it is worth the time to do additional investigating.

Many professional and general consumer publications provide descriptions and reviews of new software. Having an expert and unbiased overview of the software indicating its strengths and weaknesses is invaluable prior to purchase. An outstanding and well-established source for brief and objective descriptions of new educational/clinical software is Joan Tanenhaus' column "Diskoveries" published regularly in the *Closing the Gap* newsletter. Often, computer magazines publish an annual "Top 10" list in a variety of consumer categories that can provide an excellent starting point for updating a software collection. For example, entries deemed among the best for preschoolers or for general family entertainment are worth considering for clinical use.

Another excellent way to find out about new products is to attend professional conferences. At the annual convention of the American Speech-Language-Hearing Association, hundreds of exhibitors provide participants with a hands-on look at their products. This is an excellent source of information and preview opportunity for specialized software and hardware. For an even broader sampling of assistive technology and special software, the *Closing the Gap* newsletter and annual resource directory are useful, as is their annual convention in Minneapolis.

Software publishers often include demonstrations on their web sites. Either the demo runs via the web or a demonstration version of the software can be downloaded for temporary use. At the very least, detailed descriptions and sample screen shots are widely available on publishers' web sites. These go a long way toward conveying the essence of a particular software program and its instructional approach, so that disappointing purchases can be avoided.

PURCHASING AND REGISTERING SOFTWARE

Once a software program with good potential is identified, there are a variety of purchase methods possible. In general, purchase by mail or via the Internet is reliable and fast. This is good because many titles of clinical interest will not be widely available in software retail stores. It is wise to check the return policy of the store or company from which the software will be purchased. For example, some distributors may not refund money if the software has been opened/installed. Some educational software distributors will accept return of software within 30 days for a full refund. It is important to know in advance what the policy is, and it is important to review and return unacceptable software promptly.

Most software comes with a registration card or on-line registration option. Registering promptly is important because it frequently entitles the user to technical support if there is a problem. When a serial number is present on the CD or manual, technical support personnel may require it before they will answer questions. Clinicians should consider developing a database or filing system for keeping track of software titles, sources, purchasing dates, serial numbers, and technical support hotlines and web addresses.

INDIVIDUAL SOFTWARE LICENSING

Generally, when an individual copy of a software package is purchased, it entitles the purchaser to use the software on a single computer. Note that the purchaser does not own the software itself, but rather a license to use it. The conditions of this license are spelled out in detail in a document that accompanies each copy of the software (often on the envelope in which the software is packaged or in a file included in the installation program). Usually, the publisher of the software maintains the sole copyright, meaning no one else is legally entitled to copy it or sell it.

It is important for clinicians to understand the conditions of the software license in order to avoid unethical and illegal situations. For example, a single-copy, single-license software package cannot legally and ethically be installed for simultaneous use on a computer in the speech room as well as a computer in the special education resource room. It is a violation of single-license agreements to purchase a single copy of a therapy program and then install it on multiple computers throughout a clinic or school.

Attempts to rig software so that it is copy-protected have decreased over the years. Copy-protection schemes involve booby-trapping the software in some way so that illegal copies do not work, or legal copies only work if some "proof" of ownership is provided, such as a serial number. One well-known example of this in children's software is the copy protection device used in Broderbund's *The Playroom*. Every few times the software is launched, a combination of toys appears including a blank. The "key" to what should be placed in the blank is printed on the back page of the software documentation. Apparently it was assumed that people who made illegal copies of the software would skip the manual. It proved to be a source of much irritation to licensed users, however, who were forced to keep the manual at their fingertips at all times. No other Broderbund products include such a system, fortunately.

In defense of software publishers, however, much money is lost each year due to illegal copying and sharing of software. An independent survey commissioned by the Software and Information Industry Association (SIIA) and the Business Software Association estimated that in 1999, software piracy losses exceeded $12 billion worldwide and had topped $59 billion over a 5-year period (SIIA, 2000). As SIIA points out, such losses are translated into fewer jobs, lost tax revenue, and disincentives for publishers to develop new and better products. Just because software can be installed on multiple machines simultaneously does not mean that it is legal or ethical to do so. It is important to pay developers for the use of their software, so that it continues to improve. When discovered, illegal installation and distribution of software often carries stiff penalties.

SITE LICENSING AND LAB PACKS

When multiple copies of a software package are needed, alternative licensing arrangements may be more cost-effective than purchasing several single-copy licenses. A common solution used in educational settings is a "lab pack," which generally consists of permission to install the software on a small number of machines in a single location at a substantially discounted rate. Five-packs or ten-packs often include only one copy of the software's documentation (user manuals).

Another solution to the problem of multiple users is a site license. A site license may specify either a limited or unlimited number of legal installations at a site or within a certain institution. For example, a hospital system might purchase a site license for virus protection software. The site license might grant the hospital system 200 legal installations and a year of free updates from the software publisher. Someone in a central location must track the number and location of legal copies that have been installed.

SHAREWARE

Shareware is software widely found on the Internet and among members of computer clubs. Authors of shareware encourage people to use it and share it with others. When the shareware is found to be useful, the user is asked to register the copy by sending the author a modest fee. In return, the registered user might receive technical support, free updates, or additional software features. Note that the author maintains the copyright to the software, even though permission to copy and give away the software is freely granted to others. A recent alternative to user fees is the inclusion of advertising in free, non-registered copies of the software (e.g., the popular e-mail utility *Eudora*). If the user pays and registers the software, an ad-free, full-featured version becomes available.

The Internet provides a superb distribution mechanism for shareware, so it is appearing in an ever-increasing number of titles. In Section VI, the widespread use of shareware on handheld computers is discussed. Although shareware often has a very narrow target audience, occasionally a new utility or game will come along that becomes an instant hit or eventually a commercial product. For example, the now famous and best-selling children's paint program *KidPix* (Broderbund) began as software that a father developed for his own child and then decided to "share." Clinicians can locate shareware via the Internet in lieu of purchasing clinical software, but much time can be wasted on products that are not of good quality. Clinicians could use reviews in popular magazines and the personal recommendations of "techie" friends to find the best offerings.

PUBLIC DOMAIN (COPYRIGHT-FREE)

When creative material such as literature, music, artwork, or software is in the "public domain," it is no longer copyrighted. In other words, it is legal and ethical for anyone to copy, modify, or even sell the material. Public domain software is often available in bundles and sold at a low price by a distributor who guarantees its technical integrity. For example, clipart libraries made up of images in the public domain are widely available. Many computer users are interested in such public domain artwork, so that they can legally copy and modify the images for use in their own for-profit endeavors (e.g., advertisements, commercial web pages).

Especially when funds are limited, public domain software can be an excellent resource. However, the old caveat "you get what you pay for" definitely applies. Identifying, installing, and testing public domain software might be a good job for a volunteer assistant or computer "geek" from the local high school. Clinicians who are computer novices are unlikely to enjoy this often-frustrating process. However, with the support of a technical friend, good software may be identified for clinical use or for free distribution to clients.

Clinicians may find sources for public domain or shareware that have done the testing and selection in advance. For example, Technology for Language and Learning (TLL) is a non-profit organization in New York that has been collecting and distributing public domain and shareware for special populations for more than a decade. TLL limits its efforts to software for the Macintosh operating system.

SUMMARY

For various reasons finding good software is both easier and harder than it has ever been. Clinicians may be overwhelmed with the number of titles and products offered in the local discount store as well as by special publishers. On the one hand, using the guideline that the best software is the most widely advertised is often not successful. On the other hand, the Internet has made previewing software easier than it used to be. Many software developers make free trials available, so that unclear or misleading marketing information can be checked prior to purchase. Clinicians are encouraged to use the recommendations of colleagues and the exhibits at professional meetings to aid in finding software and other new technology products to meet their needs.

Clinicians should be clear in their own minds about the difference between licensed software, shareware, and software in the public domain. Copyright laws apply to clinicians in every work setting, and violations that are identified can carry stiff penalties.

REVIEW FOR TOPIC 14

1. List three sources that clinicians could use to find clinical software.
2. What advantages to finding software are provided by commercial web sites?
3. Why is it important to register new software?
4. How can multiple copies of software be purchased at a discounted rate?
5. Who has permission to sell a shareware product? Who has permission to copy or distribute a shareware product at no cost to the recipient?
6. How do shareware and public domain software differ?

QUESTIONS FOR DISCUSSION

1. At a state association meeting, a clinician runs into an old friend who works as an SLP in a nearby rehab center. In the course of conversation, the clinician tells the friend about a new software program that is working well for several patients on her caseload. The friend asks if she can borrow the CD for a few weeks because her center does not have money for new software. How should the clinician handle this situation?
2. Visit one of the many web sites that offer public domain software for a general audience (search for "public domain software"). From this list of titles, do you see anything that could be clinically useful? What are the pros and cons of public domain software?

RESOURCES FOR FURTHER STUDY

Software Publishers Association. (1998). Software piracy: Is it happening in your school or university? *T.H.E. Journal, 25*(9), 66–67.

Wynne, M.K., & Hurst, D.S. (1995). Legal issues and computer use by school-based audiologists and speech-language pathologists. *Language, Hearing, Speech Services in Schools, 28*(3), 251–259.

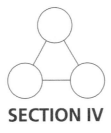

Using a Computer to Generate Therapy Materials

Introduction to Using a Computer to Generate Therapy Materials

Clinical computing competency #3: The clinician will take advantage of computer capabilities to generate personalized clinical materials to enhance intervention with specific clients.

Novice computer users and experts alike will enjoy attaining this clinical computing competency. Novices may use software templates to create reward certificates or speech homework calendars for their clients. Intermediate users may explore the use of clip art and digital photo libraries to make worksheets, games, communication aids, or computer-based mini-lessons. Clinicians with more advanced computer experience and resources could use text, sound, graphics, and digital video to create multi-media or web-based therapy materials. This competency can be achieved with a minimum or maximum investment in time and resources, depending upon the interests of the clinician and the needs of her clients.

CHOOSING AND MAKING THERAPY MATERIALS

Clinicians report that a variety of factors contribute to their selection and purchase of certain therapy materials, including recommendations from supervisors and peers, advertisements, catalog promotions, budget limitations, demonstrations at conferences, and institutional policy (Ballanger, 1996). Clinicians across work settings use homemade or individualized materials at least some of the time. Why do clinicians often create therapy materials for use with their clients? Reasons offered include small budgets, desire for more variety, difficulty finding exactly the materials needed, focus on an individual client's particular need or interest, and, for many clinicians, pleasure in the creative process.

If clinicians are already making therapy materials, how can a computer contribute to this process? Answering this question is the purpose of Section IV. Using a computer, a clinician can develop some of the same kinds of materials that he may already be making by hand; if he's lucky, using the computer makes the process faster and easier to replicate the next time he wants to create a similar item. For example, the first time a homework page is created, the computer might not be faster or more efficient than a more traditional approach, especially if the clinician is learning to use a new computer-based tool in the process. However, once the worksheet is generated and saved, it is simple to slightly change the wording, add a person's name, or adjust the size of a picture to individualize it for use with multiple clients. The advantages the computer brings to the task of making therapy materials include 1) easily made changes, 2) alternative presentation formats, and 3) professional quality output.

Besides making traditional materials such as stimulus cards and worksheets, some clinicians will pursue the use of computers to create the kind and quality of materials that would be difficult or impossible for most individuals to develop without new technologies. Granted, the way most people start is to use a computer to help do something they already know how to do without one. For example, consider the project of making a class experience story or journal about an important event. After the storybook or journal is finished, children will use the book as a jumping off point to work on speech goals, sequencing, and telling personal narratives as they work with the clinician. Using a more traditional method, it would be possible to use a Polaroid camera to take photos of preschoolers making masks and carving pumpkins. Then the pictures can be arranged in a scrapbook and accompanied by children's written comments. The clinician or teacher could write the words under each photo, and then laminate the pages.

How could a computer make a difference in this project? First, the traditional method produces a single, fragile document. If a child spills milk on it during lunch, it may or may not survive. If this was a computer-based project, multiple copies could easily be produced. In fact, books with individualized cover pages or features could be developed to focus on the interests and needs of various children in the room. Some children may require larger photos or fonts, or fewer words on a page. Some children need to practice arranging pages in the right order to help re-tell the story. The child with physical challenges needs an electronic version so that he can view it on a monitor and turn the pages by touching the screen. None of these adaptations are as feasible with the traditional homemade class picture book.

Generating materials with computers will intrigue some clinicians and will become the vehicle by which they pursue and achieve more advanced technical understanding. Some clinicians will want to go on to author new materials for use with clients during computer-based activities. Later topics in Section IV help clinicians understand the resources and skills required for creating and using resources libraries, resource editors, multimedia, and authoring tools.

UNDERSTANDING THE TECHNOLOGY

Current software products make it possible to quickly create a wide variety of individualized clinical materials. This software ranges from specialized programs that perform one task quickly and well, to general purpose authoring tools that can accomplish a variety of tasks but may require a greater time investment. An example of the first type is certificate-making software that clinicians can use to generate personalized awards that rival those produced at professional print shops. A second way to accomplish this task is to purchase "certificate paper" from an office supply store and use a word processor to add appropriate text in a beautiful font. A third way would be to make use of an award "tem-

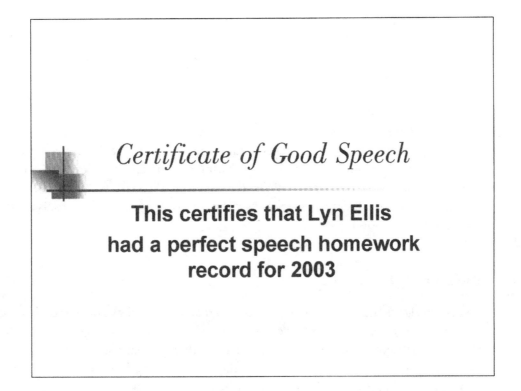

Figure 15.1. Example of computer-generated award certificate made from a *Microsoft Office* template.

plate" built into most standard business software suites. A software "suite" is a collection of programs that work together to provide a complete set of functions or capabilities. For example, a business "suite" might include a word processing software, spreadsheet software, database or address book software, and presentation or slideshow software. Microsoft Office is the most popular suite of software tools worldwide, and currently the certificate template resides in the *PowerPoint* templates that accompany Office (see Figure 15.1).

The programs used by clinicians to generate therapy materials include generic business and education software as well as software designed with special needs and communication disorders in mind. Some programs may be found in the bargain bin at the local office supply store for under $50, and some may cost several hundred dollars and be ordered only from specialized distributors.

Most of the programs mentioned or described throughout the topics in Section IV can be used successfully with a small time investment, although the more advanced authoring tools may require more time and patience to master. The primary purpose of Section IV is not to provide step-by-step instructions for a particular software tool, although some sample projects are described in how-to detail. Rather, the primary purpose is to give readers an idea of what is possible with software that is currently widely available. In each Topic of Section IV, specific materials projects will be described.

It is important to note that some of the software discussed in Section IV has obvious and important roles in administrative computing activities. Computers can greatly facilitate administrative activities such as report writing, billing, and client records. These functions go beyond the scope of this book. Readers may want to consult other sources for information about administrative applications of computers, such as *Computer Applications for Augmenting the Management of Speech-Language and Hearing Disorders* by Franklin Silverman (1997).

The decision to generate therapy materials with the help of the computer introduces choices and questions regarding not just software, but also hardware. Fortunately, this clinical computing competency can be achieved no matter what kind of computer is available. Availability of a color printer is optimal, but much can be done even with black and white/grayscale output. Scanners, digital cameras, digital video cameras, and various storage media are other peripheral devices that some clinicians will want to explore in the context of creating therapy materials. Suggestions for how to use these tools are discussed throughout Section IV.

BENEFITS FOR CLIENTS

How do clients benefit from having access to materials that have been especially designed or customized for them? Consider three real clinical materials projects that illustrate the range and the potential for computer-generated therapy materials. The first case example was developed by a student clinician in the Truman State University Speech and Hearing Clinic. A clinician used a life-size picture of a child's own face to engage an otherwise reluctant child in a discussion of body parts.

CASE EXAMPLE: Head, Shoulders, Knees, and Toes! (Using a digital camera and color printer to create a nearly life-size client portrait)

Situation: The client was a toddler with Down syndrome in her first semester of therapy. The language goals for the semester included labeling body parts, and the clinician planned to use a total-communication strategy pairing oral words and sign language. At first, efforts to engage the child in traditional activities for labeling body parts met with minimal interest or cooperation on her part.

Technology Solution: The clinician brought a digital camera to therapy one day and asked the child to pose for pictures, which she loved doing. The clinician took several close-ups of the child's face, arms, hands, legs, and feet. Later that day, the clinician looked at the photos on the computer and printed out a large picture of the child's face. Other pictures were saved for another time. The clinician trimmed the picture of the child's head and used it as the start for a nearly life-size paper doll that illustrated the basic body parts vocabulary for the week. Parts were removable so they could be taped on the wall or the mirror one piece at a time.

Outcome: The next week in therapy, the client attended well during all of the activities that involved her paper doll. She recognized herself, as indicated by her use of the words "me" and her name. She labeled her eyes, ears, and hands and feet, imitating signs and oral words to refer to her own body as well as to parts of the doll. These materials were used frequently for about a month, and then sent home with the child.

The second example is based on an account of the work of school clinician Debbie E. Brady, Columbia, South Carolina, as described in an article for *ADVANCE*, a national newsletter for speech-language pathologists and audiologists. According to the article, Brady had used a digital camera with the children on her caseload for several years (Palacio, 2001). The example below is based on just one of her many creative ideas.

CASE EXAMPLE: That's Me! (Using a digital camera and color printer to create stimulus cards)

Situation: School clinicians use stimulus cards for working with students on almost any speech or language target. Commercial stimulus cards may not include exactly the words or concepts that the clinician wants his or her students to practice, or everyone may be tired of using the same few stimulus cards for a particular sound or concept. Commercial stimulus cards may or may not adequately reflect the interests and cultural backgrounds of the students in a particular school.

Technology Solution: The clinician used a digital camera to take pictures of her students performing actions, demonstrating concepts, portraying various occupations, and completing sequences of events. Classroom activities such as feeding the class pet, working on art projects, and acting out a story were captured by the camera. Some students portrayed the characters in a nursery rhyme. In other photos, the literal and nonliteral meaning of idioms were shown, like, "You're pulling my leg" or "Quick as a wink." The clinician printed the photos in various sizes and used them to create sets of stimulus cards that "starred" the students in the school.

Outcome: The stimulus cards showing the students demonstrating the target concepts were a big hit. Students poured over them and talked about them for longer periods because they and their friends were in the pictures. The interests and cultural backgrounds of the students on the caseload were well represented on the cards. Gradually, the clinician built up a collection of custom stimulus cards that ideally suited her students.

The third example is another based on a case at the Truman State University Speech and Hearing Clinic. It is different from the first two not only in the technology used, but also in the outcome. In this final example, the clinician intended to create a computer activity itself that would be personalized for the client, not just materials for off-computer use.

CASE EXAMPLE: Electronic Memory Book (Using a scanner, clip art, and *PowerPoint* to make an electronic client family album)

Situation: A 75-year-old client with a degenerative neurological condition came to the clinic to learn to use his new communication device and practice conversation strategies. His newly assigned clinician was more than 50 years younger, and feared that they would have little in common to discuss. This proved to be true during their first few meetings, except when she asked questions about his family. He became interested in this topic and worked hard to convey information. There were several siblings and grandchildren, however, and he had difficulty remembering the relationships and keeping the conversation going.

Technology Solution: The clinician asked the client to bring in some favorite family photos and obtained his permission to scan them. They were returned to the client unharmed, and the scanned versions were incorporated into a *PowerPoint* slide show. The clinician placed a photo on each electronic page, with a prompt for a caption. The cover page identified this as an electronic memory album for this client and the date. During each therapy session, the client and the clinician together completed at least one page of the memory book. "Talking" about the photo using the communication device, the client told the clinician what to type. Sometimes it was a simple photo caption or sometimes it was a favorite memory about that person or a brief account of an adventure.

Outcome: The client and clinician enjoyed having a shared purpose for discussing the client's family photos. Both of them found this topic of conversation motivating and comfortable. After several weeks, the clinician made a color printout of the final product, which the client took home. The client's wife was thrilled by the communication this activity drew from her husband and planned to make color photocopies of the memory album for other family members.

THE ISSUE OF TIME AND RESOURCES

In many ways, the issues surrounding the use of computers to generate therapy material are no longer technical ones. That is, the key questions are no longer about whether the technology to do these things is available, reliable, or reasonably priced—it is all of these things. Now the important questions are, "What kinds of materials do clinicians need?" and "Do personalized therapy materials make a difference?" The perceived benefits will have to outweigh what clinicians perceive to be the costs in resources, time, and energy.

The three examples all involve the use of an external peripheral device such as a camera or scanner, and software tools that are generic in nature (rather than specific to communication disorders). There are substantial benefits for clinicians who have skills with general-purpose software. People who take the time to develop such skills usually find many additional ways to use them. In other words, their initial investment yields unanticipated returns.

Consider a clinician who learns how to use a generic clip-art library in order to make a personalized overlay for a child who uses a communication device. The process of incorporating clip art into a document becomes familiar to meet that initial clinical purpose. Suddenly, the clinician finds the same process useful for projects for other clients such as generating individualized homework sheets, games, bulletin boards, newsletters, and emergent literacy activities. If asked at the outset, the clinician might have denied any intention of making individualized homework materials. Once the time was invested in acquiring the necessary skills, however, new tasks seemed like a doable and beneficial extension.

SUMMARY

Many clinicians are in the habit of customizing traditional therapy materials to meet the needs of specific clients. Using computers to facilitate this process can yield exciting results for both clinicians and clients. A wide range of software and hardware components can be employed in the achievement of this clinical computing competency, although any computer with a printer can provide an adequate start. Computers bring three particular advantages to generating materials: 1) flexibility to accommodate many different clients, 2) easily adjusted features to accommodate individual needs or situations, and 3) high-quality products.

REVIEW FOR TOPIC 15

1. Describe five different items/materials that clinicians could generate using computers.
2. Is it true that computers always save time, even the first time the clinician uses one to make materials? Explain your answer.
3. Explain the three particular advantages that computers bring to the task of making therapy materials.

QUESTIONS FOR DISCUSSION

1. Discuss possible advantages for clients if clinicians can readily produce materials especially for them.
2. Describe examples you may have seen or created yourself.
3. How do you feel about the prospect of generating your own therapy materials? Is this idea attractive or not? What do you anticipate would be the drawbacks and benefits for you as a professional? What resources might you need that you don't already have?

RESOURCES FOR FURTHER STUDY

Bull, G., Bull, G., Thomas, J., & Jordon, J. (2000). Incorporating imagery into instruction. *Learning and Leading with Technology, 27.* Retrieved July 8, 2003, from http://www.iste.org/LL/27/6/index.cfm

Palacio, M. (2001, February). Take a picture, it lasts longer: Novel use of digital cameras enhances therapy in schools. *ADVANCE for Speech-Language Pathologists and Audiologists*, 6–7.

Using Utilities and Templates to Generate Therapy Materials

Clinical computing competency #3: The clinician will take advantage of computer capabilities to generate personalized clinical materials to enhance intervention with specific clients.

Using software templates and utilities to generate therapy materials is an excellent way for clinicians who have few resources or novice level computer skills to achieve this clinical computing competency. Templates and utilities generally yield impressive-looking and rewarding results from a minimum investment in time and trouble. This competency involves selecting an appropriate design for the materials and implementing the directions given in a template. The important thing for beginning clinicians is to remain focused on the targeted goals already chosen for the client. Templates and utilities for generating therapy materials are great confidence builders, whether used by the clinician outside the therapy session, or during therapy with a client as a computer-based activity (as described in Section III).

With computer templates and utilities, clinicians can make greeting cards, signs, award certificates, stickers, stimulus cards, bulletin board materials, worksheets, homework calendars, brochures, and newsletters, among many others, to use clinically. The software templates and utilities can be sorted into two groups: those designed for general purpose use by business or the public, and those especially designed for communication disorders or special education. Table 16.1 presents some software exemplars of general purpose templates and utilities. Table 16.2 provides examples that have been especially developed for use by clinicians and educators.

GENERAL-PURPOSE TEMPLATES AND UTILITIES

Most computer users have access to some of the general-purpose software listed in Table 16.1. New peripheral devices such as printers and scanners often have additional general-purpose software conveniently bundled in at no additional cost. For example, software that generates greeting cards or calendars is common.

Table 16.1. Generic templates and utilities that clinicians could use to generate therapy materials

Microsoft Office (Microsoft): Includes a project gallery of examples and clip art library for *Word, PowerPoint, Excel.*

AppleWorks (Apple): Word processor, database, spreadsheet integrated program.

Microsoft Works (Microsoft): An integrated suite of home and business software.

Adobe HomePublisher (Adobe): This or similar software is often bundled with computers, printers, scanners, and digital cameras. It includes templates for many common formats such as brochures, greeting cards, and signs.

Print Shop (Riverdeep Interactive Learning): Formerly from Broderbund, this classic software includes thousands of QuickStart Layouts and premium-quality graphics that let users produce professional quality projects such as newsletters, posters, reports, web pages, pamphlets, calendars, banners and labels. Edit and enhance photos with sophisticated tools and special effects, then incorporate them into any project.

GamePak Interactive (FTC Publishing): Offers thirteen different game *PowerPoint* templates based on popular game shows. Activities are intended to reinforce vocabulary and other specific skills.

Avery Kids Printertainment Software Kit and Supplies (Avery): Provides templates for common projects like greeting cards, invitations, and more.

The word processing software that is on a clinician's computer is likely to include templates for special projects and document formats such as newsletters, brochures, lists, envelopes, and labels. Certificate templates are commonly found in presentation software templates, such as the samples currently included with Microsoft's *PowerPoint*. Clinicians who explore these templates and examples may discover the means to create many easy-to-do projects.

Sometimes, templates are called "assistants" or "guides." Along a similar vein, "wizards" are usually automated guides that step the user through a series of choices that would otherwise be a complex process, such as installing new software. Templates may take a step-by-step approach, but often they just present an example that users edit to match their own preferences. "Utilities" are software programs designed to help the user handle a particular task or group of tasks easily, much like a wizard but without the forced sequence of events. A program that automatically moves files from digital camera media to a computer and then erases the media, or a program that converts files from one format to another are examples of a utility.

Perhaps the ultimate general-purpose template software is Microsoft's *PowerPoint*, originally designed to make it easy to put slideshows and presentations together. Creative clinicians and educators have learned to manipulate the strengths of *PowerPoint* to their advantage resulting in much more than a basic slideshow. For example, FTC Publishing (Bloomington, IL) has released several examples of templates for *PowerPoint*. The *Game Pak Interactive* CDs contain educational game templates created with *PowerPoint*. Clinicians, parent volunteers, or even older students could use the templates to create skill practice activities based on popular television game shows. The user supplies the content, so the games could be designed to correspond to an adult client's special interest or hobby or a child's curriculum unit in science or social studies.

SPECIALIZED TEMPLATES AND UTILITIES

Picture This Pro (Silver Lining) is a relatively inexpensive CD-ROM resource library of 2,900 high-quality color photographs. There are many ways these photos can be used

Table 16.2. Examples of templates and utilities especially designed and marketed for communication disorders and/or special education

Picture Express (Picture Express Software): This CD consists of templates for printing stickers, gameboards, worksheets, and picture cards, using the 600 pictures included. Drawings have been selected especially for use in phonology and articulation therapy and can be sorted by phonological features, word length, and vocabulary level.

Picture This!, *Picture This Pro!*, *School Routines and Rules* (Silver Lining Multimedia, Inc.): Each of these economical CDs consists of a large library of photos collected with special needs in mind; comes with index and template software for printing one or several photos per page, with or without text or borders.

Overlay Maker (IntelliTools): Template utility for creating alternative keyboard overlays and off-computer activities with symbols, photos, and/or text.

Brubaker on Disk (Parrot): Database of 1000+ text items that clinicians can choose to have automatically formatted into various question types. Allows quick customization of popular Brubaker-style worksheets for adults and adolescents.

Boardmaker (Mayer-Johnson): More than 3000 picture communication symbols (PCS) and 100 pre-made templates for use with popular communication devices or to create calendars, schedules. English version 5 comes with color or black and white symbols, with or without text labels in 19 languages; international language/culture versions also available.

clinically, which is discussed in later topics. *Picture This Pro* comes with a simple template interface that quickly allows the user to search for the desired photos and print them out in a chosen format, with or without text labels in English, Spanish, French, Italian, or German. For example, if medium-size pictures are needed, the clinician might select and print four pictures per page. This collection of pictures was designed with the picture needs of clinicians and special educators in mind. Clinicians with minimal computer skills or previous understanding of graphic file formats, and so forth, will feel successful at finding and printing just the right picture materials for a speech game or language board. Clinicians looking for worksheet and lotto-type game board templates to go with a library of images (drawings, not photos) will find this combination in *Picture Express* (Picture Express Software). The starter kit comes with some printing supplies (e.g., sticker sheets, card stock).

Even more specialized in intent and outcome is *Brubaker on Disk* (Parrot). This CD-ROM includes a database of language and cognitive exercises intended to help clinicians generate customized worksheets. The worksheets created with this product have the look and feel of the well-known aphasia workbooks by Susan Howell Brubaker. The difference is that users can pick and choose items that meet their exact specifications and combine them into a personalized workbook of any number of pages. According to the publisher, the CD includes 1,500 exercise items never published in the traditional format. To use the computer-based worksheet generator, the clinician specifies the concepts to be addressed, the difficulty level, response type (e.g., multiple choice, matching), print size, and font. The program automatically chooses a set of exercises that the clinician can then edit and modify as needed. Workbooks can be saved and printed or modified later.

These are just two examples of the many specialized templates and utilities available for clinicians who are interested in generating therapy materials with the help of a computer. Such software virtually guarantees that even computer novices will be successful at creating a professional looking product for client use.

UNDERSTANDING THE TECHNOLOGY: THE JOYS AND FRUSTRATIONS OF TEMPLATES

Clinicians will find that using templates and utilities is convenient and efficient most of the time. As mentioned previously, templates are a useful way to become familiar with the capabilities of the computer and sometimes the features of new software. However, the same things that make templates useful (e.g., pre-designed elements, limited choices) also make them frustrating at times.

The constraints of a template may interfere with a clinician's specific plan or design concept. This is the same phenomenon that occurs when a person follows ANY kind of template—a recipe, a sewing pattern, a map—and finds that the results do not suit. Sometimes, the templates can be modified and gradually users are able to develop their own creations or just move on to more advanced tools. The resources discussed in Topics 17, 18, and 19, such as resource libraries and authoring software, offer the next step for motivated clinicians.

PROJECT IDEAS: GETTING OFF TO A SIMPLE START

Several entry-level ideas for making clinical materials are described in Table 16.3. Most clinicians could complete these projects in 20 minutes or so, without much preparation. The goal here is to make something impressive with minimal stress. Beginners who try one of these should choose something that sounds easy and do it when they have time to enjoy it. Minimize frustration by avoiding an overly ambitious first project and resolve to live within the limitations of the template at first.

An example of a simple beginning that evolved into an extended application occurred when the *Picture This!* CD (Silver Lining Multimedia) was new in the Truman State University Speech and Hearing Clinic. It was used to develop a bulletin board about the summer Olympics (Be a Speech Champion!). From the Olympics web site, color photos of adult athletes in major events were captured and printed (with web citations). Then we paired these on the bulletin board with full-page printouts of photos from *Picture This!* that showed children doing similar activities: swimming, running, biking, and jumping. This

Table 16.3.   Easy clinical materials project ideas based on templates and wizards

Using any basic business quality word processor:

> Look through the sample template files and clip art that came with your word processor or presentation software. Using one of the templates, make a sign with an inspirational quote, a brochure about how teachers should make referrals to you, a certificate for someone who needs a boost, or a personal calendar. The templates available will depend on your software. The web site for your software will probably offer additional downloadable templates and possibly clip art, at no additional cost.

Using software such as *Picture This!* or *Picture This Pro!* (Silver Lining Multimedia) or *Boardmaker* (Mayer-Johnson):

> Using any of these programs, choose photos or symbols to go with a language or articulation goal. Become familiar with the vocabulary and images included, so you will know what is available for a particular client or group.
>
> 1. Print out a page of selected images, to use for stimulus cards or homework.
> 2. Design a bulletin board and locate images related to the theme. Make large printouts to enhance visibility.

project introduced the whole clinic to *Picture This!* and soon it was in high demand among student clinicians anxious to prepare a variety of engaging activities for their clients.

Templates found in major business software packages usually work in one of two ways. Clinicians may find that the template is self-contained and complete—more like an example users are expected to copy or modify. For instance, a brochure template may consist merely of a pre-formatted document that the user opens and edits. Inserting text or clip art further individualizes the project. Alternatively, a wizard asks for information or choices from the user, then generates a calendar or other customized document based on the chosen specifications. As with text, users can click on the art in a template document to delete it and replace it their own photo, clip art, or image copied from a web page.

THE ISSUE OF TIME AND RESOURCES: PAPER AND INK

The software listed in Table 16.2 ranges in price from about $70 for the *Picture This Pro!* to several hundred dollars for resource collections such as *Brubaker on Disk* or *Boardmaker*. Price is often directly related to the power and flexibility of the software. In the case of specialized software for communication disorders, however, a contributing factor to high price is also the relatively small size of the potential market. To recoup the development costs, small companies must charge a higher price for their products. Word of mouth and product reviews in professional publications can help clinicians find out whether the price is worth the potential benefits of a particular program.

Time and budget are omnipresent factors in clinicians' decisions to make their own therapy materials, whether or not a computer is part of the equation. Obviously, if a computer is routinely used to generate materials, a review of printer features and expenses may be beneficial. Speed of output (pages per minute in black and white and color), cost per page, image accuracy, reliability, and technical support are important considerations. For example, the purchase price of a printer may be relatively low, but the savings are lost if expensive ink cartridges need frequent replacement. Product reviews in major technology magazines and web sites can provide helpful and objective information about initial and long-term printer costs and durability.

Budgeting for paper use is another consideration. Printers (inkjet or laser) usually produce a better result if hardware-specific paper is provided. Frequent printer jams and poor quality of text and images may result when plain copy machine paper is substituted. Printer paper in a wide range of weights and finishes is also available for particular tasks, such as printing a photo or a t-shirt transfer. Discretion in selecting the right kind of paper for the printer and the task can contribute to cost containment and support administrative endorsement of customized, clinician-generated materials.

The last word of advice concerning resource management and printers has to do with making multiple copies. Most clinicians have access to a black and white photocopy machine. It is usually less expensive per page to photocopy an original than it is to print many copies of the same document from a printer. At least this is an issue to consider where budgets are tight. Sometimes the photocopy budget is different than the ink cartridge budget, and so resources should be used accordingly.

SUMMARY

Clinicians use both general-purpose and specialized templates and wizards to help them generate clinical materials. Templates and wizards that come with business software help users create specific documents such as greeting cards, calendars, certificates, posters, resumes, newsletters, and brochures. Specialized software may help clinicians produce communication boards, games, picture cards, and worksheets.

Templates and wizards help users learn the features and capabilities of complex software, allowing them to produce impressive results with a minimum of expertise. However, design templates and wizards are narrow in focus and somewhat inflexible. Users may become frustrated by template limitations, requiring them to explore more advanced tools.

Fabrication of customized clinical materials requires consideration of cost allocations for resources such as paper and printer ink. Product reviews can help clinicians identify printers that have specific desirable features. Choosing the right paper for the printer and the project will help ensure the best possible results.

REVIEW FOR TOPIC 16

1. What is the distinction made between the two types of templates and wizards listed in Tables 16.1 and 16.2?
2. Describe the uses of "templates" and "wizards." How do these applications help the user generate a product?
3. What budget and resource issues related to printers should clinicians consider?
4. Describe three projects/materials that a clinician could make with the help of a software template or wizard.

QUESTIONS FOR DISCUSSION

1. Why do some clinicians find using a template frustrating? Can you think of an example when you were constrained by something that was supposed to be helping you?
2. What templates are available with your primary word processor? Try inserting clip art into a word processor document (usually, the Insert menu). How could you use these resources to generate useful materials?

RESOURCES FOR FURTHER STUDY

Bull, G., Bull, G., Blasi, L., & Cochran, P. (2000). Electronic texts in the classroom. *Learning and Leading with Technology, 27*(4), 46–56.

Bull, G., Bull, G., & Dawson, K. (1999). The universal solvent. *Learning and Leading with Technology, 27*(2), 36–41.

Cochran, P.S., & Bull, G.L. (1991). Integrating word processing into language therapy. *Topics in Language Disorders, 11*(2), 31–48.

Creating and Using Digital Resource Libraries

Pictures, Clip Art, and Photographs

Clinical computing competency #3: The clinician will take advantage of computer capabilities to generate personalized clinical materials to enhance intervention with specific clients.

Learning to develop and use resource libraries to create therapy materials is an excellent way for clinicians who have intermediate computing skills to address this competency. In response to clinicians' strong interest in high-quality materials that can be matched exactly to a client's needs, publishers are now offering excellent digital collections of photos, drawings, symbols, and illustrations for clinical and educational use. Competency with such resource libraries should involve more than merely choosing an image and printing it from a template (as in Topic 16). A clinician who has competency with resource libraries should be able to define a therapy goal and activity, find a desired image, and incorporate it into the materials she is developing outside of a template, such as an illustrated worksheet. Some clinicians will want to take the further step of creating and using their own collections of digital resources (photos, sounds, videos).

Finding a good resource library is like finding a $100 bill—it makes a person feel rich. Luckily, publishers of materials for education and rehabilitation have become aware of the market for collections of images, symbols, sounds, and videos that clinicians and teachers can use in hundreds of ways never imagined by the person who compiled the collection. Examples of such compilations are described in Table 17.1. These resource libraries are just what they sound like—groupings of thousands of separate files, usually assembled into logical categories such as food, clothing, actions, seasons, people, animals, transportation, and more. Resource libraries are an entirely different genre of software than was discussed in Sections II and III. Typically, these products are not used directly with clients; instead, the library's assets may be tapped in advance to create digital or paper materials for therapeutic activities.

This topic focuses on using digital resources to create traditional therapy materials. In addition to discussing commercial resource libraries, this topic introduces three alternative ways of obtaining images for therapy materials: downloading web images (photos or art), scanning existing images (photos or art), and using a digital

Table 17.1   Examples of resource libraries (photos, pictures symbols, clip art, animations) available for use in generating therapy materials

Resource library and publisher	Description
Picture This!, *Picture This Pro!*, *School Routines and Rules*, *Functional Living Skills*, and *Behavioral Rules* (Silver Lining Multimedia, Inc.)	Each of these CDs consists of a library of 1,000–5,000 photos collected with special needs in mind; index and templates for printing several photos per page, with or without text or borders are included. Depending on the CD, searchable by category, phoneme, and so forth. Note that these JPEG format photo files can be accessed, copied, or inserted into other software outside of the *Picture This!* templates.
KidPix Deluxe (Riverdeep/Broderbund)	Originally a children's drawing program, *KidPix Deluxe* has many extra features that go beyond a simple paint application. Includes an array of tiny "stamp" images, easy ways to manipulate and print shapes and patterns of any size and color, and a talking alphabet. Magical screen transformations, and over 50 Wacky brushes with their own unique sound effects.
Photo-Objects Collections (Vols. 1, 2) (Mayer-Johnson)	50,000 royalty-free photos in each collection, arranged by categories; browser allows you to see thumbnail images while you search
The Big Box of Art (Mayer-Johnson)	Wide range of royalty-free digital images (350,000) including photos, clipart, animations, and illustrations organized by category; search engine included.
Boardmaker (Mayer-Johnson)	Over 3,000 picture symbols and 100 templates for device overlays or communication boards that can also be used to make things like calendars and daily schedules. English version 5 comes with text labels in 19 languages; international language/culture versions also available.

camera to create new photos. Note that Topics 18 and 19 highlight the role of resource libraries in the development of computer-based activities for use with clients and Topic 20 covers relevant copyright information.

IMPORTING GRAPHICS, PHOTOS, OR MOVIES INTO A DOCUMENT

Major word processing packages frequently include at least small collections of clip art that can be inserted into any document. Clinicians are not limited to these clip art libraries, however. A similar copy and paste process allows users to integrate images from a variety of other sources. The specific sequence of steps varies by program application and computer.

In general, images can be integrated into word processing documents in either of two ways: inserting a file, or copying/pasting to transfer an item that is part of another file. A clinician may want to use an image saved by itself as a separate file, such as a photo taken with a digital camera or one of the photos from a digital resource library such as *Picture This Pro!* Many clinicians successfully print out pages of photos using the pre-configured templates in *Picture This Pro!*, but never realize that the photo files are available for use in their own documents. To access such files, the individual employs the word processor's "import" or "insert from a file" function to read in the file and place the photo into a document. Notably, the file import procedure emanates from the productivity tool (i.e., word processor or presentation program) not the resource library application, such as *Picture This Pro!*.

Another way to find graphics is to consult a graphics or clip-art library, in which each file may include several images stored together on a page rather than individual files. Or, a clinician may create one or more original graphics using a paint or drawing tool application, such as *Kid Pix* (Riverdeep/Broderbund). This would be just like using clip art from a resource library, except the clinician designs the clipart herself. From a *Kid Pix* screen, she would select just the part of the page or image that is needed. The selection can then be copied and pasted into a working document using the appropriate Edit menu options. Note that in this process, the clinician begins in the source of the image, copies it, and then switches back to the destination document to paste in the image.

Using a digital resource library such as *Boardmaker* (Mayer-Johnson) also requires the copy-and-paste method, if the clinician is creating materials that go beyond the scope of the templates provided with the program. This popular collection of Picture Communication Symbols (PCS) is used to generate communication boards or overlays from the program's templates pre-designed to fit common communication devices. Using the copy and paste procedure, clinicians use *Boardmaker* as a resource library for developing additional support materials such as activity cards, sentence symbol strips, personalized books, and other clinical materials. The desired PCS are copied from the *Boardmaker* library and pasted into the destination document (i.e., a word processor or drawing progam document) or a *Boardmaker* template. For instance, a clinician could generate pages of illustrations intended to help the client practice action verbs, target sounds, or spatial relationships (Figure 17.1). Maximizing the flexibility of programs such as *Boardmaker* to go beyond making communication boards helps to justify the required investment of time and money.

There are many collections of resources that can either be imported or copied and pasted into word processing documents. These include copyrighted as well as public domain collections of photographs, clip art, and video segments (see Table 17.1 for resource examples, and see Topic 20 for a discussion of copyright).

UNDERSTANDING THE TECHNOLOGY: THREE MORE WAYS TO OBTAIN IMAGES

Clinicians who do not have access to commercially available resource libraries, or who need illustrations of less common concepts, will want to investigate alternate ways of obtaining and integrating images into their homemade therapy materials. Three good options include downloading images, scanning existing images, or creating new images with a digital camera.

Downloading Web Images

One convenient, cost-effective source for photos or drawings of almost anything is the Internet. Access to an international collection of images also helps to ensure that materi-

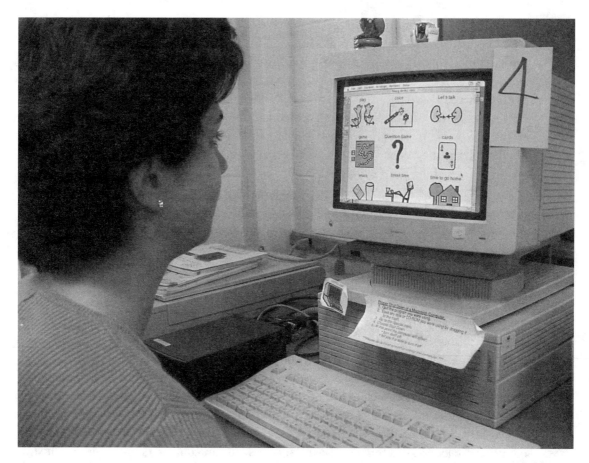

Figure 17.1. A clinician chooses picture symbols from *Boardmaker* (Mayer-Johnson) that she plans to use to make articulation therapy stimulus cards. (Courtesy of Truman State University Speech and Hearing Clinic.)

als are interesting, motivating, and culturally relevant to clients. However, web surfers need to be aware that some images—photos, drawings and designs—will not be available for downloading and/or they may be copyrighted. Clinicians should be aware of their obligations and responsibilities concerning copyright and the use of images they find on the web (see Topic 20).

A clinician begins a collection of web images to archive for future use by searching the web to find desirable photos or drawings. Once a good picture is identified, the next step is to save it as a file on the clinician's computer. From that point on, using it will be just like using the "insert file" method for photos from commercial resource libraries like *Picture This,* or a digital camera. The easiest way to "capture" a web image is to click on it—right click with a Windows browser, or hold the mouse button down when using a Mac. A menu or dialog box of choices will appear; the clinician should pick one that says something like: "Save this image to disk" or "Save as a file." Then the browser software will provide an opportunity to name the file. Consult the tips for downloading and saving images in Table 17.2.

Using a Scanner to Digitize Existing Images

Sometimes it is possible to take advantage of images that exist in non-electronic format. For example, there may be photo prints of a client's family members or special events that

Table 17.2.　Tips for downloading and saving images from the Internet

Make a folder on your hard drive or disk as a standard location for your downloaded files.

Select files in JPEG or GIF format since they import easily into most word processors and other applications.

Avoid changing the filename extension (jpg, gif, tif).

Give the image file a meaningful name (e.g., "beach.jpg", not "ima35a.jpg").

Pay attention to the directory or location where the file will be saved on your computer, so it can be retrieved later.

Note the URL (Universal Resource Locator or web address).

Give credit to sources for images you include in your work.*

Use a web browser to view the files later, if other photo or image software is not available.

*Note that crediting your source does not constitute permission to use the image in a way that violates the owner's copyright.

the clinician would like to use in generating materials. Sometimes a color photocopy will do, although it is an expensive option. Availability of a scanner and printer provides another alternative. There are advantages to scanning images. Once an image is scanned (converted to digital format on the computer), it can be manipulated, edited, or reprinted an unlimited number of times. For example, a clinician might want to resize photos of the client's family members so they uniformly fit into a communication wallet or he may need to edit a photo to emphasize just the client and crop or cut out the scenery (see Figure 17.2)

Flatbed scanners have become increasingly inexpensive and easy-to-use peripheral devices. The process of scanning an image or photo from a book is straightforward but specific to particular hardware and software configurations. Typically, an item is placed facedown on the scanner's glass surface or document plate (e.g., a photocopier). A light source and array of sensors pass beneath it and transmit data from the scanner to the computer.

Image-editing software, such as *Photoshop Elements* (Adobe) or *PhotoImpact* (ULEAD) works in coordination with the scanner's driver software to capture the image and provide editing tools for picture manipulation. As noted previously, the scanned graphic should be saved as a JPEG or GIF file. When saving the file, another consideration is the "quality" (resolution) setting. The quality choice selected by the clinician will impact the size of the file (i.e., high quality = big file) and the detail displayed in the image. Usually, a medium quality setting should produce satisfactory results for clinical materials that will be printed out. If the image is being prepared for e-mail or web posting, a low-medium quality setting is adequate since detail is not essential but smaller file size is optimal. If photos are to be printed out in extra-large format or projected on a large screen, high-quality settings are desirable. It is important to consciously choose the file format and quality setting the image is saved in, rather than assuming that the default on the image-editing software is appropriate.

Scanning text documents is different than scanning pictures. A document with text, such as a comic strip, can be scanned and saved as a graphic image. Pictures of text, such as lettering within graphics files, cannot be edited in the usual way with a word processor. A scanned document can, however, be converted to a plain text (word processor) document through a process called optical character recognition (OCR). The distinction is important because OCR documents can be manipulated and edited just like other text documents. This is the kind of scanning that is done to move forms into digital format, for example. The accuracy of OCR depends on the clarity of the text characters in the

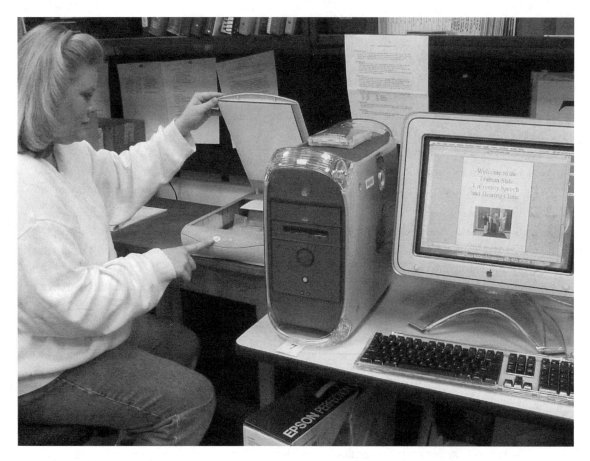

Figure 17.2.   A clinician uses a flatbed scanner to digitize a photo for use in a clinic sign she is making (Courtesy of Truman State University Speech and Hearing Clinic).

original document as well as the quality of the scanning software. Better results may be obtained through the use of specialized OCR software, such as *OmniPage, OmniForm,* or educational software such as *WYNN* (Freedom Scientific) or *Kurzweil 3000* (Kurzweil Education Systems). Completing this operation and achieving consistent accuracy in the graphic–to-text conversion is a more complex procedure than simply scanning a picture to use or import into an existing document. The use of OCR scanning to adapt text materials for individuals with physical and cognitive challenges will be discussed in Section VIII.

Making New Digital Photos with a Digital Camera

The increasing affordability and prevalence of digital cameras is an exciting development for clinicians interested in technology and in creating therapy materials. Digital still and video cameras are available with a range of features, sizes, and prices.

The primary difference between a digital camera and a regular film camera is storage of the image once the photo is taken. A digital camera, as the name suggests, "digitizes" the image—converts the light and dark and color information to numbers that a computer can interpret. This happens immediately as the picture is taken, so no film is required. The picture data is stored in special media, according to the design of the camera—floppy disks, CD-ROM, or special digital camera storage media such as a Memory Stick (Sony) or other memory card (Canon, Kodak, and others). The number of pictures that can be taken depends upon the quality of image selected and the capacity of the storage media chosen (various sizes are available).

After pictures are moved to a more permanent storage location (e.g., a computer hard drive or a CD), they can be deleted from the camera's storage media. The cable or other type of interface for transferring pictures from the camera's storage media to the computer depends on the camera model. Once pictures are saved on the computer, they can be edited and manipulated like other images from other sources discussed in this section. Some photo printers come with special slots that are media-ready and bypass the computer entirely.

THE ISSUE OF TIME AND RESOURCES: CHOOSING AND USING A DIGITAL CAMERA

Clinicians may be surprised to find that digital cameras are available for a reasonable price. Many schools and clinics which once invested in commercial film development and "instant" cameras, have switched to digital cameras that seem easier and more cost effective. Before purchasing a digital camera, individuals should consult with friends and consider product reviews and ratings (see Table 17.3).

Some clinicians will dither about whether a digital still or digital video camera will best meet all of their needs. At present, some digital still cameras can record brief videos of moderate quality, and most excellent digital video cameras can also produce still images of moderate to good quality. In settings where both kinds of photography will be routinely required, probably both kinds of cameras will be necessary until cameras become available that do both tasks equally well.

Digital cameras do not entirely eliminate the cost of making original photos, especially if high-quality photo paper and color printing are used. However, they do lower the risk/cost of taking lots of photos that are ultimately rejected. Savings come from features that allow pictures to be viewed instantly and saved selectively. Only the pictures that really match the photographer's intent are printed out. In addition, digital photo files permit the photographer to tinker with the image in many ways—cropping it, adjusting the contrast, changing the size of the image, or adding a caption.

PROJECT IDEA: MAKE A TWO-DIMENSIONAL AND THREE-DIMENSIONAL ACTIVITY BAG

The purpose of this project is to develop a kit of thematic materials suitable for a therapy lesson designed to expand the symbol vocabulary of a client (semantics) or teach the use of symbol combinations (syntax and pragmatics). These materials would be appropriate for use in a variety of teaching/therapy approaches including milieu teaching, interactive model, aided language stimulation or a system for augmenting language (for a review of these approaches, see Beukelman & Mirenda, 1998). Whether the kit is to be used with

Table 17.3. Factors to consider when choosing a digital camera

Digital resolution (maximum image quality)

Storage media

Size and weight

Power source

Recording speed

Zoom capability

View-finder

Preview capability (LCD screen)

Still photo and video options

children or adults depends on the theme/objects chosen by the clinician. The kit should include a bag or box to hold everything, small three-dimensional objects related to an appropriate therapy theme, digital photos of the objects individually and in combinations, photos or drawings of similar objects to promote generalization, and a parallel set of symbols/line drawings representing the same language concepts as the objects and photos, and word labels for each of these. This collection will allow the clinician to take a client from comprehension and use of 3-D materials to the more symbolic comprehension and use of photos, symbols, and oral or written words (see Figure 17.3 and Table 17.4).

Once the toys, photos, and other materials are collected, consider laminating all the paper items to ensure that they will withstand plenty of use. Attach the smooth side of a strip of Velcro to the outside of the canvas bag or box that will contain the materials. This makes a handy way to present the materials to a client. Put a small piece of sticky Velcro on the back of each photo/picture and the project is complete.

Clinicians can use the therapy bag to assess a client's responses to a range of closely related materials. This may speed up the selection of appropriate materials and goals for the client in future sessions. Many clients with language impairment have difficulty generalizing from "real" objects to pictures and symbols. Access to a digital camera facilitates the creation of photos that exactly match the three-dimensional materials being used in therapy, thus reducing the cognitive gap that must be crossed by the client. Once the client understands that the objects and photos match, generalization to dissimilar materials can become a goal.

SUMMARY

Readers are encouraged to investigate the digital resource libraries that are now available, or to pursue the development of their own collections of photos and other materials. The process of inserting a file (image) from a resource library into a standard word processing document is a basic skill to be mastered by clinicians pursuing the competency discussed in this topic. Expenditures on hardware such as a scanner or digital camera should be supported by consulting local expertise and researching product reviews and feature comparisons on the Internet and in trade magazines.

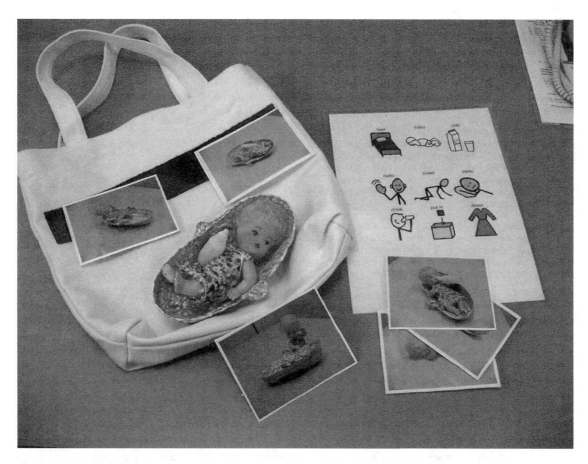

Figure 17.3. Therapy activity bag used to help clients move from three-dimensional materials to symbols. The clinician used a digital camera to create cards used in therapy. (Courtesy of Truman State University Speech and Hearing Clinic.)

Beyond accessing resource libraries, three additional ways of obtaining digital images include downloading web images, scanning existing photos or graphics, and using a digital camera to create new images. Clinicians can use combinations of digital images to create a wide variety of therapy materials such as traditional and electronic worksheets, stimulus cards, posters, games, and bulletin boards. Organizing files into meaningful categories and maintaining an index of the archive can enhance management of personal collections of digital images. For example, instead of animals, transportation, and similar categories frequently seen in commercial resource libraries, clinicians may organize their own digital archive according to other schemes, such as initial phoneme (R Folder, S Folder) concepts (Among and Between Folder, Kitchen Items Folder), or events (May Puppet Show Folder, 2004 Reading Week Folder, Special Olympics Folder, Making Pudding Folder).

REVIEW FOR TOPIC 17

1. Explain the term "digital resource library." How is a digital resource library different from CAI applications or other software to be used directly with a client?

Table 17.4. Directions for therapy activity bag project, involving digital photos and symbols

Steps for Activity Bag Project	Examples
Consider the client's age/type, goals and the therapy approach to be used.	This kit could be used with preliterate clients ages 3–8 with the aided language stimulation approach.
Find or purchase objects/toys (small, inexpensive, but NOT tiny)	Small doll baby, bottle, bed ($2.00 pkg. at discount store)
Take digital camera photos of the objects illustrating language concepts or structures that will be the goals for use of the kit (note that multiple kinds of language goals are possible with the same set of objects). Insert multiple photos into a word processing document and print them so that they are at least 2x2 inches and no larger than 3x5 inches.	Digital photos of objects in various activities (e.g., baby in bed, baby drinking bottle, baby crawling, baby waving, baby sleeping)
Find and print pictures/photos of similar objects that clearly show salient object features but that do not match these objects exactly. Sources recommended: *Picture This Pro!* (Silver Lining Multimedia) or other photo library, or the Internet. Same size requirements.	Baby, milk, crib, child drinking, baby sleeping, child crawling, adult waving
Find and print black and white or color Picture Communication Symbols (PCS) illustrating main concepts and vocabulary WITHOUT printed labels. At least 2x2. Available via *Boardmaker* (Mayer-Johnson) software.	Baby, milk, bed, drinking, crawling, bye
Make printed labels representing each major concept/vocabulary item. May be individually typed with word processing and large font (26-28 point font recommended).	Baby, milk, bed, drinking, crawling, bye

2. Briefly describe four ways that a clinician can find digital images and incorporate them into the development of clinical materials.

3. Describe two ways that clinicians can integrate a photo or graphic into a word processing document.

4. A digital camera does not use film. Explain how a picture is captured, saved, and printed from a digital camera.

5. Go to the shopping area of a search web site (such as Yahoo Shopping). Assuming you have $400 saved up to buy a digital camera, what features would you like it to have? Conduct a feature comparison and print it out and then write a brief statement explaining your top choice.

6. Re-read the directions for downloading an image from the web and try it. How did it work? Print the image that you downloaded, along with the URL from which it was obtained.

QUESTIONS FOR DISCUSSION

1. If you had the time and resources to develop your own digital image library, what clinical themes or topics would you emphasize and why?

2. What traditional photo and picture materials do you use most in your clinical practice? Discuss how they could be improved to more closely match your needs and the needs of your clients. Could the technology described in this topic help make this happen?

RESOURCES FOR FURTHER STUDY

Bull, G., Bull, G., & Dawson, K.. (1999). The universal solvent. *Learning and Leading with Technology, 27*(2), 36–41.

Bull, G., Bull, G., Thomas, J., & Jordon, J. (2000). Incorporating imagery into instruction. *Learning and Leading with Technology, 27*(6). Retrieved July 8, 2003, from http://www.iste.org/LL/27/6/index.cfm.

Palacio, M. (Feb, 2001). Take a picture, it lasts longer: Novel use of digital cameras enhances therapy in schools. *ADVANCE*, 6–7.

Multimedia Explorations

Resource Editors

Clinical computing competency #3: The clinician will take advantage of computer capabilities to generate personalized clinical materials to enhance intervention with specific clients.

The digital resources described in Topic 17 hinted at the possibilities of computer-based multimedia exploration. Competencies related to creating multimedia materials require familiarity with resource libraries (Topic 17) and an understanding of the role of resource editors (the present topic). Some clinicians will be satisfied with making use of multimedia components developed by others. They will combine them and present them in ways particularly effective for a client. Clinicians who are motivated to take the next step will develop their own multimedia by acquiring skill in changing and manipulating photos, drawings, sounds, or videos, using software tools such as resource editors. In addition, clinicians who are competent creators of multimedia will consider the specific needs of their clients and the objectives of therapy as they design multimedia materials and activities.

Traditionally, "multi-modality" therapy might include aural stimuli (the clinician's voice), visual stimuli (pictures or text), a mirror (visual feedback), and possibly tactile cues. The word multimedia also implies that more than one sensory mode has been included in an experience, event, or product. In other words, multiple media—graphics, photography, text, music, speech, animation, or video, in some combination—have been incorporated into a single result. Topics 16 and 17 emphasize the use of still images (photos and graphics) in clinician-made materials. The present topic adds sound and video to the clinician's repertoire, resulting in multimedia creations.

In previous discussions of software well suited for creating a shared context and applications intended to facilitate literacy skills, the notion of a "multimedia toolkit" was raised. For instance, this term was used in Section III to reference to the well-known *Imagination Express* series. Each program (Neighborhood, Rainforest, Ocean, Castle, Pyramids) offers a theme-related collection of backgrounds, objects, sounds, music, and reference material, from which learners can create multimedia scenes and stories. As good as this software is, however, each module is limited in scope to its theme and the available objects. Sometimes, clinicians will want to use multimedia materials that have even more flexibility in content and format.

Examples of multimedia tools that are inexpensive, easy to use, and/or commonly available on most computers are described in Table 18.1. This software makes a good beginning point for clinicians who are learning about multimedia development at an entry level. Most clinicians with computer access will find something in Table 18.1 that is already available to them, or that they could easily download and try. More advanced tools are described in Table 18.2.

EASY MULTIMEDIA PROJECT IDEAS TO TRY: MEMORY BOOK AND MOVIE SLIDESHOW

Without investing the money and time required to obtain and master a specific advanced resource editor (e.g., *Adobe Photoshop*), clinicians can get a feel for multimedia development through the use of software that is standard in most work settings—any business class suite such as *Microsoft Office* (*Word, Excel, PowerPoint*) or *Apple Works* (Apple).

These project ideas make use of *MS Word* (or other current business-quality word processor) and *PowerPoint* (presentation software), to give clinicians some experience combining sound, text, graphic, and video. To go farther in multimedia development, though, clinicians will need additional software tools. The productivity applications employed in the two project ideas presented in this chapter do NOT do the same things as either an authoring tool (Topic 19) or professional quality resource editor (discussed later in this topic and listed in Table 18.2).

PROJECT IDEA: CREATING A DIGITAL MEMORY BOOK

Project Description: Create an electronic "memory book" with or for a client using pictures, clip art, and possibly music and speech.
Software Tool: *PowerPoint*
Possible Project Topics: Family, favorite traditions, ideal adventures, proud moments, favorite places, preferred foods, top choice movie, and TV star biography.

This project can be accomplished in several ways, depending on the available resources, client, and purpose of the project. For an older client, each page could be about a family member, an important event, or favorite activity. Creating a book with a child might involve recording a routine or event/scripting (lunchtime at school) or a special occasion (birthday party, class trip). The result can be as simple or as elaborate as the clinician wants to make it. In Section III, the clinical interactions and goals that could be addressed in a shared activity are described and discussed in more detail. Recall that one reason for using the computer as a context for therapy in this way is flexibility—the activity can be perfectly tailored to the client. Having a shared purpose—like making a book—can provide a motivating context for purposeful communication attempts on the part of the client. In many instances, therefore, the clinician will want to start the project ahead of time but include the client in the many aspects of finishing the project.

Clinical experience with such projects suggests that it is a good idea to develop a framework for the memory book before the client becomes involved. Having the basic

Table 18.1. Examples of entry-level multimedia tools that clinicians could use to generate therapy materials

Multimedia tools	Descriptions
Microsoft Word (Microsoft) *PowerPoint* (Microsoft) *Microsoft Works* (Microsoft)	Explore backgrounds, color combinations, animation, sound and transition effects in *PowerPoint* or use the Picture tools in *Word* to import and roughly edit a photo or clip art item.
Adobe Photo Elements (Adobe)	The standard in photo enhancement and editing, a sub-set of the features of *Adobe Photoshop*. Even this version can seem complex for novice users, but most people won't outgrow it.
iMovie (Apple)	Setting the standard in easy-to-use video editing, this software comes with every Mac or can be downloaded.
Windows MovieMaker version 2 (Windows)	*MovieMaker* is Microsoft's answer to *iMovie* for basic video editing. Not quite as many features, but definitely useable for a free utility that comes with every Windows machine or can be downloaded.
QuickTime Picture Viewer (Apple, Mac, or Windows)	For viewing and printing photo files.
KidPix Deluxe (Riverdeep/Broderbund)	Experiment with drawing tools, animation, sound and slide shows.
Windows Sound Recorder (Microsoft)	No-frills sound recording and editing utilities included with Windows. Use to create stand-alone sound files or add spoken comments to *Word* documents.
Kodak Picture Software or a similar product (i.e., from Canon, Epson, or Sony) that provides computer-based control of a digital camera and a photo editing program	Camera vendors usually bundle a low-end photo-editing software package with the camera at no additional cost. Most scanners and printers come with similar applications.
SimpleSound (Apple)	Control panel application that permits users to record and add new alert sounds to their Mac system. The current version records but does not have editing capability.*
VirtualDub (Windows, free online through Open Source software available under a General Public License [see Topic 13 for information about GPL] http://www.virtualdub.org)	*VirtualDub* is a video/sound capture/processing utility for 32-bit Windows platforms (95, 98, ME, NT4, 2000, XP), licensed under the GNU GPL. It lacks the editing power if a general-purpose editor such as *Adobe Premiere,* but it is streamlined for fast linear operations over video.
Multiware (BeachWare, available from Don Johnston, Inc.)	Inexpensive collection of royalty free sounds, video clips, screen backgrounds. This is a resource library, not an editor, but it's a good way to get started using more than still photos and clipart in projects.

* For many years, Macs came with a microphone and audio input as standard equipment. Many newer Mac OS systems require additional purchase of a sound card and microphone or a USB microphone in order to record sound.

structure in place allows for more time to engage the client in discussing the underlying content, recalling features and details of an event, and focusing on the special touches that personalize the book. The framework could consist of a set of *PowerPoint* slides that include a title page, decorative background, and pages labeled for each important idea in the electronic book. *PowerPoint* is designed to help users quickly design and develop a set of slides. A program wizard (discussed in Topic 16) makes this a straightforward process even for a newcomer to *PowerPoint*.

Pictures can be added in any of the ways discussed in Topic 17: scanned photos, digital camera photos, or images downloaded from the web. Any kind of visual element can be inserted into a *PowerPoint* slide. For purposes such as a memory book, low to medium

Table 18.2. Examples of multimedia resource editors that clinicians could use to generate therapy materials

Multimedia tools and resource editors	Descriptions
Fireworks MX (Macromedia)	Image editor, available alone or bundled with *Dreamweaver*, Macromedia's high-end web design program.
Adobe Photoshop (Adobe) *PhotoRetouch Pro* (Binuscan)	Sophisticated, professional level photo editing and graphic design software.
Adobe Illustrator (Adobe)	Professional level graphics design software, including drawing (vector-based) and painting (bitmap) modes.
Adobe Premiere (Adobe)	Early standard-setting video editing software, includes soundtrack tools.
Final Cut Pro (Apple)	Video editing software for Mac OS computers, that receives high marks from reviewers for usability and features such as real time editing; a number of compatible hardware products (keypads, keyboards) especially for video editing are available.
BIAS Deck VST (Bias Sound Creative)	Multi-track recording and playback for Mac OS computers. Sophisticated audio recording and editing.
ArtMatic Pro (U&I Software)	Recommended for graphic designers, includes more than 3,000 templates to generate patterns, backgrounds, and abstract images.

Note: These are advanced software applications that require training, time, and practice to master.

resolution quality for photos should suffice, so that file sizes are reasonable (under 500 K). Illustrations from clipart can be added for humor or aesthetics. Special sound and slide transition effects can also be included to enhance or highlight particular pages.

Memory book designers should be sparing with special effects and visual distractions. It is important to keep the visual perceptual abilities of the client in mind when choosing font sizes and color contrasts. Usually simple backgrounds and a display with high contrast between font color and background color are effective for both children and adults.

When the basic framework is presented during therapy, the client can be invited to dictate a comment for each page. For example, the client might be asked to tell about a favorite family activity or a special memory about a family member whose picture is on the page. The clinician can type this narration onto the slide or page, making it a unique reflection of the client's interests. Depending on the goals for the session, the client might be practicing remembering or saying a family member's name, reading aloud, or recalling specific information. Even pragmatic skills such as giving and requesting clarification could be targeted (see Section III). In *PowerPoint*, spoken commentaries can also be recorded, adding a personal and multi-modality dimension. As an ongoing project, the client and the clinician might work together to complete additional pages. Speech and language skills can be reviewed and practiced by going back over the progress on the book at the beginning and end of each session. This activity is appropriate for individual and small-group therapy.

As pictures or sounds (especially speech) are added, the size of the project file needs to be considered. If the goal is to send an electronic (not just printed) version home with the client, the available storage media and associated hardware must be kept in mind. The project can be stored on the hard drive or clinic network while in progress, but to make it available to the client later, several alternatives are possible. To accommodate a project with a large file size, the clinician could save the memory book on a CD using a CD Read-Write drive. A zip disk or floppy disk provide limited storage capacity, but may be used for compatibility with the client's home system. Sending the project to the client via the Internet is also a possibility, if the client has the capability to receive it and a high speed Internet connection.

The software needed to run the memory book may or may not be available on the client's home computer. In the case of *PowerPoint*, this problem can be resolved with *Power-Point Viewer*. *PowerPoint Viewer* is a program used to run slide shows created with Microsoft *PowerPoint* on computers that do not have *PowerPoint* installed. In the current version, for example, the Viewer can be added to the same disk that contains a presentation by using the Pack and Go Wizard. The Viewer and project file can then be used together to run the slide show on another computer. Clinicians should consult the Help files that come with *PowerPoint* for specific instructions on where to find *PowerPoint Viewer* and how to prepare a *PowerPoint* presentation for viewing under these conditions. Updates and additional information are also available from the Microsoft *PowerPoint* web site.

PROJECT IDEA: SLIDE SHOWS WITH MOVIES

Besides entertainment value, there can be legitimate instructional purposes for adding video clips to *PowerPoint* slide shows. Sometimes moving pictures are needed to convey an important concept or evoke a target utterance. It is surprisingly easy to insert a video clip (movie) into a *PowerPoint* slide, following the directions that come with the software.

The first step is to choose the clinical goal or instructional objective that will be addressed by the slideshow with movies. Examples include practicing action verbs, predicting what will happen next, asking WH questions, developing script/narrative skills, or working on main idea and inferencing skills. The latter will provide the purpose for the following example.

Project Title: At the Movies

Software Resources: *PowerPoint* and video clips (sources follow)

Preparing Video Clips: Once the goal of the activity has been determined, the available movies (video clips) should be reviewed to identify the ones that will best suit the project. This can be done by downloading royalty-free clips from the web, creating brief movies with a digital video (DV) camera, or by looking through a resource library of clips, such as the collection found on the *Multiware* CD-ROM (Beachware, available from Don Johnston, Inc.). Move the clips that will be used for the project into a separate folder/directory so that they are all together and easy to find. (Note: This folder of video clips must be included with the *PowerPoint* slideshow project when it is moved to a CD or another computer.)

Creating a PowerPoint Slide Show: Begin with title slide and a second slide that briefly summarizes the activity and provides directions for clinicians who might use it. Start the activity with a new slide and insert a movie by accessing the Insert menu. Continue adding additional slides with activity components and movies until the desired length is achieved. Keep in mind that the folder with the files of video clips used in the *PowerPoint* slide show must be a travel companion when the project is moved or saved on a different media.

Activity Design: Note that in the example, two slightly different tasks are illustrated (see Figure 18.1). In the first slide, the client is invited to watch the movie of a teenager mowing the grass, then choose the best title from three choices listed on the slide: "Mowing the Yard," "Noisy Saturday," or "Earning My Allowance." In this activity, the computer will not provide feedback about whether the client's choice is justified or not. The movie and choices will merely serve as a jumping off point for conversation between the client and clinician or a group of clients. For example, the title "Mowing the Yard" might be the best for conveying the main idea shown in this short clip. "Earning My Allowance" or "Noisy Saturday," though, would be more inspiring titles as story starters for an oral or written narrative task.

The second slide in the example presents the movie segment and asks the client to name the movie, without any pre-conceived titles available. This more challenging task could be used to elicit a simple verbal response or, in edit mode, the clinician could type in the title suggested by the client, to reinforce literacy skills.

When the project is used in therapy, the clinician or client will need to click on the movie frame on each slide to make the movie run. The display of the clip may be a bit jerky depending on the quality of the video and the speed of the computer. The clinician and client may watch the clip several times and talk about it before proceeding. Flexibility is built-in when the clinician developed the materials himself and intends to use them interactively with the client. With design decisions based on client age, interests, and goals, a slide show with movies can be used effectively with children and adults, individually or in groups.

ADVANCED MULTIMEDIA TOOLS

Experiences with multimedia toolkits and projects can build the confidence of professionals who want to develop their own materials. Clinicians with this experience may want to go on to develop their own sounds, videos, and photos about a unique topic or theme. A useful analogy is the difference between a person who bakes a cake from a mix, and one who bakes a cake from scratch by gathering and measuring all of the ingredients. The results may be terrific in either case, but clearly the latter baker has more opportunity to modify and personalize the recipe. The tools described in Table 18.2 represent software that a clinician might need in order to develop multimedia materials "from scratch." Here the term *tool* correctly implies that skill and practice are required in order to achieve proficiency.

For beginners, it is a good idea to obtain some experience with entry-level projects and resource libraries before attempting to master an advanced resource editor. Many motivated clinicians will invest in learning to use one or two resource editors, but very few individuals would have the time or need to master all of them. For example, *Fireworks* (Macromedia) is ideal for preparing photos or original drawings for use on the web or in multimedia presentations. The remaining tools in Table 18.2 might never be required for a clinician interested in developing original art as part of a *PowerPoint* slide show or web

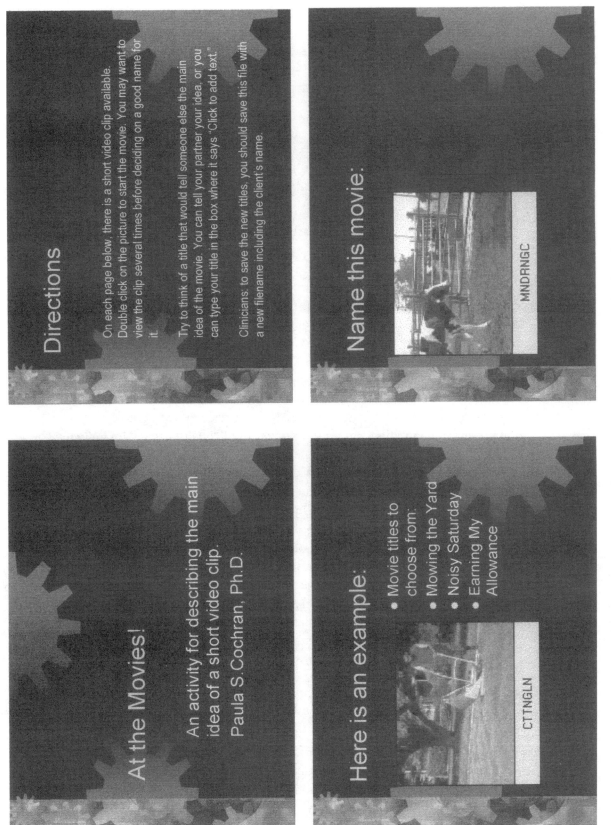

Figure 18.1. Examples of a *PowerPoint* (Microsoft) project with video clips. From the copyright-free collection *Multiware* (Benchware).

site. Other clinicians may be more interested in editing videos and have no need for *Fireworks*. The best approach is to start by identifying a specific task or purpose and choose a corresponding application to accomplish it. As mentioned previously, selecting the right tool may be expedited by reading current reviews in technology magazines and web sites, and consulting with friends.

UNDERSTANDING THE TECHNOLOGY: DIGITIZING AND EDITING RESOURCES

What does it mean to "digitize" something? Every day, people use digital cameras, listen to digitized music (CDs and MP3 recordings), and rent digitized movies (DVD). Computers are at the heart of all of these technologies. When a sound, a picture, or a video is "digitized" it is literally converted into digits—combinations of zeros and ones that a computer can store and reproduce upon command. The quality of digital media varies according to several factors, including the recording conditions, equipment, and choices made by the person in charge. High-quality digital media generally require more storage space (larger file size) than medium to poor quality. The increasing demand for high-quality sound and graphics in consumer applications such as game software has contributed significantly to the effort to make storage and memory larger and less expensive in today's computers.

Clinicians experimenting with resource editors need at least a basic understanding of the process of digitization and the consequences of "quality" variables. When a computer or other device digitizes something, it records samples based on the original. Visual materials are captured and reproduced at a particular resolution or dots-per-inch (dpi). Sound is recorded at a specified sampling rate (so many samples per second of a certain size). Digital video quality variables include the size of the movie display and the rate at which the video will be encoded and decoded during playback. Think about the dot-to-dot pictures that appear in children's coloring books. A high rate of sampling is like a dot-to-dot picture where the dots are close together and very little guessing is required in order to envision the correct shape of the drawing. A low sampling rate—like dots that are far apart—results in gaps that allow for distortion. Obviously, more digits must be stored and retrieved in order to produce excellent digitized sound, graphics, or video.

Sometimes there is a logical reason to trade quality for convenience or cost. For example, small graphics files load faster into web browsers, making the highest quality (most colors, most dpi) in art and photo files less desirable for some applications. Likewise, lower quality sound files require less storage space, permitting more speech or music or special effects to be available. A review of the resource editor's help files may explain the consequences of choosing certain digitizing parameters or quality settings. For example, the Windows ME edition of Microsoft's *Sound Recorder* utility provided a guide to various levels of sound quality and their relationship to sampling rates.

High quality (e.g., CD quality) sound files require dramatically higher sampling rates than low quality (e.g., telephone quality). This issue is especially important when the clinician is working with a client who may have auditory impairments or speech impairments that may compromise the quality of the sound and how it is perceived. Most sound recording utilities (as well as the professional speech therapy applications discussed in Section V) permit the clinician to choose a sampling rate or quality level, within the limits of the computer hardware. For most clinical purposes, the highest possible setting is desirable.

Consumers are already aware of many of the advantages attributed to digital media. For instance, playing a music CD repeatedly does not result in a degradation of the audio signal, unlike tapes or vinyl records. This is in part because digital compact disc (CD) media can be read by a laser beam and converted back into the sound waves we hear. There is no source of friction or wear (e.g., a needle, a tape head). Compared to traditional formats, digital media are easier for an average person to create, manipulate, and store, via a personal computer. Consider, for example, the process of enlarging a typical 4 × 6 photograph. Some hobbyists build dark rooms and become expert photographers and film developers. However, thousands more individuals—who would never attempt their own film development—are snapping photos with a digital camera and editing them with image editing software to create exactly the size and effects desired before printing.

Digitizing and Editing Photos and Other Image Files

Generally two steps are required to digitize and edit a photo or other image

1. Digitization (usually accomplished with a digital camera or a scanner)

2. Viewing and editing the image

As previously discussed, the most common file formats encountered while working with digital photos are JPEG and GIF. These formats are cross-platform and they are frequently used in web design applications. Other common formats are bitmap (.bmp) and .pict (Mac) that are more common in clipart and paint files created with applications like *Kid Pix* (Riverdeep/Broderbund). Most photo or image editing software can accept all of these file formats and following image manipulation the results can be converted to a wide variety of formats. At a basic level, photo editors facilitate common image manipulations like cropping, rotating, enlarging, and reducing. Even simple camera support products like *Kodak Picture Software* can do these things plus allow the user to improve the contrast or brightness levels in a photo. More advanced photo software adds functions like filters, layers, and special effects required by graphic artists.

Clinicians should be aware that photos on the computer monitor will often appear better than when they are printed. This is due to the discrepancy between the dots-per-inch (dpi) showing on the monitor, versus the dpi reproduced by the printer. Some printers are especially designated as photo printers. They achieve higher resolution (dpi) but usually at a slower speed than most people want for everyday text. Many low-cost regular inkjet printers do an excellent job with photos if special photo printing paper is used.

Digitizing and Editing Sound

Digitizing sound requires that the computer have a sound card or chip that can convert a sound signal (from a microphone or audio input jack) into digital format. If the sound card and microphone are present, often a single software tool is used to "capture" or record the sound and then to do simple editing. Sound editing can be as complex as the most sophisticated photo and video editing, which is why they still give an Oscar for the best sound editing in a movie each year. For most clinicians developing multimedia projects, the most frequent sound editing function needed is to cut dead time at the beginning or end of a recording, thus maximizing storage space and instructional effect. It is frustrating to click on a button or a slide and wait through several seconds of static before the speech or music or sound effect begins. Windows system software comes with *Sound Recorder*, a utility that permits the user to record with a microphone and then edit the beginning or end of the recording and save the file for use in other applications.

Advanced sound editing capabilities are present in some video editing packages, as well as in stand alone products intended for audio professionals such as *BIAS Deck* (Mac) and *Cakewalk SONAR 3* (Windows). Professional speech analysis software such as Kay Elemetric's *CSL* and GSI's *SoundScope* also provide some sound editing capabilities (see Section V). Recall that the quality of digitized sound is affected by many variables, including sampling rates, microphone characteristics, and sound card quality. These factors are discussed in more detail in Section V. Sound files exist in many formats, indicated by the file name extension. The most common file name extensions/format of sound files are: .wav (Windows), .aif or .aiff (Macintosh), or .mpg (Motion Picture Experts Group).

Digitizing and Editing Video

Digitizing video can be accomplished in two ways

1. Record the action with a digital video (DV) camera
2. Convert existing videotape or film to digital format

The latter process requires the computer to have video digitizing capability, which is not standard equipment in most current consumer and school configurations. Two parameters constrain the quality and file size of DV, and some technical understanding is necessary to discuss them. A brief introduction to pixels and bit rate should help amateur creators of multimedia materials understand the variations in video quality that are encountered so frequently.

The image on a monitor, a television, or a theater movie screen is made up of dots, like those over-emphasized in the cartoon-like portraits of famous people by artist Roy Lichtenstein. These dots are referred to as pixels, and the number of pixels horizontally and vertically describes the size of an image. Instead of inches or centimeters, pixels can be used to measure an image on a monitor. At a low-resolution setting, a computer monitor displays 640×480 pixels. The greater the number of pixels, the more detailed the image appears to be, and the larger the file size required to store the image.

Often a small window is used to display video on a computer monitor, because videos that were recorded with a low-resolution setting look best this way. If the window is expanded, the pixels are larger but the image looks blurred. The same thing happens to low-resolution photos when they are enlarged. Sometimes a little blurring is more tolerable than a small display, as determined by the viewer. The number of pixels available is set at the time the video or photo is digitized, irrespective of the playback settings. For example, a small dimension of 176×144 pixels might be used to create video for web consumption.

The second parameter of interest is bit rate. This is the sampling rate at which the image is digitized and the speed at which the file is later sent to a player. The higher the rate, the less an image will appear distorted, but with respectively larger file size. Bit rate is usually measured in kilobits per second (Kbps). Video for a dial-up web server might be recorded with a very low bit rate of 56 Kbps, compared to 256 Kbps for broadband usage. The significance of this information is that the display size (measured in pixels) in combination with sampling rate (measured in Kbps) determine: 1) the quality of the resulting recording and 2) the size of the resulting file.

The latest collection of video editing tools for hobbyists and professionals are designed to work seamlessly with DV camcorders. The DV camcorder records and digitizes the action until the files can be downloaded to a computer, via a cable or wireless infra-red connection. Once the files are on the computer, they can be viewed and edited with one of the growing number of applications available for this purpose. *iMovie* (Apple) set the initial standard for ease-of-use, but several advanced video editing packages have evolved for both Mac and Windows operating systems.

Basic video editing capabilities include cutting and combining clips of video, adding or editing a sound track, and adding titles and simple special effects like fade-outs. Beginners should be wary of the drawbacks to using what appear to be "simpler" software tools as resource editors. The inflexibility and limitations of these applications can actually consume more learning time and instill more frustration than a more sophisticated product.

Video and sound files most often have file extensions like .avi (Windows format) or a Moving Pictures Experts Group (MPEG) derivative such as .mpeg, .mpg, .mp3, DV, and others. Considerations for making video to use on the web or for sending to other people via e-mail relate to file size and how the video will be transmitted. Prime factors are

- Bandwidth (the capacity for simultaneous transmission of data over a network)

- Limitations imposed by the local Internet Service Provider (ISP)

- Bit rate (how fast can the video be delivered to the viewer for watching).

Recommendations and additional information about these variables are available at web sites and in help files that accompany video editing software and DV camcorders.

THE ISSUE OF TIME AND RESOURCES: MAKING YOUR OWN DVD OR CD

Multimedia projects that include video, sound, or high-quality photos are likely to become larger files than others typically created by clinicians. A detailed clinical report written with a typical word processor might require 75 kilobytes (Kb) of storage space on a disk. At this rate, clinicians take a long time to fill a 1.44 MB or 3.5 inch floppy disk. (Divide by 1,000 to convert Kb to MB.) A nine-slide *PowerPoint* presentation only requires about 244 Kb if it does not include large image or video files. A typical low quality 8-second video clip of a bicycle race (with sound) from the *Multiware* (Beachware) collection requires 1,038 Kb, or 1.01 MB of storage.) Add a 7-second video clip of children playing (about 950 Kb), and already the project exceeds the storage capacity of a 1.44 MB floppy disk. Using low-medium quality settings, a rough estimate of storage requirements for sound and video is about 1 MB of storage for every 8–10 seconds of data. Another way to say this is, a floppy disk will hold one 10-second medium quality video/sound segment; a 250 MB zip disk would hold a *PowerPoint* slideshow and about 25 short videos or voice recordings.

Clinicians who have unlimited network storage and never plan to move or distribute their projects can be less concerned about storage. However, for most enthusiasts, serious pursuit of multimedia requires thoughtful consideration of storage media. Alternatives that should be considered include portable external hard drives and creation of personal CDs and DVDs. Convenient, reliable external hard drives are available at reasonable prices, and offer an ideal solution for clinicians who need to carry large files or pre-installed software from place to place. This is an excellent choice for intensive work on video editing.

In other instances, clinicians may want to back-up or share their files on a CD-R or DVD-R. Use of this medium depends upon the clinician's access to a CD or DVD read-write (RW) drive, or a combo drive that does both. The capacity of a single recordable 700 MB (80 minutes) compact disc (CD-R) is about the same as 436 floppy disks. Software wizards are available that step the user through the process of burning a CD or DVD. Burners come rated for various speeds, which determines how long it takes to burn a new CD or DVD (i.e., 10x, 20x, 40x, where a 40x CD burner is fastest).

SUMMARY

Multimedia implies that more than just text or graphics are components of a software product. Basic multimedia software tools offer clinicians opportunities to incorporate digital images, video, and sound into computer-based intervention. Initial exploration of children's multimedia toolkits (such as the *Imagination Express* series or *Kid Pix Deluxe*) may be a precursor to development of entry-level projects from scratch, using commonly available programs such as Microsoft's *PowerPoint*. Creation of the projects illustrated in this topic allow clinicians to create interactive activities that incorporate text, speech, sounds, music, photos, clipart, video clips, and transition effects.

Developing multimedia projects "from scratch," requires the use and understanding of more advanced software tools. Resource editors allow the clinician to design materials with features customized to address the client's goals and needs. To maximize the investment of time and training involved in creating projects with resource editors, it is important to determine the desired task or purpose of the project and select the appropriate tool. Familiarization with digitizing techniques used to capture pictures, movies, sounds, and speech is essential to taking advantage of the features offered by a variety of resource editors. Development of multimedia projects also requires consideration of quality parameters, file type and size, and storage alternatives.

REVIEW FOR TOPIC 18

1. Give a definition of multimedia and describe three examples.
2. Describe three things a clinician might do in preparing to create and use a memory book project, similar to the one discussed in this topic.

3. What is a resource editor? Explain why it is important to identify a specific task or purpose before selecting an application.
4. Why does a high-quality sound file or high resolution image file require so much disk space?
5. Use the analogy of a dot-to-dot picture and to explain how sampling rates vary, use the difference between the quality of a telephone and a CD as an illustration.

QUESTIONS FOR DISCUSSION

1. Why do some photos and pictures look better on the computer monitor than they do when they are printed out? Discuss this phenomenon and possible ways to avoid being disappointed.
2. How can clinicians make well-informed choices about which resource editors to purchase and invest time in learning?
3. Describe an example of a multimedia project or materials that you would like to attempt to develop.

RESOURCE FOR FURTHER STUDY

Lambert, J. (2003). *Digital storytelling: Capturing lives, creating community.* Berkeley, CA: Digital Diner Press.

Using Authoring Tools to Develop Computer-Based Therapy Materials

Clinical computing competency #3: The clinician will take advantage of computer capabilities to generate personalized clinical materials to enhance intervention with specific clients.

Some clinicians will want to take the creation of their own therapy materials to another level. Beyond individualized materials for clients to take home or use in traditional therapy activities, some clinicians will make maximum use of computer capabilities to create their own computer-based activities. Designing original computer activities usually requires familiarity with digital resource libraries or competency in creating new multimedia resources, as well as competency with at least one computer language or authoring program. More than just proficiency with the technology, however, this competency also requires clinicians to deliberately choose the role the computer will play in their new activity and understand the impact of other important software design factors.

The concept of clinicians developing or programming their own software arose early in the discussions and explorations of the role of computers in the field of communication disorders. Generally, the word "programming" refers to developing coded instructions using a computer language. For many languages, this code is then "compiled" and "run" in order to make something happen on the computer. Popular computer languages include C++, Fortran, and VisualBasic. An analogy to programming that many people understand would be creating a web page using only HTML code. In contrast, "authoring" refers to using a development tool to design and combine software components into a novel application. This is more analogous to creating a web page using web development software like *Dreamweaver, Adobe Pagemill,* or *Microsoft FrontPage.*

Perhaps the focus on programming in the 1980s and then authoring in the 1990s resulted in part because many early clinical software products were designed and programmed by clinicians, spouses, or hobbyists with close ties to the profession. Some early adopters contended that due to lack of adequate commercial software, clinicians should learn computer programming languages (e.g., BASIC) (Ventkatagiri, 1987). Others were making the case that the programming language Logo was a way for clinicians and clients together to control the computer and create a shared context for therapy (Cochran & Bull, 1985).

Easier and faster than programming from scratch, authoring software gradually became available but early versions were primitive and focused on the development of CAI. As an alternative, the notion of mini-software programs or routines (tools) that clinicians and teachers could incorporate into larger programs was touted (Bull & Cochran, 1985, 1987). Such software tools would reduce the programming overhead, and increase the chances that clinicians would be able to tailor their applications to the client's specific needs, or so the argument went. In fact, few clinicians ever learned to use computer languages to develop their own software or computer activities, with or without the assistance of pre-programmed components.

In the 1990s, authoring software became more sophisticated and popular with the advent of *HyperCard* (Apple), the first hypermedia application. This was the beginning of the notion of "links" and making nonlinear navigation available to the computer user. Instead of following the programmer's pre-determined linear sequence of screens and events, the user could choose or avoid buttons (links) connecting various options in the software. Suddenly, it was no longer the case that each computer user would have the same experience with an instructional program, because in hypermedia the user controlled which links or buttons were activated. The new potential for individualization and flexibility of design was thrilling for amateur developers. With *HyperCard*, it was relatively easy for novices to incorporate sound, text, and graphics in ways that previously had been inaccessible to anyone except programmers with advanced skills (Cochran & Bull, 1991). In addition to an elegant authoring interface, *HyperCard* included a sophisticated programming language that accommodated the needs of more advanced users. Although limited to computers running Macintosh operating systems, *HyperCard* was widely used by hobbyists, teachers, students, and clinicians. Many applications for special populations were developed and distributed as freeware or shareware. Until the web replaced it as the primary outlet for developers, workshops, books, and articles enthusiastically encouraged clinicians to learn *HyperCard* (e.g., Lieberth & Martin, 1995).

So, the clinician today who finds herself wanting to create her own web applications or stand-alone computer activities is following in a tradition already two decades old. Fortunately, there are many excellent development tools available and an active development community to whom clinicians can look for examples and support.

UNDERSTANDING THE TECHNOLOGY: MULTIMEDIA AUTHORING PROGRAMS

The software described in Table 19.1 includes a combination of what most computer experts would call authoring tools and programming languages. There are many more possibilities available, but this table includes those tools and languages that are being widely used by educators and clinicians. This software is popular in part because new users can become competent with a reasonable amount of time and instruction. In every case, this software lends itself to inclusion of multimedia elements such as photos, clip art, animation, speech, music, and/or video. In addition, for each software package, a stand-alone player utility facilitates sharing and dissemination of projects to other users who may not own the original development software.

The newest of the software described in Table 19.1, *BuildAbility* (Don Johnston, Inc.), is being highly touted in assistive technology circles. For example, at the annual *2002 Closing The Gap* technology conference in Minneapolis, many sessions by teachers and clinicians highlighted the use of *BuildAbility* with children who have special needs. *BuildAbility* is an example of authoring software being used in two different ways: 1) as a computer activity directly involving the client in developing multimedia and 2) as the medium for an activity developed by the clinician or teacher for the client's later use. Two notable features include the ease with which accommodation to single switch users is accomplished and the availability of both synthesized and digitized speech. Developers may pre-record digitized speech to announce page titles, give directions, incorporate a client's name, or provide other important personalization especially helpful for nonreaders. Alternatively, a text-to-speech function can be engaged that will read aloud text printed on the screen using synthesized speech. *BuildAbility* comes with a tutorial and sample stories/activities. Additional support materials are available on the publisher's web site.

HyperStudio was developed by Roger Wagner with education in mind. *HyperStudio* was among the first "hypermedia" tools designed especially for use by children, not just adults. Not only is incorporation of various media easy to do in *HyperStudio*, but providing various pathways through a body of content in a non-linear way is readily possible. The "hyperlinks" can be created using buttons that users activate, or not, as they choose. There have been many books and on-line avenues for sharing projects and insights from classroom uses of *HyperStudio*. For example, *Month by Month™ for HyperStudio®* is available for purchase. According to the publisher, these monthly lesson plans provide curriculum-based projects that promote self-expression and encourage creativity.

Intellipics Studio is an updated version of a utility originally designed to allow clinicians and special educators to develop activities for use with an alternative keyboard (Intellikeys). However, it has much broader application than this, and has become a user-friendly authoring program with some sophisticated features. An extensive clip-art library is included, facilitating the rapid development of computer activities related to almost any content area. Special effects and animations are simple to create. Clinicians and teachers use *Intellipics Studio* frequently to develop accessible, electronic versions of traditional classroom materials such as children's storybooks. (This must be done with care to avoid copyright infringement; see Topic 20.)

Macromedia Flash MX is a professional-quality, sophisticated programming environment primarily marketed for development of Internet content and applications. It is often sold bundled with Macromedia's popular web development software *Dreamweaver*. However, *Flash* can be used to create activities without Internet access, that run in stand-alone mode. *Flash* includes powerful video, multimedia, and application development features.

Microworlds and *Microworlds Pro*, from Logo Computer Systems Incorporated, are based on current versions of the computer programming language Logo. Logo was originally made popular as a result of the work of a team at M.I.T. and the publication of Seymour Papert's (1980) seminal book: *Mindstorms: Children, Computers, and Powerful Ideas.*

Table 19.1. Examples of authoring tools and programming languages that clinicians could use to develop their own computer-based therapy activities

Software title and source	Description	Recommended uses
BuildAbility (Don Johnston)	*BuildAbility* is cross-platform authoring tool designed to facilitate the quick development of computer activities for use with persons who have a variety of special needs. Easy incorporation of multimedia elements, choice of using or combining synthesized text-to-speech and digitized voice. Marketed with optional libraries of photos, sounds, and backgrounds.	Teachers and clinicians working with persons who have moderate to severe impairments can quickly develop simple computer activities with graphics, colors, sounds, music, or other motivating elements for switch and touch-window users. Student's computer must have *BuildAbility* program or player utility (free download) installed.
Macromedia Flash MX (Macromedia)	*Macromedia Flash MX* is a professional quality, sophisticated programming environment. It is primarily marketed for development of Internet content but can be used to create stand-alone applications.	Used by professional web designers and amateurs alike, Flash is an excellent choice for developing and managing animation and visual effects. Easy distribution or sharing via web. End user must have *Macromedia Flash Player* installed (free download).
HyperStudio (Knowledge Adventure)	Now available as *HyperStudio 4*, this authoring tool has a long and illustrious history among educators. It has evolved as users demanded more multimedia features. Current version includes 125 new sounds and 1,800 updated graphics and photos.	*HyperStudio* can be used directly with children over 5 years old, or by adults creating their own finished activities. Excellent for developing electronic storybooks, games, and projects such as multimedia reports. End user's machine only needs *HyperStudio Player* (free download) to run projects. Some web-sharing available.
Intellipics Studio (Intellitools)	*Intellipics Studio* is an updated multimedia authoring tool that includes drawing and painting tools, a quizmaker, an expandable graphics library with more than 1,500 images and more than 200 sounds. Compatible tools sold separately for developing math and talking communication activities include *IntelliMathics* and *IntelliTalk II*.	Widely used to make literacy activities and classroom content more accessible to clients with severe impairments, however useful for developing activities for any level of user. Projects can be run on a computer without the original program if *Intellipics Studio Player* is installed (free download).
Microworlds 2.0 and *Microworlds Pro* (Logo Computer Systems Incorporated)	*Microworlds 2.0* and *Microworlds Pro* are cross-platform Logo-based multimedia authoring tools designed to have a low threshold for beginning users, and a high ceiling for advanced users. The latest version of *Microworlds Pro* includes a web authoring interface, 128 multi-colored shapes and a Fat Bits Editor to grow and shrink shapes. Shapes serve as objects that can be scripted/instructed. Easy incorporation of music (including MP3s), pictures, videos (Including MPEGs) web pages (HTML), sounds (WAV) and QuickTime VR (Mac only).	*Microworlds 2.0* is recommended for direct use by children at the second grade level to middle school. Clinicians too, may enjoy using *Microworlds* to develop their own multimedia projects. *Microworlds Pro* is recommended for junior high/high school through adult developers. A player utility is available (free download) so that projects can be viewed over the web or used on computers where *Microworlds* is not installed.
PowerPoint (Microsoft)	*PowerPoint* is a component of the familiar Microsoft Office suite of applications. It was originally designed for developing business presentations (slideshows). *PowerPoint* is generally considered easy to learn, although it has some advanced features many users rarely explore.	Ideal for linear slideshow-type activities. Older elementary students and adults learn quickly to obtain impressive results using available slide transition effects, and so forth. Can be saved in a format to run on machines without *PowerPoint* if correct player utility is installed.

Logo was designed to provide a way for children to gain control over a computer and use it to explore various concepts and principles about the world of language and numbers. From the beginning, it had both a graphics component ("turtle graphics") and impressive ability to manipulate language (called "list processing" by computer programmers).

As mentioned previously, throughout the 1980s there were Logo workshops, books, conferences, newsletters, and special interest groups for people interested in using Logo for educational and other purposes. When *HyperCard* and other powerful authoring tools became available and prevailing attitudes toward education began to value accountability more than creativity, Logo's popularity faded. As of 2004, Logo is enjoying something of resurgence in popularity, especially among educators who adopt a constructivist philosophy of instruction. For an update on various versions of Logo and consideration of its role in educational computing see Bull, Bull, Cochran, and Bell (2002).

Although various versions of Logo are available, *Microworlds* and *Microworlds Pro* are mentioned here for several reasons. They are available for both Windows and Macintosh operating systems, they have excellent multimedia capabilities, and they lend themselves to use directly with clients as well as development of activities for clients.

PowerPoint is a component of the familiar *Microsoft Office* suite of applications that is so dominant in business settings. Originally envisioned as an authoring tool for developing business presentations (slide shows), *PowerPoint* is now used by educators and clinicians as a classroom and clinical tool. Photos, clip art, movies, sounds, and voice recordings can be readily incorporated. *PowerPoint* features are discussed with examples in Topic 18. Because it is widely available and because users are not intimidated by it, *PowerPoint* can be an excellent beginning authoring tool.

As is the case with the other software described in this topic, there are active support groups for *PowerPoint* users. Not only are there resources available from Microsoft, but also there are educators, special educators, and clinicians exploring the instructional uses of *PowerPoint*. The potential of *PowerPoint* as an assistive technology has been described (Voelkerding, 2002; Walter, 2001). Clinicians, educators, and professional developers share their insights, design tricks, and favorite resources in on-line discussion groups and forums such as those available on the *Closing the Gap* web site.

For example, a group of engineers in Great Britain have developed a synthesized speech utility for *PowerPoint* presentations, called *PowerTalk* (Medical Engineering Resource Unit, 2001). *PowerTalk* is a free (downloadable) utility that automatically speaks the text of a Microsoft *PowerPoint* presentation using the Microsoft Speech API. At this time, it is compatible with Windows 2000 and Windows XP. The developers claim that *PowerTalk* was created to help those who have difficulties talking while presenting or for an audience that contains people with visual impairments. Clinicians may find it useful, however, as a way to provide additional literacy support for individual clients with or without visual impairment, who are viewing a presentation as an instructional unit.

On the Internet, the exact location of active support groups, helpful hints, and valuable resource suggestions changes continuously. In addition, each time a new version of an authoring tool or programming language is released, a new the support system develops. The important point is that such resources are readily available on line for any clinician who decides to develop competency with one or more of the possibilities described in this Topic.

PROJECT IDEA: HOW TO MAKE A *POWERPOINT* "CLICK LESSON"

Purpose: To use *PowerPoint* as an authoring tool to create a touch screen or mouse accessible lesson with pictures, words, or both

Materials: To make a lesson exactly as described in these directions, you will need *PowerPoint* Version 4 or later. These directions assume a beginner's familiarity with *PowerPoint* or similar software. Earlier versions of *PowerPoint* can be used to make variations on the ideas presented in these directions. For example, a slide show activity could still be produced with integrated text and graphics. But Action Buttons (used here to protect one side of the screen from mouseclick activation) are only available in the most recent versions of *PowerPoint*.

Pictures: These directions will take you through the steps of creating a "click lesson" using *PowerPoint*. For this exercise, you will use the clipart that comes with *PowerPoint*, however for future lessons you design you could make use of graphics from a variety of sources including picture libraries, digital cameras, or symbol software. In this way, you can adjust the content of your click lesson to match the needs of your clients.

Making a Lesson:

1. Open *PowerPoint*, and start a new blank presentation. When the Autoformat dialog box appears, choose a slide format that is blank except for a title line (see Figure 19.1A).

2. Click on the title line and type the words "Find the cat" (see Figure 19.1B).

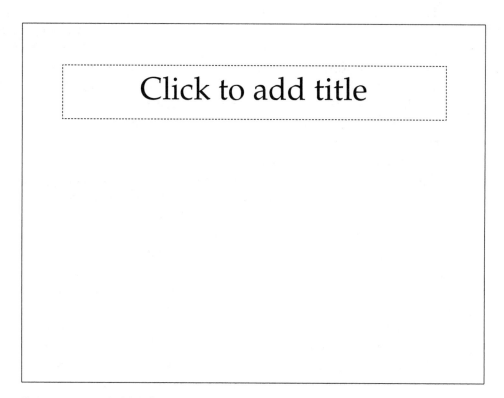

Figure 19.1A. Sample slide before text has been added.

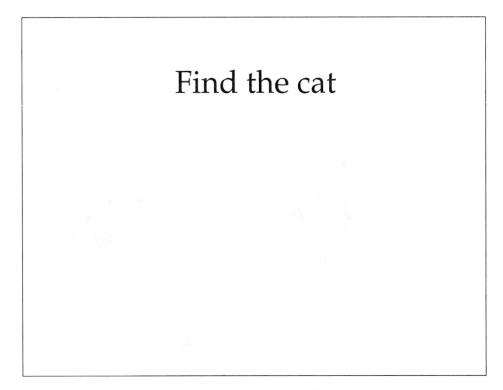

Figure 19.1B.   Sample slide after the text "Find the cat" has been added.

3. Under the Insert menu, choose to insert a picture (clip art). Find and select a cat (or any image you prefer) in the *PowerPoint* clip-art library. When the image appears on your slide, adjust its size by clicking in the corner and moving the arrows diagonally. Make the cat the correct size, then grab it in the middle and move it to the left half of the slide. Repeat this procedure to add a bat image. This will be the "prompt slide" in your lesson. Your slide should look something like Figure 19.1C.

4. Choose New Slide from the menu and repeat Steps 2 and 3, adding a second slide to your presentation (see Figure 19.1D). On this slide, put only the word "cat" in the title, and paste only a picture of a cat underneath. This will be the "reward" slide in your presentation. Make this graphic larger to fit the space.

5. Run your slide show from the beginning (slide 1). Notice that wherever you click on slide 1, it always goes on to the reward (slide 2). This is how *PowerPoint* slide shows usually work. The click of a mouse anywhere (or touch of a touchscreen) takes you to the next slide.

6. Now it's time to put the finishing touches on slide 1, so that it ignores clicks on the bat side and rewards clicks/touches on the cat side. This will be accomplished by adding a transparent action button, which covers the wrong answer and does nothing when clicked (see Figure 19.1E). In edit mode, start on slide 1. Under the Slide-show menu, choose the Action Button option. Select a "custom" or blank button. Set the action to "none." Back on slide 1, draw a large button covering the right half of the slide (over the bat); this is done by dragging the button tool from the middle of

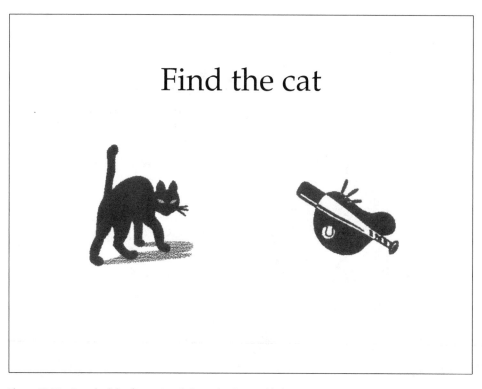

Figure 19.1C. Sample slide after text and clip art has been added.

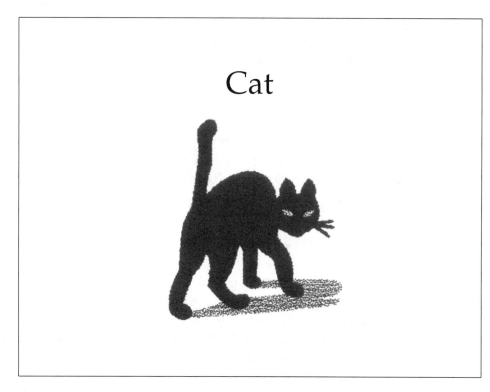

Figure 19.1D. Sample of second slide, the reward if the client guesses correctly.

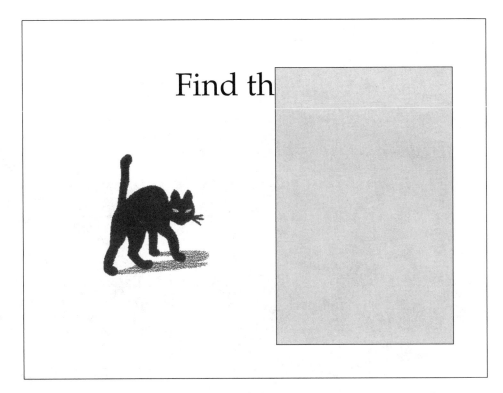

Figure 19.1E.   Sample of slide with button covering the incorrect answer.

the upper edge of the slide to the lower right corner. When you release the mouse button, the bat will have disappeared under the button–don't worry.

7. Double click on the action button you just made, so you can set its attributes. Make the fill transparent (no fill), and the line transparent (no fill), and click "OK." Now the bat will show up again and everything should look the same as before you made the button. But in reality, a transparent button is covering the bat (the wrong answer) so that if the client clicks on it, nothing will happen.

8. Try the new action button by running the slideshow a couple of times. Choose the bat and nothing should happen. Click on the cat side of slide 1 and the large cat on slide 2 should appear right away. This two-slide sequence is the basic building block of a click lesson. You extend the lesson by adding more two-slide sequences. The following are some enhancements to consider:

- Add sound or visual effects to reward slides.

- Add personalized photos or pictures from digital libraries.

- Make more than two choices available by using multiple invisible action buttons per slide.

- Consider more elaborate activities, such as stories with various endings, that make use of other *PowerPoint* features such as the ability to link slideshows.

- Develop a library of click lesson ideas as seen in Figures 19.2–19.7.

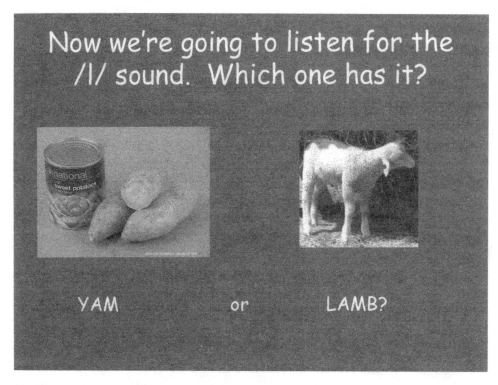

Figure 19.2. Amy's click lesson example: find the /l/ sound.

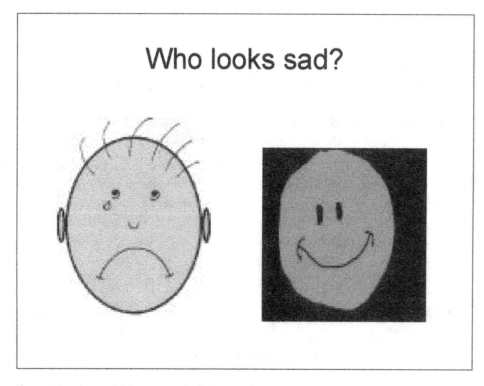

Figure 19.3. Kieren's click lesson example: find the sad face.

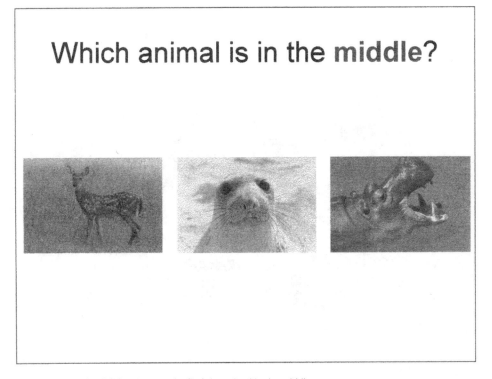

Figure 19.4.   Jori's click lesson example: find the animal in the middle.

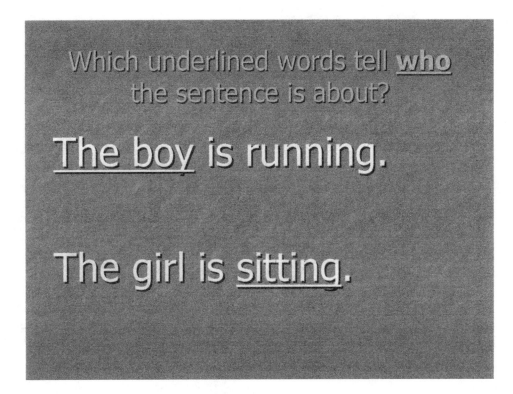

Figure 19.5.   Shana's click lesson example: find the part of speech.

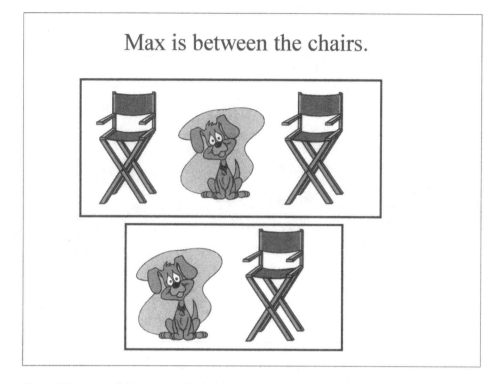

Figure 19.6.   Jenny's click lesson example: find the object between two objects.

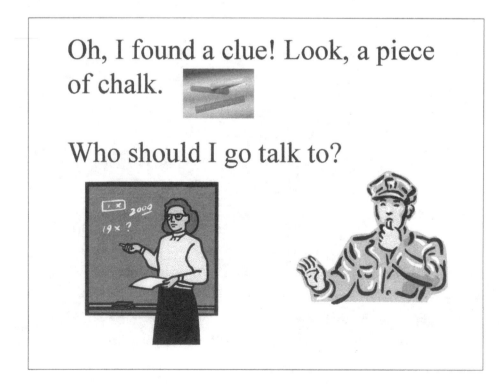

Figure 19.7.   David's click lesson example: branching story.

LOOKING AHEAD: OPEN SOURCE VERSUS PROPRIETARY SOFTWARE DESIGN

Clinicians who have been using computers with clients for several years are likely to have encountered a situation in which some of their favorite software is no longer available for the current generation of computers. Throughout this book, examples of such software that was innovative and effective early in the history of clinical computing are described. Some that have been lost are among the few software programs for our field that have been designed to match best practices and systematically evaluated by researchers. The *PepTalk* series (Communication Skill Builders) for Apple II computers, developed by Shriberg, Kwiatkowski, and Snyder, comes to mind. Why are these programs no longer available if they worked and clinicians liked them? In many cases, it is just too expensive for publishers to continuously revise and update software to match the new formats and features that customers expect. The profit margin for much clinical and educational software is low, and the commercial market for special populations is relatively small.

There are no easy solutions to this problem. One thing clinicians can do to help ensure the future of good software is to follow copyright laws and licensing regulations. Clinicians can also develop and update their own computer-based activities, using authoring tools or programming languages. Yet a third alternative exists, perhaps as a happy medium between starting from scratch in software design and losing favorite commercial software to technological progress. This alternative makes use of a different approach to software development and marketing.

The *PowerTalk* utility is made available under a special kind of license. *PowerTalk* is Open Source software. Open Source software can legally be modified to address individual needs and preferences (see a more complete explanation in Topic 13). So, *PowerTalk* is non-proprietary and is issued under a General Public License (GPL). This means that users are free to copy or modify it as long as they do not use it as part of any proprietary software (software other people may not change or copy).

The success of the Open Source movement in business and engineering raises the question of whether a similar movement might be possible in educational and clinical software development (Bull, Bell, Garafalo, & Sigmon, 2002). An Open Source approach could help clinicians and teachers develop and share exemplary clinical and educational computing models, activities, and software. This approach would make it possible to engage a widespread pool of talent in developing, improving, and sharing effective software. Newly improved software could be in the hands of clinicians quickly, via the Internet. More information about Open Source software development is available from Open Source Initiative, a non-profit corporation that operates an informative web site on this subject.

THE ISSUE OF TIME AND RESOURCES: BEING A SOFTWARE DESIGNER

Clinicians are most likely to develop new software activities or short programs for their own use in therapy. Software designed for diagnostics, speech or voice analysis, or biofeedback, in contrast, is likely to require a development team and more resources than most clinicians will have to bring to the task. Today's authoring tools make the quick development of personalized computer activities possible. However, it can be quite time consuming to go beyond the simple, individual activity level to designing a more complete unit of instruction or a series of activities that help clients practice and achieve better communication skills. Some clinicians will pursue an advanced level of software development, however, in the way that a hobbyist might pursue expertise in photography or gourmet cooking. It is especially important for such clinicians to take time to think about the rationale behind the computer activities they are designing. This rationale should include two components: 1) what clinical or educational research supports the way this content is being presented and 2) what role is the computer intended to play when this software is used?

As the *PowerPoint* Click Lesson example illustrates, it is all too easy to create basic drill-and-practice activities with most available development tools. For some clinical goals, such helping clients use their new articulation behaviors smoothly and automatically, drill-and-practice may be useful and efficient. Clinicians who choose and design CAI activities for other goals such as language learning, however, presumably believe that people learn language primarily through stimulus–response–reinforcement experiences (a behaviorist view). In contrast, many clinicians will have been taught that language is learned primarily through communicative interactions with other people (a sociolinguistic view). Clinicians who believe this about language learning but who have only drill-and-practice computer activities available for therapy will find themselves frustrated, even if they designed the CAI themselves.

It is just as easy to develop software and activities that lend themselves to use as a context for communication during a therapy session as it is to develop CAI. At first, however, this may not be apparent and may require a deliberate effort on the part of the software developer. Recall that CAI and computer-as-context applications generally place value on very different software features. It may be useful to review these priorities before beginning software design (see discussions in Topics 4, 7, and 13).

SUMMARY

A variety of authoring tools and programming languages is available for use by clinicians who are interested in developing not only quick personalized computer activities, but also more ambitious software projects. Some of these tools, such as *BuildAbility* and *Microworlds,* can even be used directly with a client in order to share the development process. Creating their own software is one way that clinicians can address the problem of good commercial software that is quickly outdated and incompatible with new generations of computers. An alternative development model, Open Source, may become more popular for clinical and educational software in the future. In this model, the development burden, as well as the benefits, are shared by volunteers who use and improve the software, then make it available to anyone under a General Public License.

Clinicians who pursue competency in designing and developing software are reminded to consider their own philosophical and theoretical assumptions about how communication skills are learned or remediated. Ideally, the role of the computer and the design of the software will reflect the clinician's values.

REVIEW FOR TOPIC 19

1. Back in the 1980s, why were clinicians encouraged to learn a programming language?
2. *HyperCard* software marked the beginning of "hyperlinks" in software design. What is a "hyperlink"?
3. Which of the authoring tools and languages discussed in this topic have "player" utilities so that programs created with them will run on computers than do not have the original development software installed?
4. Which of the authoring tools and languages discussed in this topic are noted for ease of accessibility accommodation, such as switch use?
5. Why has some early, effective clinical software disappeared from the current market?

QUESTIONS FOR DISCUSSION

1. Discuss ways in which the Open Source movement in software development could effect the development and marketing of software for communication disorders or special education.
2. Why is it important for clinicians who are developing their own software to consider their underlying views on communication development and rehabilitation before they make final design decisions?

RESOURCES FOR FURTHER STUDY

Bull G., Bull, G., Cochran, P., & Bell, R. (2002). Learner-based tools revisited. *Learning and Leading with Technology, 30*(1), 11–17.

Bull, G., Bell, R., Garfalo, J., & Sigmon, T. (2002, Oct). The case for Open Source software. *Learning and Leading with Technology, 30*(2), 10–17.

Voelkerding, K.A. (2002, Feb-Mar). PowerPoint as an assistive technology tool. *Closing the Gap: Computer Technology in Special Education and Rehabilitation.* Retrieved June 1, 2003, from http://www.closingthegap.com/ctg2/members2/search.lasso

Understanding Copyright Laws

Clinical computing competency #8: The clinician will demonstrate familiarity with legal and ethical considerations that apply to assistive technology and the use of computers in the management of communication disorders, and will adhere to appropriate standards.

Clinicians who achieve this competency will be familiar with copyright law and how it applies to their everyday experiences with technology. This includes their use of materials downloaded from the web or scanned with a scanner or inclusion of copyrighted items in materials they develop for use with clients.

Since the 1980s, new technologies have made it remarkably easy for the general public to reproduce and combine text, graphics, and other media. In the not-too-distant past, such manipulations were generally limited to the domain of professionals in fields such as public relations, graphic design, publishing, and entertainment. Among these professionals, copyright laws were well understood and routinely enforced. There was much less concern that private individuals could have a negative financial impact on a copyright owner, for a simple reason: to do so was considerably more difficult than it is now. Teenagers listening to Elvis Presley or early Motown records lacked a convenient way to copy the music and share it with friends who did not buy the original vinyl records or sheet music. They could loan their records, certainly, but they could not make multiple copies to give or sell to someone else. So, there was little chance that individual fans could do anything in violation of copyright law that would significantly impact the profits or royalties reaped by the recording studios, artists, or songwriters.

Powerful, easy-to-use technologies such as photocopiers, videocassette recorders, audiotape recorders, and, more recently, scanners, CD and DVD R/W, and the Internet have changed this. Now routine violation of copyright laws is a real, even if unintentional, possibility for the average person. This topic introduces clinicians to the key concepts in copyright law and explain how it relates to the creation of therapy materials.

WHAT ARE COPYRIGHTS?

New vigilance regarding enforcement of copyright laws has resulted from the onslaught of new technologies, along with much discussion over how they pertain to new media. The Software Publishers Association (SPA) summarized the heart of the existing law as follows:

> The Copyright Act (17 U.S.C. Section 106) gives the owner of copyrighted work the exclusive right to reproduce the work, prepare derivative works, distribute copies of the work, and perform or display the work publicly. In most cases, no one can make copies of a copyrighted work without the copyright owner's permission, and anyone who does so is an infringer of the copyright and may be held liable to the full extent of the law. (1998, p. 66)

These rights of the copyright owner pertain whether the work is text, graphics, photos, video, music, electronic media (software), or any other media. Copyright applies to both published and unpublished works. For works created after January 1, 1978, copyright lasts 70 years after the author's death. Works created before that date and still in their first renewal term are protected for 95 years after the original grant of copyright. Note that software licensing has its own set of regulations and conventions, which are discussed in Topic 14.

WHAT DOES "FAIR USE" MEAN IN THE COPYRIGHT LAW?

Many people assume that copyright law does not apply when the "cause" is a good one. So, it may seem as if church choirs and middle school marching bands should be allowed to photocopy extra copies of their music, because copies of sheet music from a publisher are so expensive. This is a perfect example of a situation where illegal reproduction occurs instead of purchase, and so the copyright owners have not received their entitled royalties or profits. Now imagine that the band director decides to play the music at a concert. The concert is to raise money for uniforms, so admission is charged to people who attend. In this case, not only has the copyright been violated, but someone has materially benefited from use of the illegally copied material. Such an infraction hardly seems worth making a fuss about; but multiplied by thousands of violations, the size of the financial impact is significant. Copyright law applies to everyone, including non-profit organizations, educators and educational institutions, religious institutions, health care providers, and government agencies.

The copyright law makes a provision for "fair use." Whether the conditions of fair use are present is determined on a case-by-case basis. The doctrine of "fair use" allows for the duplication or use of copyrighted work without prior permission under special circumstances. If the band director photocopies a trombone part for a new student to use until an original can be obtained from the publisher, this could be considered fair use. In this case, timely provision of the material to a student was justified, the photocopy included just a small percentage of the entire orchestration, and there was no intent to avoid paying legitimate fees. A similar "fair use" argument could be made when a clinician uses a photocopied test protocol just until a replacement supply is obtained (at which time, an original form should replace the photocopy). Schools have some particular privileges, as outlined in the *Agreement on Guidelines for Classroom Copying in Not-For-Profit Educational Institutions*. These guidelines were designed to cover only print material such as books, periodicals, and musical compositions, however, not other media.

It is an over-simplification, but the essence of the "fair use" provision is the purpose to which the copy will be put, and the loss or potential loss of profits or royalties. A school clinician who reproduces copyrighted images for a take-home activity sheet for particular children is probably safe within the "fair use" provisions. For example, commercial logos or slogans are frequently included as part of survival vocabulary and community awareness lessons. A less clear case is a clinician in private practice who may charge clients for services such as homework materials. If copyrighted materials are included without permission, this could be perceived as "reselling" someone else's property. Similarly, it would be inappropriate for a clinician to include images scanned in from famous children's books in a collection of homework materials intended to become a commercial product. Such images could only be included if the clinician could obtain permission to use the copyrighted material in this way. Some companies, such as the Disney Corporation, are notorious for aggressively protecting their copyrights by prosecuting offenders.

HOW CAN I BE SURE THAT I AM IN COMPLIANCE WITH COPYRIGHT LAW?

The safest way for clinicians to find out whether they may reproduce, modify, or distribute copyrighted material for clinical use is to contact the copyright owner and ask for permission. Often permission is generously granted, especially for non-profit educational purposes. Occasionally, permission is granted within the work itself, in order to save end users this step. Thus, permission to make unlimited photocopies of forms or activity sheets may be included within an activity book or printed on the forms themselves. Many educational and professional publications grant subscribers advance permission to photocopy or use excerpts by stating such in the publication information at the front of each issue.

Some software resources, such as clip art, sound effects, photo libraries, and movies, come packaged in "copyright free" collections. Items from such collections can be incorporated into therapy materials without concern about copyright violation. When resources are downloaded from the web, clinicians should assume they are copyrighted unless expressly told otherwise. Many web photos include a small copyright notice in the corner of the image, to ensure that the source remains known even if it is downloaded to a private computer, or re-used without permission.

The important thing is for clinicians to be aware of the issues surrounding copyright and to do their best to use their resources in a manner that is both legal and ethical. Not only is this the best practice ethically, but it also models appropriate behavior for clients, their families, and fellow professionals.

SUMMARY

Clinicians are advised to ensure that they are making appropriate use of media such as text, symbols, photos, drawings, music, or any other copyrighted materials. Citing sources of images and other resources is good practice, but even citation does not mean that the copyright holder waives any right to profits to which they are entitled. Clinicians should interpret the notion of "fair use" conservatively.

REVIEW FOR TOPIC 20

1. Why are publishers more concerned now about copyright laws and violations by the general public than they were in the 1980s?
2. What are holders of a copyright entitled to?
3. Describe how a clinician can ensure that copyrights are not being violated.

QUESTIONS FOR DISCUSSION

1. Describe a clinician's responsibilities with regard to copyright laws—give an example of a clinical situation in which copyrights were violated and explain how it could have been avoided.
2. Explain the notion of "fair use."

RESOURCES FOR FURTHER STUDY

American Psychological Association (2001). *Publication manual of the American Psychological Association (5th ed.)*. Washington, DC: Author.

American Library Association (2003). Copyright web site. Available at http://www.ala.org/Content/NavigationMenu/Our_Association/Offices/ALA_Washington/Issues2/Copyright1/Copyright.htm (September, 2003).

Hoon, P. (Ed.). (1997). *Guidelines for educational use of copyrighted materials.* Pullman: Washington State University Press.

Note: The information provided in this topic should not be construed as legal advice.

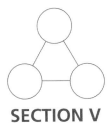

Using a Computer as a Feedback Device

Introduction to Using a Computer for Feedback or Biofeedback

Clinical computing competency #4: The clinician will demonstrate the ability to plan and implement activities in which performance feedback to the client from the clinician is supplemented by feedback (visual, and/or auditory) from the computer.

Perhaps more than any other clinical use of computers, this one requires clinicians to have a technical understanding of what the computer is doing. Clinicians using computers to help provide feedback to clients must invest time in learning the correct setup and use of such tools, as well as their limitations. Competent clinicians will help clients make use of the full range of feedback options, low-tech and high-tech, that are available in the modern clinic.

Computer-based feedback and biofeedback are among the most compelling of the available clinical applications of computers. Once they see these applications, clinicians usually understand immediately why they can be valuable for some clients. Depending upon their typical caseload, clinicians pursuing this clinical computing competency should explore the use of computer-based feedback for voice parameters, speech sounds, fluency, or disorders of resonance or swallowing. Some of the tools available for this clinical application of computers arose from the long-standing effort to make speech "visible" for persons with hearing impairment. Thus, some clinicians will find computer-based biofeedback useful in their work in aural rehabilitation. Another frequent application of this technology is to reward and encourage vocalization from non-oral children with developmental delays. Computer-assisted speech and voice sample analysis for diagnostic purposes is a close companion to computer-assisted biofeedback. In some cases, the same hardware and software tools are used, with minor changes either in software selections or procedures.

DEFINING FEEDBACK

A person with a repaired cleft palate may nonetheless continue to use inappropriate hypernasality while speaking. An attorney making frequent presentations under stress may use hard glottal attack and eventually develop a vocal pathology such as contact ulcers. A person with hearing impairment may use inappropriate pitch or volume while talking. Like most people, speakers who have speech or language disorders are often unaware of the characteristics of their own speech. Anyone who has tried to learn a second language can identify with this situation. It is easier for speakers to improve when they can understand and identify the problems in their own speech. Then, some speakers can make use of consistent feedback to change the way they talk.

Feedback is information. Whether it is about a behavior, a product, or a situation, feedback tells people how close to a desired target they are. So, developers seek feedback from consumers about a new product, and politicians respond to feedback from voters about their political actions. Likewise, course evaluations give faculty feedback about what students believe was effective and ineffective about a class; tests give students feedback about what was effective and ineffective about how they studied. Clinicians provide many kinds of feedback to persons with communication disorders. Usually, clinical feedback focuses on information about the characteristics of a client's speech or language that the client finds difficult to monitor. Clinicians provide an external source of information, or feedback, that clients sometimes must trust more than their own perceptions.

TYPES OF FEEDBACK

The types of feedback of interest here consist of ways that humans obtain and understand information about their behavior, particularly speech behavior. Generally, types of feedback can be categorized according to which senses they stimulate; thus, auditory feedback (hearing), visual feedback (vision), kinesthetic feedback (movement), proprioceptive feedback (position), or tactile feedback (touch). Body actions generate their own internal feedback.

> For example, an articulator like the tongue would generate tactile feedback as it contacts another articulator and proprioceptive feedback as it changes position within the oral cavity. (Ruscello, 1995, p. 284)

The comments that clinicians make about a client's production could be described as "external auditory verbal feedback." Likewise, the thumbs-up a person gets from a friend after making a clever retort would be an example of "external visual non-verbal feedback."

Auditory feedback and imitation of a clinician's model have long been the cornerstones of many therapy procedures. For example, "ear training" was considered an essential element in the treatment of voice disorders for decades. Until audio taping equipment became widely available in the 1960s, most clinicians were limited in the ways they could help clients employ auditory feedback about their own speech. Even then, the more convenient audiocassette technology was still several years away. Meanwhile, equipment such as the Language Master (see Figure 21.1) was enthusiastically adopted in classrooms

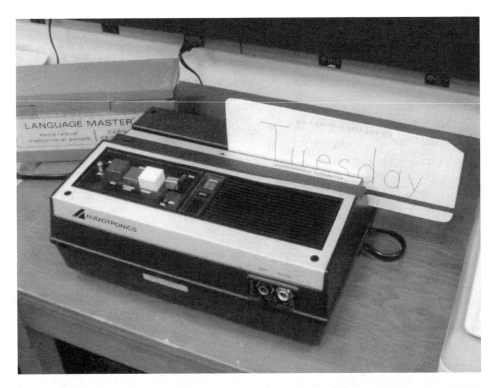

Figure 21.1. A Tutorette (Audiotronics) shown with Language Master cards from Bell and Howell, c. 1967. To record or play back, cards with a strip of audiotape were inserted into the Tutorette or a Language Master (Courtesy of Truman State University Speech and Hearing Clinic).

and clinics. It represented a vast improvement in portability and ease of use compared to large and heavy reel-to-reel tape players.

Note how such equipment was used in the following account of how to help a client learn to use a new pitch for everyday speaking. The excerpt below emphasizes the reliance on auditory feedback that characterized intervention three decades ago. But it also documents an ongoing interest in use of new technologies to provide effective feedback to clients. Morton Cooper wrote it for the 1971 edition of Lee Travis' classic *Handbook of Speech Pathology and Audiology*:

> Tape replays have always been employed in our therapy and have been of great use and assistance in altering the individual's inadequate voice production . . . Of the 1,261 patients seen [for vocal rehabilitation by Cooper and his associates over a 10 year period], only a minuscule number initially objected to the tape replay of their voices, but this negative reaction was minimal and temporary. It is surprising that little mention is made in the literature of the effectiveness of automated tape replay in vocal rehabilitation . . .
>
> Because the vocal cords cannot be touched or viewed by the patient, he must rely basically upon auditory monitoring of the vocal cord function. Intensive ear training is carried on until the optimal pitch is isolated, identified, discriminated, and established. For this training the patient used recording devices, which provide an instantaneous comparative playback (Bell and Howell Language Master). Thus, automation has been instrumental in expanding the field

of vocal rehabilitation. It enables the patient to instantaneously compare and monitor the habitual and optimal pitch levels. We employ intensive and extensive use of automation with highly directed positive vocal guidance that adheres closely to the needs of each patient's voice. (Cooper, 1971, p. 600)

One wonders what Bell, Cooper, and other pioneers in the treatment of voice disorders and aural rehabilitation would think of the alternatives to auditory feedback that are available today. Certainly, the technology for recording and playing back speech has changed remarkably, having gone through revolutions including audio cassette recorders, digital recorders, and now the ultra-portable recording capabilities of a variety of handheld digital devices (See Sections IV and VI for more about sound recording.)

Sometimes the sound of an external model or the sound of a person's own speech—*auditory feedback*—is not sufficient to help the person make changes. When possible, therefore, clinicians bring to bear additional forms of feedback, most often including visual and tactile. Clinicians and clients today benefit from the important work and technological progress that has gone on before. For more than a century, inventors, scientists, and clinicians have been developing new technologies to analyze speech and provide improved feedback to speakers (Potter, Kopp, & Green, 1947). Alexander Bell, for example, was working on making speech "visible" for the deaf when he became diverted and invented the telephone.

Currently computers can analyze certain aspects of a person's speech and/or voice and display those features visually. When the visual display provides simultaneous information about a person's physical behavior, it may be labeled *biofeedback*. For example, the computer can trace a line on the monitor to reflect the pitch or loudness of a speaker's voice as he speaks. Games in which objects move and events happen in response to certain speech parameters make the process more attractive to children and adults alike (see Figure 21.2). The speech behaviors noted in the examples at the beginning of this topic (hypernasality, voice onset, pitch, and loudness) can be reliably displayed in real time by today's technology. The addition of computers to speech science instruments has increased their power and flexibility and made them cost-effective for widespread clinical use.

DEFINING BIOFEEDBACK

Biofeedback is the provision of information about a person's physiological behavior while it is happening. So, the key differences between regular feedback and biofeedback are immediacy and the direct link between physical change and the delivery of information about that change. A person using biofeedback experiences control over the feedback mechanism. More traditional feedback in therapy often consists of a clinician evaluating each response or the client listening to a tape or watching in a mirror. The clinician, tape, and mirror do not change during the client's speech. Important though they may be, they are not providing biofeedback.

Biofeedback does not require a computer. Examples of low-tech biofeedback often provided by clinicians to help their clients monitor airflow include straws, nasal mirrors, and pinwheels. Low-tech biofeedback for voicing and loudness include voice-activated

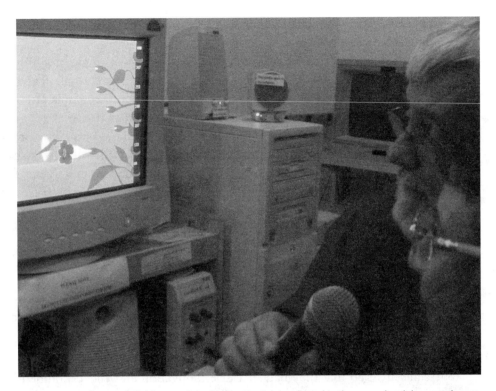

Figure 21.2. A client and clinician watch as the client's pitch is reflected in the upward and downward movements of the hummingbird shown on the computer display. They are using the *Visi-Pitch III* from Kay Elemetrics (Courtesy of Truman State University Speech and Hearing Clinic).

toys and lights. The key characteristic here is that while clients are speaking, they experience consequences that help them modify their speech. Whether the feedback is visual, auditory, or tactile, if it happens during the speech act and changes as a result of the speech act, it can be considered biofeedback.

Biofeedback has been used in many contexts other than therapy for communication disorders. For example, counselors may help clients learn stress management or relaxation techniques using biofeedback. Biofeedback associated with muscle contraction is used in muscle rehabilitation and pain management.

CLINICAL RESPONSES TO BIOFEEDBACK

A rich literature documents the efficacy of computer-based feedback in aural rehabilitation (Bernstein, Goldstein, & Mahshie, 1988; Boothroyd, Archambault, Adams, & Storm, 1975; Kewley-Port, 1994; Nickerson, Kalikow, & Stevens, 1976; Povel & Wansink, 1986; Watson & Kewley-Port, 1989), the treatment of various speech and voice disorders (Bakker, 1999; Blood, 1995; Bouglé, Ryalls, & Le Dorze, 1995; Dagenais, 1995; McGuire, 1995; Ruscello, 1995; Thomas-Stonell, McLean, Dolman, & Oddson, 1992; Volin, 1998; Watson, & Kewley-Port, 1989) and swallowing problems (Crary, 1995; Crary & Baldwin, 1997; Crary & Groher, 2000). For an extensive sampling of clinical studies using biofeedback in the management of speech disorders listed by disorder, number of subjects, design, and type of biofeedback, see Volin, 1998. In addition to published literature, there are many anecdotal accounts and unpublished papers that describe clients' responses to computer-based biofeedback.

Cochran (2000) summarized an account of an early example of a microcomputer-based visual feedback system for speech therapy presented by Rushakoff and Edwards at the 1982 ASHA convention. They described how a modified Apple II computer was used to significantly improve the attitude and speech performance of a 20-year-old college student receiving therapy for distorted sibilant sounds. As therapy progressed for this client, she was shown how to use the computer for practice and feedback. She then scheduled herself to use the computer independently several times a week. Her reluctant attitude in therapy improved appreciably, and she was soon dismissed from the clinic. According to Rushakoff and Edwards, the computer's ability to provide appropriate biofeedback and self-paced practice was the primary reason for the successful outcome for this client.

In a qualitative master's thesis study, Woods (2000) observed four client/clinician pairs as they first started to use biofeedback in articulation therapy. Woods interviewed the clinicians after their first session using computer-based biofeedback. Although their reactions were generally positive, when asked if they had observed the change in behavior that they had expected from their clients, all four clinicians reported that they had not. When asked if their clients thought the biofeedback activities were effective, three out of four clinicians said that they had. Because motivation and client attitude toward treatment is known to affect the outcome of therapy, this may be another important consideration in the use of biofeedback.

Clients may benefit from having alternative forms of feedback about their speech. They may view the computer as a more objective, less personal "judge" of their performance. Using biofeedback from the computer, clients can see when their attempts are approximating the goal, even though they may not have succeeded entirely. Working with the computer this way motivates some clients to make greater effort, produce repeated attempts, and modify their behavior in new ways.

RESEARCH PAST, PRESENT, AND FUTURE

When a client is succeeding with computer-based feedback, it could be used to extend therapy sessions and provide more time on task than otherwise could be provided. From the beginning of computer-based feedback, developers have been interested in this potential for independent client use (Boothroyd, Archambault, Adams, & Storm, 1975; Nickerson, Kalikow, & Stevens, 1976; Povel & Wansink, 1986). Researchers have already begun exploring whether the Internet can serve in this capacity. As a motivating factor, they cite the limited access to qualified clinicians that people in rural and remote communities often experience (Morawej, Jackson, & McLeod, 1999). Examples of remote monitoring of medical status and patient recovery at home are already in the literature (c.f., Swan, 1996) and books are being written about telemedicine.

According to a survey of clinicians in the United Kingdom and Ireland, they would value the increased practice and morale boost that computer applications used by clients in home-based therapy programs could potentially provide (Petheram, 1992). In his description of the "cyber clinic" of the future, Tanner (2001) envisioned that on-line feedback from computers to clients about their speech and language will be routine. Clients will sit at home and receive feedback about their productions that is highly reliable—someday. Why shouldn't we expect new technologies to make practice at home more convenient and effective? Morton Cooper, quoted at the beginning of this chapter, described such use of analog tape equipment by his patients in the 1960s:

> Automated equipment is appropriate and advisable as a helpful device for home use. The Language Master allows precise carry-over from the therapy situation to the patient's practice sessions at home. Home practice is more frequent of necessity than office sessions, and is therefore extremely pertinent to the carry-over of the very elements of voice presented and practiced under guidance in the office. The optimal pitch level and tone focus is recorded on an automated card in the office by the patient and is used as an example for comparative purposes by the patient during practice at home. (Cooper, 1971, p. 600)

But what about the present? Telepractice is a hot topic, which ASHA is embracing and facilitating through workshops and other continuing education opportunities. For the most part, the services being provided or supervised with telecommunications technologies do not yet involve replacing a clinician with a computer. Rather, the clinician works with the client or consults with a family via audio or video connection through a computer or satellite, or through e-mail/discussion groups on line (for more information, see on-line documents about telepractice on the ASHA web site).

Researchers warn that computer-based feedback during speech therapy remains far from infallible (Fitch, 1989; McGuire, 1995; Thomas-Stonell et al., 1992; Volin, 1991, 1998) and continues to require the involvement of skilled clinicians. Although many published and unpublished studies have explored these new technologies, there are still gaping holes in our understanding of how well they work and with whom. Experimental research is still lacking and training in appropriate use of such tools is unavailable in many university programs. Echoing what Cooper pointed out in 1971 about lack of documentation regarding the efficacy of the technology of his day, Dagenais reiterated this point at the 1999 ASHA convention, commenting that, "It is strange that we have all of this instrumentation, but we have no proof that it works" (Dagenais, Costello-Ingham, & Powell, 1999). Using it successfully with clients is one thing; "proving" that it works is something else.

Between the early 1990s and the early 2000s, student researchers in the Truman State University Speech and Hearing Clinic have completed eleven single-subject computer-based biofeedback studies. A summary of these studies can be found in Woods (2000). In ten of these studies, subject improvement was noted, possibly in response to biofeedback conditions. In only two studies, however, was control over extraneous variables sufficient to claim a treatment effect. A retrospective examination of these studies suggests that research design flaws were likely responsible for failure to document that it was the biofeedback (rather than other factors) that primarily caused client progress.

Exploring and documenting the efficacy of computer-based biofeedback has revealed that positive results may occur quickly, and that research designs must be adjusted accordingly. In addition, more research concerning the role of the clinician in the success of biofeedback treatment approaches is much needed.

As Volin cautioned, "None of these machines knows how to choose a target; not one of them knows how to select an appropriate task" (1991, p. 77). Many factors influence the accuracy of computer-based feedback during speech and voice tasks, including microphone placement, software settings, and model files the computer may be using to compare correct productions. Any one of these factors and others can cause a mismatch between the client's production and the computer's analysis and subsequent feedback. Clinicians should be confident about using their own judgment regarding the client's performance. They should be cautious about recommending unsupervised practice with computer applications in which the computer "judges" the client's speech. At present, computers often do not provide sufficiently reliable biofeedback about the articulation of most speech sounds to justify recommending them for independent use (no clinician available) by persons with speech problems (Masterson & Rvachew, 1999; Thomas-Stonell et al., 1992).

In contrast, some computer applications merely record and replay speech and voice, much as Coopers's Language Master did. These applications still depend on auditory feedback and require the client or clinician to determine whether the client's production was acceptable. These computer programs present a low-risk for faulty feedback and therefore high potential for independent use, once the client is certain of the task being practiced.

SUMMARY

Feedback is an important component of human communication. Speakers use various kinds of feedback to facilitate successful interaction. Speakers who have communication disorders may require more intensive, more frequent, or more specific feedback about their behavior than "usual," in order to improve their speech or language. Clinicians make an effort to provide the kind of feedback that clients find most effective for helping them change. Common types of feedback emphasized in clinical and educational activities include auditory feedback, visual feedback, and tactile feedback.

Biofeedback is a special category of feedback that can be auditory, visual, or tactile. The key idea that distinguishes "biofeedback" is that the person controls the feedback device by behavior in real time. Biofeedback is used in many fields and in many different ways in communication disorders. There are low-tech and high-tech biofeedback methods.

Computer-based feedback can be used to help speakers identify and modify aspects of their speech that are problematic. For example, computer-based biofeedback applications for articulation, fluency, and voice therapy have become economical and convenient to use. Computer-based feedback is fallible, however, and should be used by clinicians who understand the limitations of the technology.

REVIEW FOR TOPIC 21

1. Give a definition of biofeedback.
2. List three examples of "low-tech" biofeedback used in speech therapy.
3. Try it yourself: Write two sentences, one with no nasal sounds (/m/, /n/, /ng/) and one with many nasal sounds. Hold a mirror under your nostrils as you say each sentence. Does the fogging of the mirror show you when nasal emissions are occurring?
4. Does research suggest that currently available computer-based biofeedback can replace a clinician?

QUESTIONS FOR DISCUSSION

1. Consider the difficulties that clinicians face when trying to provide feedback to a client about every attempt at a therapy target. For example, consider and compare the feedback that might be provided to a child attempting correct production of /r/ and an adult who uses inadequate loudness.
2. How do clinicians provide effective incentive and feedback to a toddler who should be vocalizing more?
3. How could a computer assist with the feedback challenges you described in discussion questions 1 and 2?

RESOURCES FOR FURTHER STUDY

Case, J.L. (1999a). Technology in the assessment of voice disorders. *Seminars in Speech and Language, 20*(2), 169–184.

Case, J.L. (1999b). Technology in the treatment of voice disorders. *Seminars in Speech and Language, 20*(3), 281–295.

Masterson, J.J., & Rvachew, S.(1999). Use of technology in phonological intervention. *Seminars in Speech and Language 20*(3), 233–250.

McGuire, R.A. (1995). Computer-based instrumentation: Issues in clinical applications *Language, Hearing, Speech Services in Schools, 26*(3), 223–231.

Volin, R.A. (1991). Microcomputer-based systems providing biofeedback of voice and speech production. *Topics in Language Disorders, 11*(2), 65–79.

Computer-Based Analysis and Feedback for Voice

Clinical computing competency #4: The clinician will demonstrate the ability to plan and implement activities in which performance feedback to the client from the clinician is supplemented by feedback (visual, and/or auditory) from the computer.

Assessment and treatment of voice in the past relied on high levels of ear-training for clinicians and low-tech tools like pitch-pipes. A full range of powerful voice analysis and treatment tools are now available in computer-based applications. Effective use of computer-based feedback or biofeedback with clients requires the clinician to understand the factors that can influence the accuracy of such feedback, including for example, hardware features, program setup, and the quality and placement of the microphone. Competent clinicians will take time to become informed about the recommended preparation and procedures required in order to obtain valid and reliable results.

Prior to the availability of computer-based tools, routine measurement of voice parameters such as frequency and amplitude was clumsy at best. Some researchers had access to sophisticated tools like oscilloscopes and sound spectrography. In most work settings, however, clinicians depended on pitch pipes and ear training to evaluate a person's voice. Now even oscilloscopes and dedicated sound spectrograph equipment have been replaced by software and hardware such as the Computerized Speech Lab (CSL) (Kay Elemetrics) that has a personal computer at its core (see Figure 22.1).

New computer-based tools have made the measurement of speech and voice characteristics more objective, more precise, and more reliable. The technology that allows for excellence in measurement can also be employed as an intervention tool in many cases. See Table 22.1 for examples of computer-based tools that provide feedback to the speaker about voice parameters such as frequency and amplitude. In this topic, some basic concepts pertaining to voice are reviewed, computer-based feedback is described, and clinical examples illustrate why this aspect of clinical computing is attracting much attention from clinicians in all work settings.

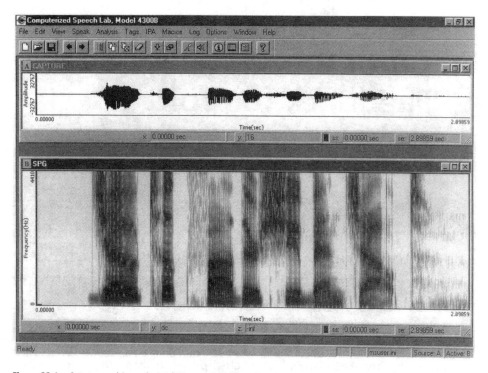

Figure 22.1.   Spectographic analysis of "Joe took father's show bench out," produced by Computerized Speech Lab (Courtesy of Truman State University Speech and Hearing Clinic).

VOCABULARY REVIEW: PITCH (FREQUENCY) AND LOUDNESS (AMPLITUDE)

The careful study of how the human voice works and the ever-improving technological advances in speech science have allowed experts to identify many parameters of phonation that can be reliably measured. At the most basic level, researchers and clinicians are interested in *frequency* and *amplitude*. Recall that frequency is the term used to refer to a physical reality–the measure of how many times a vibration occurs in a given amount of time. Frequency in reference to the human voice usually refers to the basic rate at which the vocal folds are vibrating (times per second), or their *fundamental frequency*. Human perception of changes in sound frequency is not perfect. We are more sensitive to some frequencies than to others. The term *pitch* refers to the psychological correlate of frequency. So, pitch is what humans perceive about the physical reality of frequency. Although frequency and pitch are often used interchangeably in everyday conversation, they are used precisely in speech science.

The same distinction holds true for the terms *amplitude* and *loudness* or *volume*. Amplitude refers to a physical reality of a sound wave–how much energy is present as measured by how far molecules are vibrating away from their position of rest. The amplitude of a sound wave has loudness as its psychological correlate. Humans perceive changes in amplitude as changes in the loudness or volume of a sound.

Some computer-based clinical tools include displays and settings that use the terms pitch instead of frequency and loudness or energy instead of amplitude in an attempt to be more comprehensible to clients and clinicians.

Table 22.1. Examples of computer-based analysis and feedback programs for voice

Software Exemplar	Source	Special Hardware	Product Features
Computerized Speech Lab (CSL) Model 4300B (Win)	Kay Elemetrics, Lincoln Park, NJ www.kayelemetrics.com	Yes—external hardware box and internal card from Kay (Signal-to-noise performance is typically 20–30dB better than that achieved with generic plug-in sound cards)	CSL is a high-end input/output audio device for a PC that complies with the robust specifications and features required for reliable acoustic measurements. It is a research-quality instrument, also frequently used for clinical purposes. The CSL has long been the "gold standard" in speech processing equipment. Application modules available separately for Windows include Real Time Pitch, Sona-Match, Real-Time Spectrogram, Multi-Dimensional Voice Program, Motor Speech Profile, Disordered Voice Database, Phonetics Database, Palatometer Database, Video Phonetics.
Computerized Speech Research Environment (CRSE) (Win)	AVAAZ Innovations, Inc., Ontario, Canada www.avaaz.com	User provides sound card—either Creative Laboratories Sound Blaster or Tucker-Davis Tech System II sound card are recommended. User provides compatible microphone.	CSRE is a DOS-based speech processing system for the PC that runs on Windows 95 or 98 Pentium machines. Features include signal capture, editing, spectral analysis, pitch estimates, interactive spectrograms, Klatt speech synthesis, signal manipulation utilities.
Dr. Speech v. 4 (Win)	Tiger DRS, Inc. Seattle, WA www.drspeech.com	IBM PC or compatible desktop or notebook (Pentium 133 or higher) Windows 3.1 or Windows 95 or higher, color monitor. Hard drive with at least 20MB of free space 16-bit sound card with Line-in input (Sound Blaster 16 or AWE 32 recommended) User must provide high-quality microphone (unidirectional dynamic or condensed recommended)	Dr. Speech is a Windows-based collections of software utilities for the measurement of speech and voice parameters, and real-time feedback intervention activities. Modules include: Real Analysis, Speech Therapy, Vocal Assessment, and others.
IVANS (Win)	AVAAZ Innovations, Inc., Ontario, Canada www.avaaz.com	User provides sound card—either Creative Laboratories Sound Blaster or Tucker-Davis Tech System II sound card are recommended. User must provide compatible microphone.	IVANS was designed as a voice assessment tool for Pentium PCs. It offers advanced acoustic voice measures (47 in total), which the developers claim are accurate, robust, and highly-relevant to clinical needs. Voice measures include fundamental frequency, jitter and shimmer, glottal noise, and related, derived measures. IVANS is not marketed with a primary emphasis on feedback to a client.

(continued)

Table 22.1. *(continued)*

Software Exemplar	Source	Special Hardware	Product Features
ProTrain I (Win)	AVAAZ Innovations, Inc., Ontario, Canada www.avaaz.com	No—any Windows compatible sound card (including laptops)	*ProTrain* is designed for treatment of articulation, phonology, voice, and foreign accent reduction. Specified parameters of speech are displayed in real time on the screen; client can compare productions to a target.
SoundScope (Mac) *SuperScope II* (Mac)	G.W. Instruments, Somerville, MA www.gwinst.com	Check Macintosh for audio input/output capability; *SuperScope II* is instruNet hardware compatible	*SoundScope* is a 3rd generation speech and sound analysis product line. Includes ability to record, view, analyze, play, store sound files. Provides full color spectrograms; calculates Fo, jitter, shimmer, frequency spectra (FFT), and more. Integrated text editor allows user to enter notes and observations attached to sound file. *SuperScope II* is a software design tool that can digitize, analyze, calculate, graph, and database waveform data. Used in many fields of science.
SpeechViewer III (Win)	IBM Direct or Psychological Corporation, San Antonio, TX www-3.ibm.com/able/	No—PC must have compatible sound card in computer (such as *Sound Blaster* from Creative Laboratories)	*SpeechViewer III* is a collection of 13 software modules designed primarily for biofeedback during speech and voice production. Originally designed to make speech visible to hearing impaired children, the *SpeechViewer* is now used with a wide range of clients who have speech and voice disorders. Modules include games for practicing vocalization, pitch control, volume control, voice onset, and phoneme accuracy. Look and feel is appropriate for most adults as well as children.
TalkTime with Tucker (Win/Mac)	Laureate Learning Systems, 110 E. Spring St., Winooski, VT 05404-1898	No—computer must have sound card and microphone	*TalkTime with Tucker* is a voice-activated program designed for use with young children. Five activities are included such as experimenting with loudness, sustaining phonation, and imitating animal sounds. The computer responds to child's input (for example, animal performs stunt in response to vocalization).
Video Voice Speech Training System (Win/Mac)	Micro Video, Ann Arbor, MI www.videovoice.com	Yes—external hardware box and microphone provided with software.	*Video Voice* includes approximately 20 different activities/games designed to help clients practice pitch, volume, voice onset, duration and breath control, vowels, /r/ and /s/ production, intonation and stress, fluency. Data management options permit records, reports, model files, scores for up to 120 different clients. Guaranteed free software updates, rent-to-own option.

Product	Company	Requirements	Description
Visi-Pitch II and *Visi-Pitch III* (Win)	Kay Elemetrics, Lincoln Park, NJ www.kayelemetrics.com	Yes or No—choose between versions that require external hardware box and sound card from Kay versus generic sound card user provides. *Visi-Pitch III* requires a Pentium II processor or higher with speed greater than 400 MHz. One PCI slot is required for the system's plug-in card. The computer's video graphics card should include accelerators for high-speed graphic display.	*Visi-Pitch II* consists of 8 modules for measuring and displaying frequency and amplitude of speech and voice. Based on the same high-quality hardware and software components as the CSL, but designed with a more clinically-oriented appearance and operation. The *Visi-Pitch III* expands the set of analysis tools and game-like activities suitable for children or adults, including several features previously available only on the CSL and Facilitator, including Real-Time Pitch, MDVP, and metronomic pacing. Modules also include sibilant/vowel training and delayed auditory feedback. Software-only version, Sona-Speech, works with generic sound cards and is not recommended for research purposes.
Visual Voice Tools (Win)	Riverdeep www.riverdeep.com	Win 95/98, 486 Pentiums or better (66 MHz recommended) with sound card. Microphone and headset included with software.	*Visual Voice Tools* is a collection of seven tools that help students and clients develop control of their voices. Beginning with simple sound awareness, activities include control of pitch, loudness, voicing, and breath control for phonation. Marketed as good preparation for use of the *SpeechViewer*.
Visivox	RSQ, LLC www.visivox.com	No additional hardware required – no PC required.	*Visivox* is a small, table-top device that provides visual feedback about voice volume in real time. A series of multicolored lights are differentially activated by changes in the loudness level.

ADVANCED VOCABULARY: JITTER AND SHIMMER

The *Computerized Speech Lab* (CSL) (Kay Elemetrics) includes a module entitled the Multi-Dimensional Voice Program (MDVP) which dramatically illustrates just how many measures can quickly be calculated based on a voice sample captured and digitized by the computer. Graphical presentation of analyses instantly produced by the MDVP is shown in Figure 22.2.

Some of the information provided by the MDVP is primarily of interest to researchers. This analysis is generally done after the voice sample is obtained, not simultaneously, so the MDVP does not provide biofeedback to a client. In addition to fundamental frequency and amplitude, two measures obtained through this analysis should be mentioned here. These measures help clinicians understand the natural variation that occurs in the human voice, even within the voice of a single individual: *jitter* and *shimmer*.

Even when a person is trying to sustain steady phonation, a certain amount of unsteadiness, or variation in frequency and intensity, will occur. Jitter or frequency perturbation is a measure of the cycle-to-cycle variation in frequency. In other words, the computer looks at the data collected about each cycle of opening and closing of the vocal folds and calculates how much change in rate is happening—how much variation is there—from cycle to cycle. The more stable the frequency, the lower the measure of jitter will be. However, some variation, or jitter, is inevitable. "A normal speaker without laryngeal pathology should be able to generate vowel prolongations with very little jitter, usually less than 1%" (Case, 1999a, p. 171).

Shimmer is a measure of cycle-to-cycle variation in amplitude. The more constant the amplitude is, the lower shimmer will be. According to Case, "Shimmer of more than 1 dB of variation across cycles is likely to sound dysphonic, particularly when interacting with abnormal jitter values" (1999a, p. 174). Jitter and shimmer are measured during the production of sustained vowels (not during conversational speech). There is not complete consensus about the clinical value of measures such as jitter and shimmer, but these measures are generally interpreted as indicators of vocal quality. There is still much to learn about how these measures, based on physical reality, translate into perceptual correlates that correspond to individual voice characteristics or pathologies.

COMPUTER-BASED VISUAL BIOFEEDBACK FOR VOICE

The computer applications listed in Table 22.1 confirm that the role of computers as feedback devices in speech therapy is no longer tentative. Researchers and clinicians continue to explore the possibilities with a wide range of clients. One of the earliest computer-based biofeedback systems was the *Visi-Pitch* from Kay Elemetrics. First developed and clinically established in the form of an enhanced oscilloscope, the Visi-Pitch made its transition to the Apple II platform in the early 1980s. The DOS-based *Visi-Pitch II* is still in wide distribution. Now available exclusively for Windows systems, the *Visi-Pitch IV* continues the tradition as one of the most familiar and reliable computer-based tools for voice assessment and remediation.

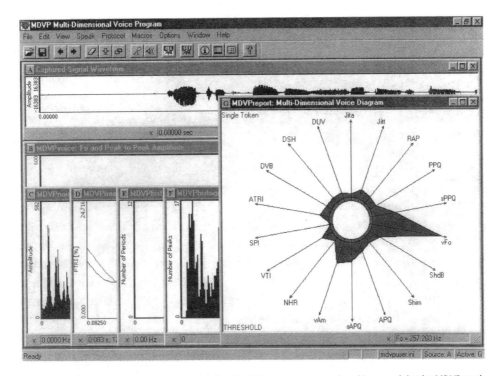

Figure 22.2. Analysis of the voice of an adult female. This analysis was produced in seconds by the MDVP module of the *CSL* (Courtesy of Truman State University Speech and Hearing Clinic).

The *Visi-Pitch II* to *IV* include modules ideal for voice assessment as well as games/utilities that are useful for voice therapy, articulation therapy, accent modification, and fluency therapy.

CASE EXAMPLE: Practicing Pitch Control and Sustaining Phonation Using Pitch and Energy Games module of the *Visi-Pitch II*

Computer display: Shows flower blossoms along the right edge of the computer screen that appear higher or lower depending upon the target vocal frequency. On the left side of the display, a hummingbird waits to fly to the blossom.

Clinician: Okay, Larissa, this bird is going to fly to the flower when it hears your voice. I want you to say /a/. I want you to take a good breath and focus on trying to get the bird to the flower.

Larissa: I'll try.

Clinician: (showing Larissa how to hold the mic, and turning it on) Ready?

Larissa: Yeah, okay.

Clinician: All right, take a breath using your good breathing and go ahead. (presses spacebar to start program)

Larissa: (shallow clavicular breath) "a"

Computer display: Hummingbird briefly moves toward open blossom.

Larissa: Oh shoot, I didn't make it. Let me try again.

Clinician:	Okay, whenever you're ready.
Larissa:	Okay.
Clinician:	Breathe deep. (presses spacebar)
Larissa:	(deep breath from diaphragm) "Ah-a-a"
Computer display:	The bird moves all the way to the blossom.
Larissa:	Yeah!
Clinician:	Way to go! You used good breathing and good voice that time.

In this example, several notable things are happening. First, three-way interaction is occurring between the client, the clinician, and the computer. The clinician's role is to choose an appropriate task, explain it to the client, and provide models or reminders that will help the client succeed ("breathe deep"). The clinician is also crucial for helping the client understand the cause of success ("You used good breathing and good voice that time"). Because the client's behavior is represented visually on the computer screen, the client can judge the adequacy of the response ("I didn't make it"). Having performance feedback that seems more objective and less judgmental, may help motivate some clients ("Let me try again").

UNDERSTANDING THE TECHNOLOGY: SIGNAL-TO-NOISE RATIO AND MICROPHONES

The *Visi-Pitch IV* currently consists of an external analog-to-digital converter box for audio input, a high-quality microphone, and collection of software modules that respond to the speaker's voice. A less costly software-only version, called *Sona-Speech*, requires an off-the-shelf audio card analog-to-digital converter, such as one that might come as standard equipment in a new PC. The *SpeechViewer III* (IBM), *CSRE, Dr. Speech, IVANS, Pro-Train* (AVAAZ) and *E-Z Voice* (Parrot) systems also depend on sound cards, speakers, and microphones provided by the user. Therefore, in contrast to the *Visi-Pitch* and *CSL*, these systems may be chosen less often for research purposes. The performance of the sound card and microphone are critical to the integrity of the signal captured by the computer. When this performance is unpredictable (because the quality and conditions of the sound card are unknown) and uncalibrated (there is no way to adjust or check sound card performance and microphone sensitivity), precise and reliable measurement cannot be guaranteed. For some everyday clinical tasks, such as visual feedback about voicing/no voice, exact measurements are not crucial, and less precise instrumentation may be sufficient. For some clinical tasks and research, measurement accuracy is crucial, such as documenting the effect of medical treatments. Clinicians should be aware, therefore, of the limitations of speech or voice analysis systems that depend on generic multimedia sound cards and consumer-quality microphones.

Clinicians may wonder why systems like the *CSL* and *Visi-Pitch* are so highly regarded because they are more expensive than tools based on off-the-shelf computer systems and take up more space on the computer cart with their special external hardware. There are several concepts relevant to this discussion, including calibration, VU meter, signal-to-noise ratio, and analog-to-digital signal conversion (A/D). A discussion of some of these follows.

Signal-to-Noise Ratio (SNR or S/N)

Everyone with hearing becomes accustomed to background noise. As I type this sentence, I am listening to music on the nearby radio. But if I concentrate, I can also hear the hum of my computer, the click of the keys, and the rhythmic thud of the clothes dryer in the background. All the time, listeners are challenged to pick out the sounds of interest from others that surround them. In some situations, speech is difficult to discriminate because of competing background noise. In such situations, the signal-to-noise ratio is said to be "low." So, S/N refers to

> The relative intensity of a signal compared to the intensity of background noise . . . Large positive values of this number are preferable because they indicate a strong signal relative to the noise background. Small positive values or negative values are less favorable for detection of signals because the noise rivals or exceeds the signal in intensity. (Kent, 1997, p. 32)

S/N is a concept that comes up frequently in audiology and aural rehabilitation. For example, one of the challenges of fitting a hearing aid is to achieve as good a signal-to-noise ratio as possible for the wearer. If all sound is equally amplified, detection of the speech signal may continue to be quite difficult.

The concept of S/N is important to the topic of selecting a computer-based system for the measurement and display of human speech and voice. If a computer is used to capture and then analyze a sample of human voice or speech, clinicians want to be sure that the sound analyzed is what the person produced, not all of the background sounds in the environment and the noise of the computer itself. In other words, the S/N should be as high as possible, so that irrelevant noise interferes with the analysis as little as possible.

Although there are exceptions, many consumer-quality sound cards and speaker systems that come with personal computers have been designed primarily to meet the needs of computer game players, not professionals recording speech for detailed analysis. "Typically, a sound card plugged into a computer has very poor signal acquisition signal-to-noise specifications when compared to professional sound acquisition systems" (Kay Elemetrics, 1999, p. 2). Game players rarely use their computers to input sound—instead, they are interested in good sound output from the sound card and speakers (so that special effects, music, and speech in the game will sound realistic). Game soundtracks sound realistic to most people because they were originally generated using professional recording equipment, just like music CDs; the personal computer system merely has to reproduce or "play" these high-quality recordings.

The external hardware box of the *CSL* or *Visi-Pitch* converts the electronic signal from the microphone into digits. It does take up space at a computer station. But it also ensures that "noise" from the computer itself does not compromise the signal as it is digitized. Kay claims that as a result, the *CSL* and *Visi-Pitch II* have an input signal-to-noise ratio "of greater than 80 dB," compared to the 40–60 dB input S/N of a typical multimedia sound card (Kay Elemetrics, 1999, p. 2). Obviously, "typical" sound cards are changing rapidly, and it may be that this gap decreases as consumer-grade technology improves. Nevertheless, today S/N is one of the reasons that computer-based analysis and biofeedback tools vary so much in price, reliability, and desirability, depending upon the needs and priorities of the user.

Microphones

The microphone specifications are also important—all mics are not created equal, especially when it comes to speech processing. Here is how one classic speech science text describes how microphones work:

> Microphones are responsive to pressure waves (e.g., sound waves) and convert the pressure variations into time-varying electrical signals . . . A unidirectional microphone placed several centimeters from the lips of the speaker transmits a higher signal-to-noise ratio than a multi-directional microphone that is equally responsive to the speaker and to sounds coming from other directions in the room. (Borden & Harris, 1984, p. 226)

The same factors that are important to computer-based analysis and feedback systems are important to a clinician attempting to obtain a good recording of a speech or language sample of a new client. Microphones come in a wide range of designs and specifications. Choice and location of microphone and S/N will affect the quality of any recording.

Some of the voice analysis and feedback programs described in Table 22.1 normally include a professional quality microphone, and some do not. Clinicians using speech recognition software or computer-based speech and voice analysis programs may find that investment in a better quality microphone significantly improves success. Consultation with distributors of the computer application may yield excellent microphone recommendations. Otherwise, look for at least a moderately priced, unidirectional, condenser-type microphone with noise cancellation.

> Because the diaphragm of a condenser microphone can be very light, compared with the more massive dynamic microphone, it is able to respond faster and at higher frequencies. Consequently, condenser microphones generally have better linearity and a greater frequency range than dynamic microphones. (*Encyclopædia Britannica,* 2004)

Good-quality mics may be damaged by abuse such as being dropped, being left turned on when not in use, or being exposed to sudden loud noise or moisture.

In addition to microphone quality, clinicians should be concerned with microphone placement. Directions that accompany systems and microphones vary in their description of the ideal placement of the microphone in relation to the speaker, in part because the microphones themselves have different design specifications. The clinical manual accompanying the *Speech Viewer III,* for example, recommends that the microphone be held approximately one inch from the speaker's mouth. As a practical way of implementing this, the manual suggests taping a pencil to the shaft of the microphone so that the eraser tip extends beyond the mic about an inch. This provides a continuous reminder of correct placement for clients and clinicians. Clinicians are responsible for familiarizing themselves with optimal microphone placement, just as they are responsible for learning how to operate software. The impact of microphone quality, accuracy of placement, and consistency of placement on the success of computer-based voice assessment or therapy activities cannot be exaggerated.

Obviously, financial constraints may prohibit the purchase of only high-end technology. Fortunately, there are less expensive alternatives available. Kay Elemetrics suggests, for example, that a combination of high-end specialized hardware systems and lower cost software-only systems may best meet the needs of larger facilities. So, a university program might have one computer equipped with the *CSL* for best-possible capturing of speech and voice samples. The less costly *Multi-Speech* from Kay could be installed on other machines that will only be analyzing, not recording, speech or voice samples.

Other options include traditional treatment approaches and computer-based applications that have less rigorous control over variables that may affect signal recording and analysis. The important thing is to realize the factors that influence the performance of computer-based tools and to be aware of their limitations. As the research examples that follow indicate, much clinical success can be had even when control over technical variables may not be ideal.

RESEARCH FINDINGS AND CLINICAL EXAMPLES OF BIOFEEDBACK FOR VOICE

In an alternating treatment study, Bouglé, Ryalls, and Le Dorze (1995) compared the use of traditional voice therapy to the use of the *Speech Viewer*. The subjects were two young adults with traumatic head injury and difficulty using appropriate pitch control and variation. The goal was to improve fundamental frequency modulation in both subjects. For these subjects, both treatments (auditory feedback from the clinician and visual feedback from the computer) seemed to be equally effective.

Testimonials regarding the efficacy of computer-based biofeedback abound in non-refereed periodicals for speech-language pathologists. An article about computer applications in *ADVANCE*, a weekly publication for SLPs and audiologists, includes the account below of a stroke patient, reported by Candace Gordon, a clinical supervisor at Portland State University.

> Prior to working with the software, the patient could not sustain a vowel for more than two seconds, Gordon recalled. "She couldn't control the respiration." Nothing seemed to work until the clinician decided to try some drill work on the computer. Using the [*SpeechViewer's* Kaleidoscope] module, the patient and clinician kept track of how long a vowel was sustained. The patient got a rewarding visual pay-off because the image changed along with the vocalizations. They continued to work together on the program until the patient got a feel for it and assumed control. The patient was able to produce vowels, then diphthongs, words, and short phrases. "A significant part of what happened with her was a result of being able to use a computer and see what was going on with her voice. She is continuing to make progress several years post stroke," Gordon reported. (Palacio, 2001, p. 11)

Both of these examples from the literature attest to the efficacy of computer-based visual biofeedback for helping someone achieve or practice an aspect of vocal performance, such as changing pitch or sustaining phonation.

The use of visual feedback (e.g., a voice-activated light) to adjust and monitor vocal intensity has been well documented (e.g., Brody, Nelson, & Brody, 1975; Lancioni, Brouwer, & Markus,1995). Visual feedback for vocal intensity is one of the most common features available among the computer-based tools described in Table 22.1. Lancioni, Van Houten, and Ten Hoopen (1997) argued that visual feedback would probably be the strategy of choice for helping persons with excessive loudness, for example, especially if they were just beginning intervention and/or had low cognitive function. However, Lancioni et al. pointed out that carry over may be limited from the desktop computer-based activities in a clinic, especially for persons with limited cognitive functioning. Once the behavior is learned and established in a clinical setting using a computer-based tool, other strategies for generalization may be necessary. Lancioni et al. (1997) demonstrated a possible solution to this limitation through the use of an inexpensive, portable auditory feedback device.

SUMMARY

Scientists have long been working on the challenge of making speech and voice "visible," for the purpose of analyzing and understanding it better, and for the purpose of helping people who have communication problems. From the stand-alone oscilloscope and the sound spectrograph to the computer-based recording and analysis systems available now, researchers and clinicians in communication disorders have continued to seek and use improved technology.

Basic acoustic analysis of the human voice focuses on frequency and amplitude and their perceptual correlates, pitch, and loudness. More detailed measures, such as jitter and shimmer, have also become readily obtainable through computer-based analysis, although there is lack of agreement regarding their clinical value.

Several computer-based tools for assessing voice parameters and providing biofeedback about speech and voice behaviors are commercially available. These tools vary not only in price, but also in their degree of technical sophistication and reliability. The role of signal-to-noise ratio, microphone quality, and placement are all factors about which some clinicians may not be well-informed. Systems that depend on consumer-quality microphones and generic multimedia sound cards may not provide the acoustic integrity that some research and clinical purposes require. Nevertheless, clinicians using the full range of available computer-based tools have reported many successes.

REVIEW FOR TOPIC 22

1. The psychological correlate of frequency is _____. The psychological correlate of amplitude is _____.
2. Define *jitter* and *shimmer*.

3. Name an example of one of the earliest systems for providing biofeedback for voice, which is still commercially available in updated form.
4. Define signal-to-noise ratio and explain how it relates to the configuration and cost of computer-based voice recording and analysis.
5. Describe the role of the clinician during therapy activities that involve computer-based biofeedback for voice.

QUESTIONS FOR DISCUSSION

1. Discuss the importance of the microphone in computer-based voice recording and analysis.
2. Consider low-tech and high-tech ways that clinicians could give a client feedback about voice parameters such as pitch, loudness, or breaks in phonation. Discuss the pros and cons of all of theses possibilities.

RESOURCES FOR FURTHER STUDY

Case, J.L. (1999a). Technology in the assessment of voice disorders. *Seminars in Speech and Language, 20*(2), 169–196.

Case, J.L. (1999b). Technology in the treatment of voice disorders. *Seminars in Speech and Language, 20*(3), 281–295.

McGuire, R.A. (1995). Computer-based instrumentation: Issues in clinical applications *Language, Hearing, Speech Services in Schools, 26*(3), 223–231.

Volin, R.A. (1991). Microcomputer-based systems providing biofeedback of voice and speech production. *Topics in Language Disorders, 11*(2), 65–79.

Computer-Based Feedback for Speech Sounds

Clinical computing competency #4: The clinician will demonstrate the ability to plan and implement activities in which performance feedback to the client from the clinician is supplemented by feedback (visual and/or auditory) from the computer.

Competency with computer-assisted articulation or phonology therapy requires many skills. The challenges faced by clinicians in using a computer this way depend somewhat on the exact software/hardware package under consideration. Currently available programs may provide auditory feedback, visual feedback, or a combination of both. They may or may not provide reliable feedback about the accuracy of a client's production, depending on the basic quality of the program, whether or not it is configured correctly, microphone quality and placement, and other factors. Clinicians and others will find it easy to operate most computer-assisted speech therapy programs. As with other clinical uses of computers, however, the clinician's role is crucial. Competency involves understanding the limitation of such programs and the factors that affect their results.

Speech therapy for articulation and phonological disorders constitutes a mainstay in the clinical practice of many clinicians. What contributions can the current generation of computer applications make to this core activity in our field? Depending on the program selected, the computer may assist with the following speech therapy tasks:

- Organizing and presenting stimuli (pictures and/or text)
- Presenting auditory models of correct production
- Presenting visual representations of correct production
- Making a recording of the client's production
- Providing an opportunity for clients to compare their productions to a model
- Providing visual or auditory feedback about the client's accuracy
- Tallying responses and keeping individual client records

Not every program does each of these tasks. Some programs may not do these tasks in a way that meets the professional standards of a particular clinician. Nevertheless, this impressive list of capabilities suggests an area of clinical computing about which many clinicians will want to become better informed.

Clinicians will find that available software/hardware packages represent a wide range of intended uses, types of feedback, and prices. Some run on almost any computer system after merely installing software from a CD. Some require more significant hardware resources or additional components that are bundled with specialized software. Examples illustrating the range of available applications for speech therapy are described in Table 23.1

The operation of certain speech therapy applications is deceptively simple. In some cases, clients themselves quickly learn how to operate the program. Why is this a problem? Although ease of use is always a highly valued feature of software, there can be drawbacks. When speech therapy software seems easy to operate, it may imply to administrators, supervisors, client families, or even clients themselves, that speech therapy itself is simple. Good speech therapists know otherwise. Further discussion regarding the professional issues raised by use of computers as feedback devices can be found in Topics 21 and 25. In this topic, the focus is on introducing the capabilities of currently available software/hardware systems for speech therapy and the factors that affect results.

UNDERSTANDING THE TECHNOLOGY: ANALOG TO DIGITAL SIGNAL CONVERSION

When someone speaks into a microphone attached to a computer, the energy from the sound they make has to somehow get converted into information the computer can use (store, analyze, or reproduce). Likewise, when a computer is asked to produce a sound (speech, music, sound effects), the code for that sound has to be converted into a sound wave that human ears can perceive. This process of going back and forth between sound waves in the air and code in a computer is called *analog-to-digital* or *digital-to-analog* conversion. The phrase *analog-to-digital conversion*, or A/D as it is often abbreviated, may sound intimidating at first. Most clinicians do not need to know all of the gory details of this process. However, general familiarity with the basic concepts and terms is part of being competent with computer technology that involves recording, displaying, and reproducing speech.

Recall from Section IV that the term "digitize" refers to the process of taking information in some format and converting it to digits so that a computer can store it, manipulate it, or reproduce it. So, a scanner digitizes photos or documents, a digital video camera or video card digitizes moving images, and an A/D converter, usually in the form of a sound card or chip in a computer, digitizes sound (music, speech, sound effects). When sound is recorded and stored in digital format, generally the sound quality is better than with analog recording devices such as regular (not digital) tape recorders. Digital sounds can be accessed, manipulated, and reproduced in ways that are not available with analog recordings.

Table 23.1. Examples of computer-based feedback programs for speech sounds

Software exemplar	Source	Special hardware	Product features
Articulation I (Consonant phonemes) *Articulation II* (Consonant clusters) *Articulation III* (Vowel + R and R clusters) *Phonology I, II*	LocuTour Multimedia Software Learning Fundamentals 1130 Grove Street San Luis Obispo, CA 93401	Mac OS (Power PC) and Windows (Pentium) versions available. Not compatible with Windows CE or NT. Requires internal sound card and microphone provided by user.	Combines **auditory feedback** with visual and auditory cuing. Uncluttered screen design features a photo of a target word, phrase, or sentence and buttons to control stimulus presentation. Digitized speech presents stimuli in exaggerated, sound-by-sound, or normal speech modes. Client can record production and compare to computer's model. Client and clinician judge accuracy of client's production, which can be tallied as correct, incorrect, or distorted. Suitable for children and adults.
HearSay (modules for Mandarin Chinese, Japanese, or Spanish) or *HearSay for All* (24 different language backgrounds)	Communication Disorders Technology, Inc. Indiana University Research Park 501 N. Morton, Suite 215 Bloomington, IN 47404	Requires a PC with a 200 MHz Intel Pentium processor running Windows 95 or higher with 130 MB of free disk space, a CD-ROM drive, and a Sound Blaster-compatible sound card with microphone and speakers (or earphones).	*HearSay* and *HearSay for All* use speech recognition technology for foreign accent reduction. The interactive game environment is designed to teach English pronunciation through **auditory and visual feedback**. Individuals work independently on English sounds that are most likely to compromise intelligibility according to research with speakers of the first language. Not recommended for beginning speakers of English, but is marketed for ESL classrooms or home use.
Indiana Speech Training Aid (ISTRA)	Communication Disorders Technology, Inc. Indiana University Research Park 501 N. Morton, Suite 215 Bloomington, IN 47404	Requires a PC with a Pentium-level processor and SoundBlaster-compatible sound card. A high-quality, noise-cancelling microphone is supplied with the system at no extra charge.	Originally intended for use with the hearing impaired (Kewley-Port, 1994), *ISTRA* has also been used in training programs with normal-hearing, misarticulating, and developmentally delayed children and adults. *ISTRA* training has been shown to be clinically effective to improve speech intelligibility (Kewley-Port, Watson, Elbert, Maki, & Reed, 1991). **Evaluative feedback** to a client is based on comparison to the client's best production (template). Judgements of correctness have been shown in research to correlate with SLP judgments (Watson, Reed, Kewley-Port, & Maki, 1989).
ProTrain I (Win)	AVAAZ Innovations, Inc., Ontario, Canada www.avaaz.com	Any Windows-compatible sound card and microphone (including laptops).	Combines **visual and auditory feedback**. *ProTrain* is designed for treatment of articulation, phonology, voice, and foreign accent reduction. Specified parameters of speech are displayed in real time on the screen; clients can record and compare their productions to a target. Suitable for children or adults, depending on activity choice
Super Nasal Oral Ratiometry System (SNORS+) (Win)	Medical Electronics University of Kent (U.K.)	(details of product availability and requirements are uncertain) Uses standard sound and video capture cards.	*SNORS+* allows objective and simultaneous assessment of the function and coordination of key articulators, according to its developers. Besides assessment capability, **visual feedback** is provided for therapy in two formats: trend waveforms over time or 2-D dynamic displays (Sharp, et al., 1999).

(continued)

Table 23.1. (continued)

Software exemplar	Source	Special hardware	Product features
SpeechPrism Pro, Speech Prism, & Vowel Target (Win)	Language Vision, Inc. P.O. Box 1361 Idaho Falls, ID 83403-1361 www.langvision.com Fully functional trial versions available via free download.	Window 95, 98, and ME multimedia PC. User must provide microphone and speakers.	*Speech Prism Pro* is intended to be a very low-cost **visual feedback** system for speech therapy. It provides six different ways to visualize speech: two kinds of real-time spectrograms; two kinds of color-based representations; an animated mid-sagittal head cross section; and a real-time vowel histogram.
SpeechViewer III (Win)	IBM Direct or Psychological Corporation, San Antonio, TX www-3.ibm.com/able/	Any Windows-compatible sound card (Sound Blaster from Creative Laboratories is recommended)	Offers primarily **visual feedback.** *SpeechViewer III* is a collection of 13 software modules designed primarily for biofeedback during speech and voice production. Originally designed to make speech visible to hearing impaired children, the *SpeechViewer* is now used with a wide range of clients who have speech and voice disorders. Phoneme Accuracy modules designed to compare client's production of a particular phoneme to pre-recorded target files are the most controversial and often the favorites of clinicians. Suitable for children or adults, depending on activity choice.
Video Voice Speech Training System (Win/Mac)	Micro Video, Ann Arbor, MI www.videovoice.com	External hardware box for analog-to-digital conversion and microphone are provided with software.	Offers primarily **visual feedback.** *Video Voice* includes approximately 20 different activities/games designed to help clients practice pitch, volume, voice onset, duration and breath control, vowels, /r/ and /s/ production, intonation and stress, fluency. Suitable for children or adults, depending on activity choice. Compares client production to model file created by clinician, client, or similar speaker. Guaranteed free software updates, rent-to-own option.
Visi-Pitch III and IV	Kay Elemetrics, Lincoln Park, NJ www.kayelemetrics.com	Choose between versions that require external hardware box, microphone, and sound card from Kay versus generic sound card and microphone user provides	Newly updated, the *Visi-Pitch IV* consists of eight standard modules (and optional programs) for measuring and displaying parameters of speech and voice. Based on the same high-quality hardware and software components as the *Computerized Speech Lab* (CSL), but designed with a more clinically-oriented appearance and operation. *Visi-Pitch III* and *IV* added some of the capabilities of Kay's *CSL* and portable *Facilitator*, including masking and metronomic pacing for speech. Software only version, *Sona-Speech*, works with generic sound cards and is not recommended for research purposes. Suitable for children or adults, depending on activity choice.

Speech, music, and other natural sounds are made up of complex sound waves that contain frequency and amplitude components across a range of values. When they are produced by a speaker, instrument, or other source, such sound waves can be called "analog" signals. The range of values represented in an analog signal must be converted (coded) into digits (binary code made up of 0s and 1s) in order for a computer to store or analyze the sound. In most speech and voice therapy applications, this conversion takes place at the moment of recording the sound, using a microphone directly connected to a computer. The analog signal is conveyed in the form of electrical pulses to the A/D converter (computer) via the microphone. The A/D converter takes samples of the signal and converts them to digits. This sampling occurs at a rate of several thousand times per second, in order to obtain an accurate recording. When a digitized sound is played back, a digital-to-analog converter reverses the process (for a more detailed description, see Ventkatagiri, 1996).

As discussed in Topic 22, sound card and microphone specifications can dramatically impact the quality of a digital recording. These two factors are often the source of difficulties that clinicians encounter when speech recognition or computer-based feedback programs are not performing as expected. The third factor for clinicians to keep in mind is sampling rate. The higher the sampling rate, the higher the fidelity of the recording. A high sampling rate results in more data points for the computer to use and less opportunity for distortion.

Often clinicians can choose the sampling rate used during A/D conversion. As a rule, they should choose the highest available sampling rate when high fidelity playback is important or when the computer will be analyzing the recording. When would a lower sampling rate be desirable? In a situation in which a client is adding speech to the pages of a story or a memory book being created on the computer, file size may become an issue. Small degradation of sound quality may be an acceptable trade for more available recording time. The sampling rate (or sample rate conversion quality) setting may have to be changed within the system software of the computer (look in sound control panels) and/or within the clinical software being used. High sampling rates result in larger files that require more memory and storage space. Older computers may have only relatively low sampling rates available.

CLINICAL EXAMPLE: RECORDING SPEECH WITH EDUCATIONAL SOFTWARE

As sound cards, speakers, and microphones have become standard equipment in the computer configurations sold for business, school, and home use, software applications are taking more advantage of speech recording and playback capability. Clinicians will find much educational and clinical software designed to allow clients to record their own speech to label objects, tell a story, or add sound effects. Several programs described in Section III include this capability as an add-on feature rather than a central focus. For example, if a microphone and sound card are available, users can record their own labels for objects in *Usborne's Animated First Thousand Words*, or their own symbol captions in *Kidspiration*, or character voices in the *Imagination Express* series (Edmark/Riverdeep). Clinicians take advantage of this recording option to give clients the opportunity to hear their own speech. Clients may expend extra effort to make themselves understood when being recorded. Repeatedly playing back this best effort and asking the client to practice matching it may be an effective exercise and represents the most basic use of computer-based auditory feedback.

Recording and reproducing the client's speech has a more central role in the objectives of *Tiger Tales* software from Laureate Learning Systems. This software presents a series of dramatic moments in a story featuring animal characters. Each dramatic moment calls for a character to say something that suits the situation. At these moments, the story pauses so that the client can record what the story character should say. Clearly, this kind of activity could be a motivating way to stress speech, grammar, and/or pragmatic skills. Clients experience external auditory feedback about their speech as the recordings are made and checked during story creation. When the tale is complete, clients hear their speech as it occurs in a "movie" of the story.

If a self-recorded digitized recording is used as a model for an articulation client, it is critical for the clinician to listen to the recording to ensure that the client is not internalizing a distorted model. Generic, low-quality microphones and sound cards may produce recordings that are acceptable for a business executive adding a voice note to a document for the secretary to act on. However, for children or adults who have possible hearing impairment, auditory discrimination difficulty, or speech problems, better audio quality may be required. This can be obtained with equipment (e.g., microphones, speakers, sound cards/analog-to-digital converters) especially designed for recording and analyzing speech, such as many of the programs listed in Table 23.1.

CLINICAL EXAMPLE: SOFTWARE ESPECIALLY FOR ARTICULATION THERAPY

Software that is especially designed for speech therapy employs auditory feedback in a different way. For example, the *Articulation I, II, III* series from LocuTour Multimedia, facilitates quick, easy auditory comparisons between a client's production of a key word and a spoken model provided by the computer. Models consist of exaggerated and normal articulation productions that originated with a human speaker and were digitized for use on the CD. The client or clinician presses buttons on the screen that play the exaggerated or normally produced target word. Optionally, they can choose to record the client's imitation. Then the computer model and the client's attempt can be played and compared as many times as desired (see other features in Table 23.1). Playing client recordings and computer models at a slightly increased volume may help some clients "hear" the difference for the first time.

In an unpublished single-subject research study, Ball (2002) successfully used one of the *Articulation* (LocuTour) modules with an adult ESL client. Although the client was motivated and cooperative, traditional articulation approaches had failed to have much impact on his articulation of certain English sounds. According to Ball, by repeatedly listening to his recording compared to the exaggerated computer model, the client came to understand that he just was not producing the correct sound. He had an "ah-ha" moment when he declared as much to the clinician, and from then on made rapid progress.

CLINICAL EXAMPLE: COMPUTER-BASED VISUAL BIOFEEDBACK

Visual feedback is an important component of most approaches to speech therapy, whether new technology is used or not. Taking visual feedback to a new level with the aid of computers, visual biofeedback about particular speech sounds is possible. As described in Table 23.1, tools such as *ProTrain I, SNORS+, SpeechViewer III, Video Voice,* and the *Visi-Pitch III* represent this category of clinical applications of computers. Recall from Topic 21 that biofeedback is distinguished by the fact that it occurs concurrently with the behavior, rather than subsequently. Feedback from clinicians is generally limited to comments and suggestions that occur after a client has attempted to imitate or produce a target. In the presence of biofeedback, the client receives information about the accuracy of articulation during the production (see Figure 23.1).

For the most part, computer-based biofeedback for speech is used to help clients work on continuant sounds: primarily vowels, fricatives, and liquids (for an exception, see Thomas-Stonell et al., 1992). Plosives and affricates have acoustic characteristics, such a brief duration, that do not lend themselves to computer-based biofeedback. Computer-based tools for monitoring and modifying resonance and nasal sounds are discussed in Topic 24. Here is the basic sequence of events that occurs during the use of computer-based visual biofeedback for speech sounds:

- Clinician chooses correct software settings, model files, and microphone placement.
- Clinician explains the task to the client and demonstrates if possible.
- Client attempts target production while watching the computer screen.
- Simultaneously, computer screen adjusts the display in response to the client's speech.
- In response to the changing computer display, the client adjusts articulation.
- As the target production ends, the client observes and interprets the screen display.
- Client and clinician together decide whether the computer feedback was accurate.
- Clinician adjusts program settings, if necessary, and prepares client for another attempt.

CASE EXAMPLE: Using the *SpeechViewer III* to Work on Production of /s/

Preparation: Prior to the session, the clinician familiarizes herself with the operation of the *SpeechViewer III*, the recommended microphone placement, the operation of the Phoneme Accuracy module, and program settings that are used to adjust the pitch range, volume range, and the sensitivity of the feedback provided. For some clients, the clinician will want the computer to respond positively to any production that even grossly approximates the target, with the intent of encouraging closer and closer approximations. For some clients, the clinician will want the computer to respond positively only when the production closely matches the target sound. The clinician has recorded a model file for /s/ for today's lesson. If the feed-

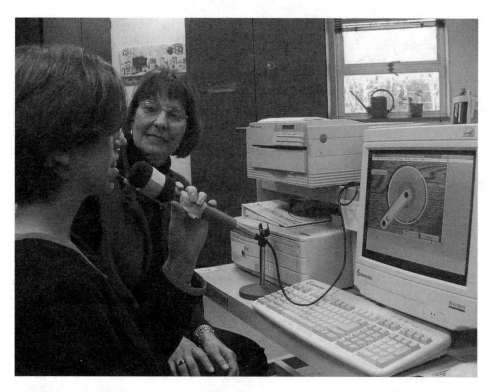

Figure 23.1. Using the IBM *Speechviewer* Phoneme Accuracy module to work on articulation of /s/. Note correct microphone placement. (Courtesy of Truman State University Speech and Hearing Clinic.)

back is not accurate, the clinician is prepared to create a model file using the client's best production.

Clinician:	Angela, today we're going to try something new. You're going to say your sound into the microphone and watch the computer screen. The better your sound is, the closer this ball will get to the center target here, see? [points to target on screen] Watch while I do one. [Clinician takes microphone and produces a clear /s/. The ball on the screen moves to the center of the target and disappears with a satisfying ker-plunk!]
Client:	Okay, let me try.
Clinician:	Keep the microphone right here when you are making your sound.
Client:	Okay. Now?
Clinician:	Yes, now. Go ahead and say /s/.
Client:	/sh-sh-sh/. Oh, man. I didn't get very far.
Clinician:	That's okay. Try again.
Client:	/sh-s-sh/. [ball on screen moves a little toward the center] Closer that time. One more, okay?
Client:	/sh-s-s-s/ [ball on screen moves to center of target and goes ker-plunk!]
Client and clinician:	Yeah!
Clinician:	That was great! Do it again!

RESEARCH PAST, PRESENT, AND FUTURE

Researchers have established the importance and efficacy of various kinds of visual feedback in speech therapy (Dagenais, 1995; Higgins, McCleary, & Schulte, 2000; Povel & Wansink, 1986; Shuster, Ruscello, & Toth, 1995). Boothroyd et al. (1975) and Ruscello (1995) provided excellent historical reviews of this research. Some tools that researchers have used to provide visual feedback to subjects include not only newer microphone-to-computer display systems for biofeedback as described previously (Pratt, Heintzelman, & Deming, 1993; Sharp, Kelly, Main, & Manley, 1999; Thomas-Stonell, McLean, Dolman, & Oddson, 1992; Watson & Kewley-Port, 1989) but also videoendoscopy (Witzel, Tobe, & Salyer, 1989), laryngography (Abberton, Hu, & Fourcin, 1998), electropalatography (Dagenais, 1995), and speech spectrography (Shuster, Ruscello, & Toth, 1995).

Ruscello (1995) and Shuster and colleagues (1995) put forth a case for using visual biofeedback in speech therapy, especially with clients who have made inadequate progress with traditional therapy. They contend that older children and adults who have failed to acquire correct production of sounds like /r/ may be experiencing a mismatch in auditory discrimination skills. Although such clients may detect correct production of sounds in another person's speech, auditory discrimination of their own productions is faulty. The rapid success experienced with visual biofeedback may be explained because it allows the client to circumvent the faulty auditory information and gain important cues in a different way. Two interesting observations that support their theory include 1) their subjects reported that initial correct productions of the target during biofeedback conditions did not "sound" correct to them and 2) subjects tended to prolong correct productions at first when they were transitioning away from biofeedback conditions. The researchers suggest that subjects were establishing different, non-auditory "sensory inputs for establishing correct production of the target /r/. It may have been a necessary transitional phase between the biofeedback condition and appropriate spontaneous use of the phoneme" (Ruscello, 1995, p. 296).

Several studies done in an effort to evaluate or improve technologies for speech therapy have shown that computer-based feedback was helpful but not sufficient for maximizing client success (e.g., Boothroyd et al., 1975; Nickerson, Kalikow, & Stevens, 1976; Povel & Wansink, 1986) or not reliable enough for clinical success (e.g., Fitch, 1989; Pratt et al., 1993). Topic 25 further addresses the issues of validity and reliability of computer-based feedback for speech. There is no doubt that this area of clinical computing will continue to undergo rapid change.

Clinical tools for providing biofeedback will become increasingly portable, inexpensive, and reliable. In all likelihood the "cyber clinic" of the future will provide speech therapy clients with computer-based analysis and biofeedback in the comfort of their own homes. As their role in speech therapy management changes, clinicians will need to stay informed about new technologies. Although they are powerful tools, computers are not yet able to understand or explain why a client may be having difficulty or when a client should be working on an easier or more challenging task. New technologies are helping physicians provide better care, but no one wants an appointment with a computer when they are sick. Likewise, new technologies won't make clinicians obsolete; they will make them more effective.

SUMMARY

Computers can assist with many traditional speech therapy tasks, including organizing and presenting stimulus items in various formats, providing an auditory model of the target, recording a clinician's model or a client's oral productions, reproducing the client's production, providing feedback about production accuracy, and tallying accuracy data. Although it may sound like the computer is taking over the duties of a clinician, important clinical tasks remain for the clinician—such as choosing a goal, motivating the client, and helping the client understand the goals and procedures of therapy. Clinicians must make sure that the computer is configured correctly, that the client understands the task, and that the computer is providing accurate feedback to the client. The clinician may need to step in at any time to help the client understand why his or her production is not accurate enough or to increase or decrease the computer's sensitivity.

Feedback is an important component of every method of speech therapy. Research has confirmed the value of visual feedback provided by a wide range of sophisticated instrumentation. Visual biofeedback tools are now reasonably affordable to clinicians in most work settings, and should especially be considered for use with clients who have not made sufficient progress with traditional therapy approaches.

REVIEW FOR TOPIC 23

1. List five speech therapy tasks that computer programs can help clinicians do.
2. What does the abbreviation A/D stand for?
3. What does "digitize" mean?
4. List three factors that influence the quality of digital recordings.
5. Describe the basic sequence of events that characterizes the use of biofeedback during a speech therapy session.

QUESTIONS FOR DISCUSSION

1. Discuss the role of the clinician versus the computer during biofeedback therapy activities.
2. Should clinicians feel threatened by the continuous improvement of technology that seems to be doing some of the same tasks the first clinicians and then paraprofessional speech aides once did? Why or why not?
3. Interview a clinician who has used computer-assisted feedback or biofeedback with clients. What does he or she think about its efficacy?

RESOURCES FOR FURTHER STUDY

Kewley-Port, D. (1994). Speech technology and speech training for the hearing impaired. *The Journal of the Academy of Rehabilitative Audiology, (Monograph), XXVII*, 251–265.
Masterson, J.J., & Rvachew, S. (1999). Use of technology in phonological intervention. *Seminars in Speech and Language 20*(3), 233–250.

Pratt, S.R., Heintzelman, A.T., & Deming, S.E. (1993). The efficacy of using the IBM Speechviewer vowel accuracy module to treat young children with hearing impairment. *Journal of Speech and Hearing Research, 36,* 1063–1074.

Ruscello, D.M. (1995). Visual feedback in treatment of residual phonological disorders. *Journal of Communication Disorders, 28,* 279–302.

Computer-Based Feedback for Fluency, Resonance, and Swallowing

Clinical computing competency #4: The clinician will demonstrate the ability to plan and implement activities in which performance feedback to the client from the clinician is supplemented by feedback (visual and/or auditory) from the computer.

Clinicians who explore the use of computers in the assessment and treatment of disorders of fluency, resonance, or swallowing should have substantial expertise in the traditional assessment and treatment of clients with these disorders. Competency may require special training with some software/hardware systems and will include familiarity with available tools and the research that has guided their development. Competent clinicians will be aware of both the strengths and the limitations inherent in the current generation of tools designed for working with clients who have these disorders.

Many of the same advantages and cautions that are described in Topics 21–23 apply to using computer-based feedback during the treatment of the disorders of interest in this topic. Clinicians may find that clients respond quickly and positively to the new information provided by the computer, or there may be difficulty adjusting the program's sensitivity, microphone placement, or some other setting in order to ensure that feedback about the client's speech is accurate and helpful.

Especially since the widespread availability of microcomputers in the early 1980s, clinicians and researchers have been exploring the use of computers in the assessment and treatment of stuttering (e.g., Bakker, Ingham, & Netsell, 1997; Brosch, Haege, & Johnson, 2002; Healey & Scott, 1995; Onslow, Costa, Andrews, Harrison, & Packman, 1996), resonance (e.g., Dalston, Warren, & Dalston, 1991; Dalston & Seaver, 1992; Nellis, Neiman, & Lehman, 1992) and swallowing disorders (e.g., Crary, 1995; Crary & Baldwin, 1997; Logemann & Kahrilas, 1990; Martin, Logemann, Shaker, & Dodds, 1994). Table 24.1 describes examples of relevant software/hardware systems. Some applications are dedicated applications for fluency/stuttering, resonance, or swallowing. Other examples

Table 24.1. Examples of computer-based feedback programs for fluency, resonance, and swallowing

Software exemplar	Source	Special hardware	Product features
Digital Swallowing Workstation	Kay Elemetrics, Lincoln Park, NJ www.kayelemetrics.com	Integrated PC-based system provided on a customized portable cart.	The *Digital Swallowing Workstation* is a second-generation integrated system for dysphagia assessment and treatment. This workstation includes the addition of digital video recording. Capabilities include **visual feedback** tools for therapy, physiologic data acquisition/measurement capabilities, and a complete fiberoptic endoscopic evaluation of swallowing (FEES) system for bedside patient assessment.
Dr. Fluency v6.1	Speech Therapy Systems Ltd., 641 Lexington Ave., New York, NY 10022 www.drfluency.com	Requires PC—Pentium 166 or higher, Super VGA graphics card with at least 16 bit color and screen resolution of at least 640 × 480, one free serial port, sound card (a PCI card is recommended).	Originally copyrighted in 1996, version 6.1 of *Dr. Fluency* was released in 2001. Intended primarily for use by teens and adults, developers suggest that some aspects of the program can be used with children if sufficient clinician assistance is provided. The full package of *Dr. Fluency* includes a patented *Dr. Fluency Breathing Monitor* and microphone. The breathing monitor is worn around the chest and attached to the computer via a serial port (COM1 or COM2). Modules take users through an intensive sequence of lessons modeled after Webster's Precision Fluency Shaping Program.
Dr. Speech v. 4	Tiger DRS, Inc. Seattle, WA www.drspeech.com	Requires IBM PC or compatible desktop or notebook (Pentium 133 or higher) Windows 3.1 or Windows 95 or higher, color monitor. Hard drive with at least 20MB of free space 16-bit sound card with Line-in input (Sound Blaster 16 or AWE 32 recommended) User must provide high-quality microphone (unidirectional dynamic or condensed recommended)	*Dr. Speech* is a Windows-based collection of software utilities for the measurement of speech and voice parameters, and real-time feedback intervention activities. Modules include:Real Analysis, Speech Therapy, Vocal Assessment, and others. Resonance is addressed with the module called NasalView. NasalView displays measurements of hypernasality and nasal emission.
Facilitator	Kay Elemetrics, Lincoln Park, NJ www.kayelemetrics.com	Not PC-based; self-contained unit with no additional hardware required.	Developed by Daniel Boone in conjunction with Kay Elemetrics, the *Facilitator* is a portable/wearable multi-purpose clinical tool that does several useful things. It can be used as a playback loop recorder, as a **delayed auditory feedback** (DAF) device providing between 10 and 500 ms delay, or it can provide either continuous or voice-activated masking. It can provide metronomic pacing (50-150 beats per minute) or speech amplification for frequencies between 70 and 7000 Hz.

ProTrain I	AVAAZ Innovations, Inc., Ontario, Canada www.avaaz.com	Combines **visual and auditory feedback.** *ProTrain* is designed for treatment of articulation, phonology, voice, and foreign accent reduction. Specified parameters of speech are displayed in real time on the screen; clients can record and compare their productions to a target. Suitable for children or adults, depending on activity choice	Any Windows-compatible sound card and microphone (including laptops).
Nasometer	Kay Elemetrics, Lincoln Park, NJ www.kayelemetrics.com	The *Nasometer II* provides real-time **visual feedback** during therapy tasks. The headset design is crucial to the product's function. It contains sensors that separately measure the acoustic energy from the oral and nasal cavities during speech. It is easy to clean between patients. The real-time display of Nasometer II enables clients to monitor their velopharyngeal control during speech. The statistical analysis of collected data on standardized passages/phrases can be compared to published normative data.	External hardware box and headset (microphone) are provided. The *Nasometer II* requires a Pentium II processor or higher with speed >400 MHz. One PCI slot is required for the system's plug-in card. The computer's video graphics card should include accelerators for high-speed graphic display.
OroNasal System	AVAAZ Innovations, Inc., Ontario, Canada www.avaaz.com	According to developers, the OroNasal System uses a patented method for measuring nasalance that reduces dependence of results on specific vowels and voiced consonants. Real-time **visual feedback** allows clients to practice with a sound and to watch the nasalance vary as they experiment with different postures of velar closure.	User provides multimedia PC, including sound card and speakers. AVAAZ supplies patented, voice-transparent pneumotach mask which user wears during program activities.
Pocket Fluency System	Casa Futura Technologies, Boulder, CO www.casafuturatech.com	Casa Futura Technologies devices have been found to reduce stuttering by 60%–80% (Zimmerman, S., Kalinowski, J., Stuart, A., Rastatter, M. (1997). *Effect of Altered Auditory Feedback on People Who Stutter During Scripted Telephone Conversations. Journal of Speech, Language, and Hearing Research, 40,* 1130–1134). DAF, **frequency-shifted auditory feedback** (FAF), and **masking auditory feedback** (MAF) are available.	The *Pocket Fluency System* is a small feedback device that provides sound to both ears. It is designed for use with traditional stuttering therapy. The *Pocket Fluency System* uses noise-canceling directional microphones to eliminate all background noise.
Super Nasal Oral Ratiometry System (SNORS+)	Medical Electronics University of Kent (U.K.)	SNORS+ is a Windows 95 version of the University of Kent SNORS airflow system. As well as being a stand-alone SNORS system, SNORS+ includes nasendoscopy, videofluorscopy, electropalatography, nasal anemometry, and electrolaryngography capability. SNORS+ allows simultaneous assessment of five important parameters of speech production, in real-time. For **visual feedback** purposes, parameters can be displayed as trend waveforms over time, or as 2-D dynamic displays.	(details of product availability and requirements are uncertain) Uses standard sound and video capture cards. Requires Windows 95® or better.

(continued)

Table 24.1. *(continued)*

Software exemplar	Source	Special hardware	Product features
SoundScope (Mac)	G.W. Instruments, Somerville, MA www.gwinst.com	Check Macintosh for audio input/output capability.	*SoundScope* is a speech and sound analysis product line that also includes some **visual feedback** capability. Users can record, view, analyze, play, and store sound files. Users can view intensity contours and measure duration of phonation. Most suitable for teens and adults.
SpeechViewer III	IBM Direct or Psychological Corporation, San Antonio, TX www-3.ibm.com/able/	Any Windows-compatible sound card (Sound Blaster from Creative Laboratories is recommended)	Offers primarily **visual feedback**. *SpeechViewer III* is a collection of 13 software modules designed primarily for biofeedback during speech and voice production. Originally designed to make speech visible to hearing impaired children, the *SpeechViewer* is now used with a wide range of clients who have speech and voice disorders. Includes activities that emphasize stopping and starting phonation and sustaining phonation among others. Suitable for children or adults, depending on activity choice.
Swallowing Signals Lab	Kay Elemetrics, Lincoln Park, NJ www.kayelemetrics.com	External box with hardware to interface to a PC, and all transducers.	The *Swallowing Signals Lab* is considered an ideal therapy tool for acute care and rehabilitation facilities. It provides quantitative measures of various parameters of swallowing and real-time **visual feedback** for the patient. It is available as a stand-alone module or as part of Kay's complete *Swallowing Workstation*.
Video Voice Speech Training System	Micro Video, Ann Arbor, MI www.videovoice.com	External hardware box for analog-to-digital conversion and microphone are provided with software.	Offers primarily **visual feedback**. *Video Voice* includes approximately 20 different activities/games designed to help clients practice pitch, volume, voice onset, duration and breath control, vowels, /r/ and /s/ production, intonation and stress, fluency. Data management options permit records, reports, model files, scores for up to 120 different clients. Suitable for children or adults, depending on activity choice. Guaranteed free software updates, rent-to-own option.
Visi-Pitch III	Kay Elemetrics, Lincoln Park, NJ www.kayelemetrics.com	Choose between versions that include external hardware box, microphone, and sound card from Kay versus generic sound card and microphone that the user provides. *Visi-Pitch III* host computer requirements are the same as for the *Nasometer* described previously.	Offers primarily **visual feedback**. *Visi-Pitch III* consists of modules for measuring and displaying frequency and amplitude of speech and voice. Based on the same high-quality hardware and software components as the Computerized Speech Lab (CSL), but designed with a more clinically-oriented appearance and operation. Modules also include **delayed auditory feedback**, masking, and a metronomic pacer. Suitable for children or adults, depending on activity choice. Software-only version, *Sona-Speech*, works with generic sound cards and is not recommended for research purposes.

include broader-based tools, some parts of which may be clinically applicable for these disorders as well as others. This topic describes examples of available products and summarizes current research for all three of these important areas of clinical focus.

COMPUTER APPLICATIONS DEDICATED TO FLUENCY DISORDERS

During the 1980s and 1990s, many clinical applications for computers have been developed, used, and discarded. Often this was not because they lacked efficacy, but because developers and publishers could not afford to redesign them for rapidly changing technology. For example, one product of the 1980s was an Apple II-based hardware and software system called *Computer Aided Fluency Establishment Trainer* (CAFET). Developed and field-tested at the Annandale Fluency Clinic in Annandale, Virginia, the system was eventually converted to DOS and made available for purchase. Still in use at Annandale, but no longer a commercial product, *CAFET* included a unique set of features that reflected the clinical approach to fluency of its developer, Martha Goebel.

CAFET was designed to give the user simultaneous biofeedback about several aspects of speech: 1) rate of onset of phonation, 2) timing of phonation related to respiration, and 3) continuity of phonation. The Annandale Fluency Clinic web site describes the hardware components of *CAFET* as follows:

> A respiratory sensor is fitted around the patient's lower chest (exact position varies from client to client.) Air pressure changes inside the tube as the chest wall expands and contracts, providing an indirect (non-invasive) measure of airflow. A pressure transducer converts the relative air pressure changes to an electrical signal. A microphone produces an electrical signal from voice input; CAFET provides a tie-clip microphone to give the patient maximum freedom of movement. A circuit board accepts signals from the microphone and transducer, and converts them to digital, computer-ready data. (Retrieved October 15, 2003, from http://www.afccafet.com/cafetoverview.htm)

Wearing the respiration monitoring tube around the chest, the user watches the computer monitor and speaks into the microphone. Real-time feedback, consisting of line tracings of various colors, appears on the computer monitor as the client speaks. Error messages also remind the client of target behaviors. As the user is introduced to the various feedback components, speaking tasks gradually increase in complexity from simple vowel prolongation to conversational speech. Users practice and adjust specific behaviors in order to obtain fluency. These behaviors include diaphragmatic (abdominal) breathing, continuous airflow (not breath-holding at the onset of phonation), gradual expiration, pre-voice exhalation, gentle onset, continuous phonation, and using adequate breath support.

Excellent initial results and maintenance of gains 2 years post-therapy have been claimed by Annandale, which has treated more than 1,200 teens and adults with *CAFET* over the past 20 years (Martha Goebel, personal communication, April 2003). Healey and Scott (1995) described the use of *CAFET* in an integrative approach to therapy for children who stutter. In a multiple-baseline treatment study of four adults who stuttered (ages 20–25), Blood (1995) combined *CAFET* with a relapse management program for counseling and attitude change. Results showed that subjects reduced their disfluencies to below a criterion of 3% stuttered syllables and maintained improvement at 6- and 12-month follow-ups. Increased positive feelings and attitudes were also documented.

In an unrelated study of clients with hyperfunctional voice disorders, Blood (1994) incorporated *CAFET* into a voice treatment protocol that also included relaxation training. The *CAFET* practice sessions focused on learning correct breathing and gradual rise of air volume, and easy onset of voice. Results suggested that, "selected aspects of the *CAFET* program were useful methods of biofeedback in conjunction with more traditional voice treatment approaches" (p. 64).

In the early 1990s, *Dr. Fluency* (Speech Therapy Systems, Ltd.) appeared on the market. According to the company web site, *Dr. Fluency* was developed by its president, Arye Friedman, who stuttered severely from a young age. It is based on the Precision Fluency Shaping program (PFSP) at Holland College (Webster, 1974) as well as the intensive fluency treatment courses at the Hadassah University Hospital Speech and Hearing Clinic, Jerusalem and the Ontario Speech Foundation Stuttering Centre, Toronto, Canada. Like *CAFET, Dr. Fluency* is able to provide feedback about both the acoustic (voice-onset, phonation duration) and physiological (speech breathing) parameters of speech. The computer program is available in four languages: English, German, Hebrew, and Swedish. The distributors claim that it is used by speech-language pathologists and communication disorders specialists in clinics, hospitals, schools, and universities around the world.

Examples of lesson topics in the *Dr. Fluency* program include prolonged syllables, correct breathing, gentle onsets, reducing air pressure, gentle transitions, continuous speech, and rate. Researchers who beta-tested the system pointed out that clinician supervision was essential while clients were learning these basic skills in order to prevent frustration. Once a particular skill was established, some clients could use the computer independently (Kuntz & Bakker, 1997). Because *Dr. Fluency* is based on an intensive therapy approach, a home version is available for clients to use for independent practice and maintenance.

The efficacy of both *CAFET* and *Dr. Fluency* have been established primarily by anecdotal evidence rather than research designed with ideal experimental controls. However, these self-contained, dedicated software/hardware packages represent important points in the history of clinical computing for fluency. Both programs also have limitations. Critics have suggested that some of *CAFET*'s technical specifications and measurements were absent or too crude to be reliable; *Dr. Fluency* is strongly tied to a single, intensive approach to fluency shaping that may frustrate clients unless there is sufficient clinician input and instruction (Bakker, 1999). In both cases, it may be difficult to obtain a version that is compatible with newer computers and operating systems. As an alternative to dedicated software for clients who stutter, some clinicians are using the components of a wide variety of computer-based tools (e.g., *SpeechViewer, VideoVoice, Visi-Pitch*) to address individual parameters of fluency (e.g., easy onset or modified rate), or to create speaking conditions that promote fluency (e.g., altered auditory feedback). A discussion of such applications follows.

COMPUTER-BASED FEEDBACK: ALTERNATIVES TO DEDICATED PROGRAMS FOR STUTTERING

Voice onset is frequently a clinical target for both voice and fluency clients. Assessing, monitoring, or changing voice onset behavior can be assisted using several of the tools described in Table 24.1, including *ProTrain*, *SNORS+*, *SpeechViewer III*, *Visi-Pitch II* and *III*, and *VideoVoice*. In general, these programs provide visual biofeedback to a client through real-time representation of amplitude. Whether voice onset has been jerky and abrupt or smooth and gradual is usually evident in an amplitude tracing.

Such an amplitude tracing, for example, is possible using the "Pitch and Loudness Patterning" activity of the *SpeechViewer III*, or the "Real-Time Pitch" module of the *Visi-Pitch III*. Although helpful for teens and adults, abstract shapes like line tracing may not keep a child's attention. The *SpeechViewer III* module entitled "Voice Onset" provides a game in which a graphic item of choice moves on the screen in response to the detection of voicing (e.g., a car moving a short way down the street, then stopping). For some clients, the goal might be to practice counting or making sentences with increasing numbers of syllables—in other words, seeing a response to phonation that motivates repeated phonation initiations. In contrast, for a young disfluent client, a clinician might set up this same *SpeechViewer* module differently, and use it in nearly an opposite way to promote "easy speech."

CASE EXAMPLE: Using *SpeechViewer III* to Provide Visual Feedback About Voice Onset

The *SpeechViewer III* allows the clinician to change how many voice onsets are required in order to reach the target in the "Voice Onset" module (put cursor on the target spot, hold down the left mouse button, then slide the target to the desired location, making either more or fewer responses necessary in order to reach the target). Some experimentation may be required in order to get this setting right for the client. Instead of working for speed, a disfluent client might be encouraged to work for increasing the time it takes to reach the target by avoiding a sudden or loud voice onset.

Clinician:	Watch. I'm going to use my easy speech to make the car move slowly. I'm gonna use the word "hello."
Clinician, with easy onset:	"Hello, hello, hello." [car moves slowly across screen]
Clinician:	Your turn, Chris. See if you can make the car go that slow.
Chris, with abrupt onset:	"Uh-Ello! hello!" [car jerks quickly in response to hard attack]
Chris:	Uh-oh. I-I-I went t-t-too fast, huh?
Clinician:	It's okay—try again.
Chris, with easier onset this time:	"Hello, hello" [car moves slowly two times] "Look, I-I-I did i-i-it!"
Clinician:	Yes, you did it! Let's practice some more.

COMPUTER-BASED DELAYED AUDITORY FEEDBACK

Researchers and clinicians report success in using delayed auditory feedback (DAF) for fluency therapy (Bakker, 1999a) and for slowing speaking rate in clients with a variety of speech disorders. Some approaches to fluency therapy involve establishing the experience of fluent speech under altered speaking conditions, such as DAF, speech masking, or metronomic pacing. Multiple techniques and technologies are available for implementing each of these conditions.

The *Visi-Pitch II* and *III* (Kay) systems include a DAF module. Clinicians would be unlikely to purchase the *Visi-Pitch II* primarily for this function, because there are other more portable and less expensive alternatives. However, if a *Visi-Pitch* system were available for working on other speech and voice goals, having DAF included in the same system would be convenient. For example, this would permit a quick trial of DAF with any client for whom slowed rate might be desirable, or in situations where other DAF equipment was not available. Perhaps this is the reason that the newer *Visi-Pitch III* includes not only DAF, but also masking and a metronomic pacing capabilities, all of which can be used to modify the auditory feedback received by a disfluent speaker.

One device described in Table 24.1, the *Facilitator* (Kay), is independent of a large desktop or laptop computer system. That is, the *Facilitator* is a portable, wearable, self-contained box that has no external computer parts (a smaller, less noticeable headset could be used instead of earphones).

An advantage of the *Facilitator* is its portability, which allows clients to move around and use altered speaking conditions (DAF, metronomic pacing, speech amplification, tape loop, or masking) in a variety of situations and locations. The five functions of the *Facilitator* make it a flexible clinical tool (see Table 24.2).

The *Visi-Pitch III* includes most of the *Facilitator* functions, which is useful when portability is not an issue. The *Facilitator* can be purchased with a case to be worn like a fanny pack around the waist (see Figure 24.1). It represents an early step forward in portable speech therapy technology that paved the way for future applications that may be even more portable, more flexible, and more widely available to the general public. Pocket-sized, hand-held devices such as those described in Section VI are becoming popular and affordable around the world. Soon clinical applications similar to those provided by the *Facilitator* are likely to be available for palm or hand-held computers, or even tinier formats. Already, Casa Futura Technologies offers a series of DAF and frequency altered feedback (FAF) products in small, convenient formats for office and personal use, such as the *Pocket Fluency System*. The *Pocket Fluency System* can be used with either a headset or a wireless earset. It provides DAF, FAF, and a masking (MAF) manual button that, according to the Casa Futura web site, is used to pull the user out of silent blocks.

Another case in point is the *SpeechEasy*, a device for control of stuttering developed by a team at East Carolina University. The *SpeechEasy* is worn like a hearing aid, either behind or in the ear. Through the use of DAF

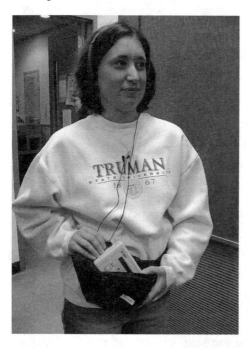

Figure 24.1. The *Facilitator* (Kay Elemetrics) can be used as a table-top or portable, wearable, therapy tool. (Courtesy of Truman State University Speech and Hearing Clinic).

Table 24.2.   Clinical applications for the *Facilitator* portable, wearable device (Kay Elemetrics)

Clinical problem	Facilitator function				
	Amplifier	Loop	DAF	Masking	Pacer
Child articulation	X	X			
Dysarthria	X	X	X	X	X
Preschool language	X	X			
Learning disabilities	X	X			X
Accent reduction	X	X		X	X
Voice disorders	X	X	X	X	
Stuttering	X		X	X	X
Aphasia	X	X		X	X
Adult right hemisphere	X	X			X
Speech/voice improvement	X	X	X	X	X

Adapted from the on-line manual Section 2, *Facilitator Model 3500, and Application Notes* by Daniel R. Boone, Ph.D.

and frequency altered feedback (FAF), *SpeechEasy* creates the illusion of another person speaking in unison with the user. According to the developers, by emulating this "choral speech" pattern, a *SpeechEasy* user can become 50%–95% more fluent.

COMPUTER-BASED FEEDBACK ABOUT RESONANCE

With regard to the computer-based assessment and treatment of resonance problems, a single product has led the way in both research and clinical settings: the *Nasometer* from Kay Elemetrics. A functional description and picture of the *Nasometer* can be found in Topic 30: Introduction to Using the Computer as a Diagnostic Tool.

While using the *Nasometer*, the client wears a headset that includes two microphones separated by a small plate. When speech is produced, the upper microphone records acoustic energy from the nasal cavity and the lower microphone records acoustic energy from the oral cavity. The computer calculates the proportion of nasal to nasal-plus-oral acoustic energy multiplied by 100 to arrive at a "nasalance" score. Nasality is the perceptual correlate of nasalance, so in theory, a higher percentage of nasalance corresponds to more nasality perceived by listeners.

On its corporate web site, Kay Elemetrics maintains an extensive bibliography of independent studies that have tested the *Nasometer* or used it as an essential instrument in documenting treatment effects. The *Nasometer* has been frequently used for diagnostic purposes and for objectively measuring the pre and post status of various treatments for velopharyngeal insufficiency, such a surgeries and oral appliances. Normative data have been collected for many languages and dialects. The *Nasometer*'s method for computing nasality has been shown to correlate well with other instrumental techniques (e.g., pressure/flow measurements, photodetection) according to the manufacturer.

As with other speech and voice analysis applications described in Section V, however, the validity and reliability of data and feedback from the *Nasometer* depends on many factors. For example, some clients with a partially repaired cleft palate or a pharyngeal flap, may produce misleading results when speaking into the *Nasometer*. The pharyngeal flap may result in the presence of both hyponasal and hypernasal elements in the speech of the patient. The nasometer averages the data, which may yield a misleading nasalance ratio, even though listeners are likely to perceive decreased nasality (Janet Gooch, personal communication, May 2003; Nellis, Neiman, & Lehman, 1992). This phenomenon illustrates why it is so important for clinicians to understand what the computer is doing/measuring in biofeedback applications. Adequate clinician involvement is an essential part of any treatment plan involving biofeedback for speech. See Topic 25 for further discussion of this issue and this example.

During treatment with the *Nasometer*, various computer-based tasks/games are available that provide real-time visual feedback to the speaker. The clinician can set a target value that the client attempts to match while speaking and monitoring the computer screen. Although some clients may balk at wearing the helmet-like headset, the *Nasometer* has been found useful with many children and adults. As described in Table 24.1, the *Nasometer* includes an external A/D conversion box similar to the *CSL* and *Visi-Pitch III* from Kay. AVAAZ, Inc. has made an alternative product available, the *OroNasal System,* which relies on standard multimedia PC hardware.

BIOFEEDBACK IN THE TREATMENT OF DYSPHAGIA

Although videofluorography is frequently used in the assessment of swallowing disorders, it has some distinct disadvantages for repeated use, as might be necessary to monitor the success of treatment. As pointed out by Katz and Hallowell, due to radiation risks, the use of repeated videofluorography is limited, and many patients may be too fragile to travel to a secondary medical site or to undergo the modified barium swallow procedure. According to these authors,

> *Fiberoptic Endoscopic Evaluation of Swallowing* (FEES), first introduced in dysphagia management in the late 1980s (Langmore, Schatz, & Olson, 1988), is quickly becoming widely used at bedside and in clinics . . . to monitor the effectiveness of specific intervention strategies during treatment. (Katz & Hallowell, 1999, p. 260)

The *Digital Swallowing Workstation* (Kay Elemetrics) includes a complete FEES unit for assessment, as well as several components especially designed for swallowing treatment. These intervention features constitute the *Swallowing Signals Lab*, which is also available as a stand-alone unit. The *Swallowing Signals Lab* includes two channels of surface electomyography (sEMG) normally used for visual feedback in teaching swallowing, a multi-channel tongue bulb array for quantifying tongue strength and symmetry as well as visual feedback in therapy, a nasal cannula channel for displaying respiratory phase, multi-channel pharyngeal/UES manometry, a laryngeal microphone, and two auxiliary channels (see Figure 24.2).

Crary and Groher presented a tutorial on the basic concepts of sEMG biofeedback in the treatment of dysphagia, to introduce clinicians to its potential. These authors concluded:

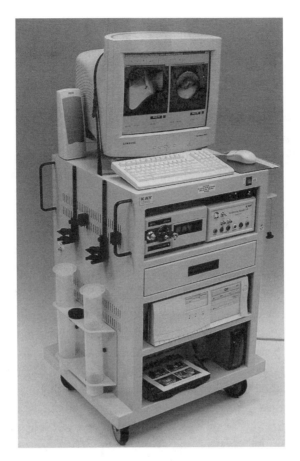

Figure 24.2. Digital swallowing station, including FEES (Courtesy of Kay Elemetrics).

We have learned through experience that some patients do better than others using this approach. For instance, those with poor laryngeal elevation secondary to radiation treatment have not responded as well as those patients with similar swallow patterns secondary to neurologic deficit. Unfortunately, we do not yet have a sufficient clinical database to make objective decisions about which patients will benefit most from the applications of this sEMG-assisted treatment approach. Our initial clinical impressions are that patients with sufficient cognitive status to understand the technique, adequate sensory and motor abilities enabling interaction with the technology, and a reasonable prognosis for improvement in impaired pharyngeal components of swallowing will have the best chance for success using this approach. We are encouraged to see that even patients with chronic dysphagia requiring long-term gastronomy feedings are able to return to oral food ingestion using sEMG biofeedback-assisted treatment. (2000, p. 124)

Thus researchers have documented the positive effect of combining biofeedback with behavioral techniques to facilitate swallowing (Crary, 1995; Logemann & Kahrilas, 1990). Equipment such as the *Swallowing Signals Lab* provide clinicians with objective information and provide patients with real-time visual feedback about their swallowing behavior. Clinical observations of improvement over time, therefore, can now be supported with data, but without the risk of repeated radiation exposure.

Crary and Groher (2000) cautioned clinicians not to be over-reliant on sEMG biofeedback as a primary treatment approach. These researchers urged clinicians to obtain appropriate training, to become aware of technical issues that may limit success of sEMG with particular patients, and to develop a comprehensive swallowing treatment plan for each individual. sEMG biofeedback, then, would be introduced specifically to "facilitate enhanced learning of novel or difficult-to-monitor swallowing movements" (p. 124).

SUMMARY

Many computer-based tools are available for addressing goals associated with disorders of fluency, resonance, and swallowing. It may be difficult to find a dedicated program for stuttering therapy compatible with the latest generation of personal computers. Several programs that provide visual biofeedback about voice amplitude can be used to help clients monitor voice onset and sustaining phonation, which are frequent goals in therapy for fluency disorders. In addition, computers can be used to modify auditory feedback about the speaker's own speech, including masking, delayed auditory feedback, or timing cues. Modified auditory feedback may enhance fluency in some speakers.

The *Nasometer* from Kay Elemetrics has dominated the area of computer-based applications for assessment and treatment of resonance disorders. A large body of independent research has documented the strengths and limitations of the *Nasometer*, which calculates a physical measure called "nasalance." In most cases, nasalance correlates well with human perceptions of nasality.

The use of biofeedback in the treatment of swallowing disorders is becoming more popular. Sophisticated, portable tools for bedside swallow evaluation and treatment are available for use by clinicians with appropriate training. Preliminary research suggests that even chronic dysphagic clients may respond positively to sEMG biofeedback if they have other important characteristics and skills.

REVIEW FOR TOPIC 24

1. Name one computer-based product dedicated to fluency, resonance, and swallowing.
2. List three specific speech/voice parameters related to fluency that can be monitored with computer-based biofeedback.
3. List three ways that computers can modify auditory feedback about a person's speech.
4. What is *nasalance*?
5. What does the abbreviation *sEMG* stand for?

QUESTIONS FOR DISCUSSION

1. Consider the features and uses of the *Facilitator* outlined in Table 24.2. Which of these possibilities sounds most interesting and useful to you, and why?

2. Explain why it is important for clinicians using biofeedback with clients having difficulty with resonance or swallowing to be familiar with existing efficacy research.

RESOURCES FOR FURTHER STUDY

Bakker, K. (1999). Clinical technologies for the reduction of stuttering and enhancement of speech fluency. *Seminars in Speech and Language, 20*(3), 271–280.

Blood, G. (1995). A behavioral-cognitive therapy program for adults who stutter: Computers and counseling. *Journal of Communication Disorders, 28*, 165–180.

Crary, M.A., & Groher, M.E. (2000). Basic concepts of surface electromyographic biofeedback in the treatment of dysphagia: A tutorial. *American Journal of Speech-Language Pathology, 9*, 116–125.

Katz, R.C., & Hallowell, B. (1999). Technological applications in the treatment of acquired neurogenic communication and swallowing disorders in adults. *Seminars in Speech and Language, 20*, 251–269.

Human Perceptions Versus Computer-Based Feedback

Clinical computing competency #4: The clinician will demonstrate the ability to plan and implement activities in which performance feedback to the client from the clinician is supplemented by feedback (visual and/or auditory) from the computer.

What happens when the client speaks into the microphone and feedback from the computer is incorrect? Have available computer-based speech therapy tools been developed on the basis of sound theories and confirmed best practices? How do computer judgments and human perceptions of a person's speech compare? Are available tools accurate and reliable enough to be effectively used independently by clients? Competent clinicians should be aware of the ongoing attempts to improve such tools as well as the issues and controversies surrounding the use of computer-based feedback in speech/voice/swallowing therapy.

People often expect computers to be more accurate and reliable than humans, and for some purposes—such as mathematical calculations—they usually are. It's a mistake, however, to attribute such infallibility to every possible function of a computer. Clinicians should be aware that many factors affect the validity and reliability of feedback produced by computer-based tools. This topic outlines criteria that could be used to evaluate such tools, summarizes research that compares human judgments to computer-based speech analysis, and suggests how clinicians can optimize the dependability of the computer-based tools that they use. The heart of the message is simple: Although some computer-based tools are excellent, the human ear is better. When evaluating a client's performance, clinicians should rely on their own perceptions and not assume that the computer is right.

The advances that have been made in the area of computer-assisted speech therapy and computer-based feedback systems are impressive. However, not all tools are developed and updated with the same level of professional expertise, and not all tools do what they claim to do. When a test actually assesses what it claims to assess, it is said to have good "validity." Likewise, valid computer tools do what they claim to do. Valid tools for speech therapy measure what they say they measure, yield data and feedback that are accurate, and agree with other dependable sources, such as clinician judgments.

In addition to validity, reliability must be present if clients are going to receive consistent information about their speech. Tests or tools are reliable if similar results occur consistently in response to similar circumstances. It could be argued that some clinicians may not be as reliable as they would like to be when it comes to judging client behaviors such as articulation productions (Axmear & Poeschel, 2001). Reliability requires that two productions that are similar in quality are judged similarly by the clinician or clinicians.

Because clinicians are subject to human frailties such as fatigue and distraction, they are not perfectly reliable. Although computers are not vulnerable to the same weaknesses, their reliability and accuracy depends on a whole range of other factors unlikely to affect a human clinician. These factors must be taken into account even during supervised therapy, and especially prior to consideration of independent practice with a computer "judging" client performance.

DESIGN FACTORS THAT INFLUENCE VALIDITY AND RELIABILITY

Watson and Kewley-Port (1989) described four design parameters by which computer-assisted speech training or feedback systems could be judged and compared. Their observations and suggestions have held up well, in spite of dramatic changes in computer technology. Consideration of these factors may be useful to clinicians trying to better understand their clinical computing tools and how their clients may respond. These factors may also be useful for reviewing various systems for purchase and for designing new systems in the future.

Physical Source of Feedback

Does the system base feedback about a person's speech production on electrophysiological signals, articulatory or swallowing movements, or the acoustic waveform produced? A wide range of articulatory movements may result in acoustic signals that humans would judge to be adequate or "normal" for intelligibility purposes. In other words, there are a lot of ways to produce a phoneme that "sounds" right. So, should feedback to a client be based on the sound (acoustic waveform) or how the sound was articulated? Watson and Kewley-Port (1989) acknowledged that for some populations, feedback based on the actual movement of articulators has been shown to be useful. Such populations include persons with cerebral palsy or adults learning a second language. On the whole, however, they favor the use of the resulting acoustical waveform as the basis for articulation feedback. "The validity of the acoustic waveform of speech as a final criterion for speech production, its relative ease of measurement, and the considerable body of literature on the recognition of speech waveforms favor this physical dimension over the other two" (p. 36).

Clinical Implications

When using a feedback system that bases feedback on the acoustic waveform produced by the client, the clinician must be responsible for monitoring and correcting important articulatory mistakes or bad habits. For example, say a client with a lisp uses computer-based visual feedback to create an /s/ that is reinforced by the computer. The clinician notices, however, that the client is still using less than ideal placement, with the tongue still slightly protruding. The computer will not know this, and so stabilization of /s/ or generalization to other sounds may be compromised unless the clinician corrects the client's articulatory placement.

Standards of Evaluation

What criterion is used by the computer to judge the accuracy/acceptability of the speaker's production? (Does it compare the production to a previously stored model file, to a predetermined ideal for the person's age and gender, or to the clinician's speech?) Watson and Kewley-Port (1989) pointed out that it is common practice for clinicians doing traditional therapy to change their criteria for what is considered to be a "correct" response, as the client's behavior improves. A successive approximation approach (e.g., that's better) is usually employed during therapy, rather than an absolute standard (e.g, that's right/that's wrong). This is consistent with commercial computer-based speech training tools that require users to record and store a "best effort" model against which later productions are compared for "goodness of fit." As skills improve, model files can be upgraded.

Alternatively, an "ideal standard" could be employed by some systems. Advantages of this approach include not losing the time it takes to acquire a suitable client-generated model and the fact that in the initial phases of therapy when computer-based feedback may be the most useful, the client may not be capable of producing an acceptable model. However, early in training, a client's "productions may be so distant from the normative standard that it is difficult to determine whether small changes in his or her speech represent a movement toward the standard or away from it" (p. 35). This can be a source of error that affects the validity and reliability of feedback to the client.

Clinical Implications

It is important for the clinician to understand what standard for performance the computer is using when feedback is provided to a client. Most currently available tools for computer-based articulation training, for example, require the clinician to create a model file using her own speech, the client's best effort, or the speech of a peer. However, some products include default model files that clinicians continue to use without realizing the consequences. Clearly, the validity of feedback from the computer will depend enormously on the quality and appropriateness of the model file.

Type and Level of Detail Reflected in Feedback

How much detailed information is included in the feedback provided? Is more information helpful or distracting for a client? For example, much detail about the speech act is included in a spectrogram, and much less by a line tracing representing pitch and/or amplitude. The type of feedback could be strictly informational, as when a contour on the computer display goes up or down as the client's pitch changes. Alternatively, the feedback could be more evaluative as when a target is or is not reached, a cartoon graphic does or does not move, or a model is or is not matched on the computer display.

Clinical Implications

Much of the research that has confirmed the efficacy of biofeedback in speech, voice, and swallowing therapy has involved complex feedback from complex tools, such as speech spectrography (Ruscello, 1995; Shuster, Ruscello, & Toth, 1995), electropalatography (Dagenais, 1995), nasoendoscopy (Case, 1999), and surface electomyography (Crary & Groher, 2000). Many working clinicians are more likely to have access to less complex, less expensive, and less fragile tools in their clinics and schools. These tools may provide simple or complex responses to client input. Will the feedback from such tools be as effective as has been demonstrated in research contexts? Some clients will be stressed by feedback that always sets a standard to be reached (e.g., matching a model, hitting a target value), and others will be motivated by such apparent goals. Although user–computer interface and feedback is the subject of intensive research in technology circles, this research has yet to be widely applied to speech or language therapy applications. The single exception that comes to mind is the early discovery that negative consequences (buzzers, gremlins, groans) were so entertaining to some children that they would deliberately answer incorrectly when using CAI. That software designers took this to heart is apparent in the no-response or minimal feedback consequences for wrong answers that is often seen in today's instructional software. So far, we know little about the exact types and levels of biofeedback or other feedback that are most useful for particular types of clients. Clinicians should watch out for new findings in this regard; meanwhile, it may be useful to try various types and levels of computer-based feedback with clients to obtain a good match.

Form and Content of Feedback

Does the form of the feedback consist of a moving cartoon, a single dot, or a line tracing? Does the content of the feedback depend on a clinician or teacher for interpretation, or is it intended for a client's independent comprehension and use?

Clinical Implications

Clinicians will have to consider the form and content of feedback their tools provide their clients and whether or not a good match is possible. For some clients, extremely simplified visual feedback may be ideal, and for some, it may be confusing. For some children, a game-like interface will be compelling and effective, and for some children it will merely distract them from the important focus of therapy. To date, there is little guidance in the literature regarding this important aspect of feedback design.

RESEARCH FINDINGS AND CLINICAL EXAMPLES

Reviews and descriptions of pioneering computer-based speech training systems have been published elsewhere (see, e.g., Nickerson, Kalikow, & Stevens, 1976; Watson & Kewley-Port, 1989). In this section, the purpose is to present examples of research that have attempted to systematically compare the feedback or measurements produced by computer-based speech tools to the perceptions and judgments of human listeners.

Interestingly, Fitch (1989) and Watson, Reed, Kewley-Port, and Maki (1989) were comparing human judgments of speech accuracy to those of two different computer-based therapy programs at about the same time. Their results, however, were strikingly different. Fitch (1989) evaluated *Computer-Aided Speech Production and Training* (CASPT), which was developed by Cooper and Neilson (1986). It is no longer a commercial product. *CASPT* was marketed as an articulation and phonology practice program designed for use by children or adults, with or without clinician supervision. *CASPT* used a speech recognition paradigm in which the users "trained" the computer to recognize their own models of the target sounds. Once model files were established, in theory, independent practice could begin. The clinician could set the degree to which an individual production would have to match the model file to be counted correct by the computer. In Fitch's study of normal speech, the "very demanding" level was used. Six young adults and six school-age children with normal speech served as subjects. After following the computer training procedures, they produced target phonemes from four groups of sounds, including fricatives, plosives, and liquids/glides. Unfortunately, the results showed poor performance on the part of *CASPT* for recognizing the correct productions of these speakers who had no articulation deficits. In conditions that should have resulted in 100% correct recognition according to native speakers' perceptions, most sounds were discriminated by the computer program correctly in only 20%–40% of trials, with the highest correct discrimination being 62% (for the sound /j/).

The same year, Watson et al. (1989) took a distinctly different approach to comparing computer and human judgments of articulation. Over several years, this Indiana University research team developed and evaluated the *Indiana Speech Training Aid* (ISTRA), which is still available for purchase (see Table 23.1). The purpose of the 1989 study was to determine whether "computer-based, speaker-dependent evaluations of individual utterances might be considered as a reasonable alternative to human judgments normally used as feedback in clinical speech drills" (p. 250). "Speaker dependent" means the computer was comparing input from a known speaker to templates created by that speaker. Stimuli for the study were provided by three adults with normal speech who were asked to say selected three-syllable words with normal articulation and with deliberately distorted speech (clear, medium-clear, medium-distorted, very distorted). The same targets were elicited from a 9-year-old with moderate to severe sensorineural hearing loss.

The taped speech samples were rated by the speech recognition component of *ISTRA* and by two groups of people: naive listeners (untrained) and expert listeners (certified SLPs). The correlation results from this data were extensive and not easy to interpret. In general, results indicated that the human judges were slightly more accurate than the computer in judging various levels of distortion, but that the computer was more reliable. Although the authors expressed some concern about the lower accuracy obtained by the computer, especially when rating the speech of the child with hearing impairment, they concluded that the advantages (such as reliability and record keeping) were worth the disadvantages during supervised use of computer-based feedback during speech therapy. They also cautioned, however, that "Unless carefully collected data support the substitution of computer-based feedback for human judgments, the [independent] use of such systems clearly might do more harm than good" (p. 251).

A third example of research comparing computer judgments to human judgments of speech adequacy illustrates the role that specific client characteristics may play in whether or not computer-based feedback is valid or reliable. Nellis, Neiman, and Lehman (1992) compared human listener's perceptions of nasality to nasalance measurements obtained from the *Nasometer* (Kay Elemetrics). The subjects of the study were 16 patients with velopharyngeal insufficiency who had had pharyngeal flap surgery. They ranged from 8 to 18 years of age and had an overall speech intelligibility rating of "good." They were asked to repeat seven sentences three times each. Listeners included 10 trained graduate students in speech-language pathology. Listeners rated each sentence production for the presence of hypernasality and hyponasality on 6-point scales.

Recall that the *Nasometer* is often used to obtain objective data for the purpose of documenting nasality before and after treatment. It is also used to provide biofeedback in treatment when it is suspected that the client may need to practice making better use of the oral mechanism in order to reduce nasality. Since "nasality" is a perceptual characteristic, the *Nasometer* cannot measure it directly. Instead, as the subject speaks, it compares energy from the oral and nasal cavities to calculate a measure called "nasalance."(See Topics 24 and 30 for more information.) Nellis et al. found that the presence of a pharyngeal flap may have interfered with the accuracy of data produced by the *Nasometer*. It is hypothesized that the flap partially obstructed airflow and energy coming from the oral cavity, which likely distorted the calculation of nasalance. In addition, the authors stated, human listeners may have had difficulty with rating both hypernasality and hyponasality in the same sentences. As a result, "For all sentences, the correlations between [human] ratings of hypernasality and nasalance scores and between [human] ratings of hypernasality and hyponasality failed to reach significance" (p. 159).

Volin (1998) considered the notion that individual characteristics may cause people to be selectively responsive to computer-based feedback (1998). In a study of 36 young adults without communication disorders, Volin examined the relationship between task stimulability and the efficacy of visual biofeedback. Subjects were taught a respiratory control task, using the respiration biofeedback component of *CAFET* (see Topic 24 for a description of *CAFET*). Volin found that biofeedback was most effective at helping those who had relatively poor response to initial training (stimulability), that verbal guidance and biofeedback were equally effective for those with midrange stimulability, and that subjects with relatively high stimulability did not benefit from biofeedback. This is the kind of information that has yet to be confirmed regarding most clinical populations. (Recall design factor three, regarding the type and level of feedback provided and how little is known about the relationship between these factors and specific client attributes.)

In summary, researchers have taken various approaches to comparing human perceptions of speech adequacy to computer-based judgments. Other research (summarized in Topics 21–24) documented the fact that computer-based feedback systems may be quite effective during therapy, under the supervision of qualified professionals. Much research remains to be done regarding the interaction of feedback design factors and client characteristics. As yet, the high levels of accuracy (validity) that one would hope for in a feedback tool used for guiding a client independently through speech therapy exercises has not been confirmed in the published literature.

IMPLICATIONS FOR INDEPENDENT USE

The effort of many to make speech "visible" for people with hearing impairment has been a well-documented quest (e.g., Bernstein, Goldstein, & Mahshie, 1988). Many attempts have been made to design and implement a device that would provide a person with a speech problem a way to practice and improve speech production independently. This was the goal behind impressive pioneer work in the development of computer-based feedback programs for speech and voice, such as that of Arthur Boothroyd and his colleagues (Boothroyd, Archambault, Adams, & Storm, 1975) and the team from Bolt Beranek and Newman, Inc. (Nickerson, Kalikow, & Stevens, 1976). In the mid- to late 1970s, Boothroyd's team evaluated the use of self-instruction sessions using computer-based speech training with children at the Clarke School for the Deaf. They were pleased with student effort and motivation, but also observed problems such as "the difficulty of preparing sufficiently extensive and carefully graded exercises" and "the tendency for the students to develop bad speech habits unrelated to the specific skill involved in the drill. A live tutor would immediately spot the error and attempt to correct it. The computer system provided no feedback about features not involved in the exercise" (Boothroyd et al., 1975, p. 190). Nevertheless, they remained committed to the notion that "unsupervised drill has much to recommend it" (p. 190).

Currently, whether a particular computer-based feedback or speech training system is appropriate for independent use by a particular client will have to be determined on a case-by-case basis by clinicians. They will consider the design of the computer system, its apparent accuracy and reliability, and the individual characteristics of the client. Competent clinicians will be cautious about believing manufacturer claims regarding independent use, unless research from disinterested parties backs up such claims.

WHAT CLINICIANS CAN DO TO ENHANCE THE EFFICACY OF COMPUTER-BASED FEEDBACK TOOLS DURING THERAPY

The following list details some of the things clinicians can do to ensure that feedback tools meet the needs of their clients.

- Choose the best quality computer-based feedback system that budget constraints will permit, including good quality peripherals (mic, speakers)
- Become familiar with program settings and how to personalize them for individual clients
- Learn and use the recommended microphone placement
- Monitor the environmental conditions (noise, glare)
- Choose appropriate goals and tasks for therapy that lend themselves to computer-based feedback

- When choosing goals for computer feedback activities, consider the attributes of the client such as vision, stimulability, cognitive status, and oral mechanism characteristics that may limit success

- Give clear instructions and demonstrate what the client should do, using the computer if possible

- Help the client focus on the computer feedback; don't compete by drawing the client's attention away from the monitor too often

- Create and reinforce a positive client attitude

- Believe the perceptions of human speakers, especially trained clinicians, over the judgments of any computer

- If the computer's response or feedback to the client is not accurate, adjust settings and try again or discontinue use

SUMMARY

From the beginnings of computer-based feedback and training in the field, there has been keen interest in developing a system that clients could use independently to improve speech skills. In many ways, this interest has paralleled the notion in educational technology of replacing teachers with computers. Just as in education, however, replacing a professional with a computer has turned out to be more challenging than developers expected. Many factors affect the validity and reliability of the feedback provided by computer tools, some related to design and some related to implementation during therapy. When there is lack of agreement between computer judgments and human listeners, clinicians should always trust their own perceptions over what the computer reports.

Having clients use computers for independent speech or voice therapy is not just a matter of replacing the clinician's "ear" with an accurate speech recognition system; it's also a matter of substituting a computer for the clinician's experience, intuitions, expertise, and flexibility. As discussed in Section II, there is scant research indicating that this has been successfully accomplished with any clinical software to date, including computer-based feedback systems. There are, however, many actions that clinicians can take to optimize the success of computer-based feedback systems used in therapy.

REVIEW FOR TOPIC 25

1. Although some computer-based feedback tools are excellent, the human ear is _____.
2. When the same results are obtained over and over again, an instrument or procedure is said to be _____.
3. When an instrument or procedure measures what it claims to measure, it is said to be _____.
4. List 4 design factors that influence the validity, reliability, and client reaction to computer-based feedback.
5. List 5 actions clinicians can take in the implementation of computer-based feedback to optimize its potential for a client.

QUESTIONS FOR DISCUSSION

1. When a client speaks into a microphone attached to a computer-based feedback program for speech or voice, and the computer's response does not seem right to the clinician, what should the clinician do?
2. What are the arguments for or against independent client use of computer-based feedback tools?

RESOURCES FOR FURTHER STUDY

Kewley-Port, D. (1994). Speech technology and speech training for the hearing impaired. *The Journal of the Academy of Rehabilitative Audiology (Monograph), XXVII,* 251–265.

McGuire, R.A. (1995). Computer-based instrumentation: Issues in clinical applications. *Language, Hearing, Speech Services in Schools, 26*(3), 223–231.

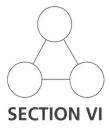

SECTION VI

Getting Connected

Telepractice, the Internet, and PDAs

Introduction to Telepractice and Using the Internet in Clinical Practice

Clinical computing competency #9: The clinician will demonstrate awareness of resources that provide continuing education, research results, technical support and information about availability, funding, efficacy, and efficiency of new clinical computing products as well as assistive technology devices and services.

The Internet has opened a new world of resources for professionals in every field, including communication disorders. At present, we have barely begun to recognize the potential changes in professional education, consumer education, and clinical practice that may eventually result from the "information highway." The possibilities are exciting and extensive. Competent clinicians should be knowledgeable about the concept of telepractice and the use of the Internet for a variety of professional purposes.

Section VI introduces several topics related to the central idea of using technology to be more connected to clients, fellow professionals, a central work place, and professional resources. New technologies continue to make it easier and less costly for clinicians to have uninterrupted access to the Internet, e-mail, discussion groups, and phone service. Wireless options are eliminating the previous barriers created by the need to retro-fit older buildings with the cabling necessary to provide high speed Internet access. The increased power and affordability of handheld computers are keeping access at the fingertips of itinerant clinicians or of those who may be providing most of their services within the confines of a client's bedside. There is increased professional attention on the capabilities of electronic communication (audio, video, data, text) and how these capabilities might be used to enhance health care services. A new patient–caregiver dynamic in communication disorders—telepractice—has resulted.

What are the clinical implications of clinicians "getting connected?" No one knows yet, but most in the field agree that the impact is going to be deep and wide (Tanner,

2001; Wynne, 2001). One thing is certain, however. The rapid changes in technology may impact how services are delivered, but many of the principles of good practice and effective use of computer-based activities will remain essentially the same. In other words, clinicians who have developed competencies using computers face-to-face with clients will be in a much better position than those who have not, to implement and assess the remote use of new clinical applications. Topic 26 provides a taste of what is here and what is coming.

WHAT IS TELEPRACTICE?

Telepractice and the advanced use of web-based technology were declared a focused initiative of the American Speech-Language-Hearing Association for 2001–2003. Several special projects and efforts were put into place as part of the Association's concentration on this topic. These efforts included major reorganization and enhancements to ASHA's web page for professionals, consumers, and students. In addition, a report on the current state of telepractice in our field was developed and disseminated via ASHA's web site (the actual URL for this report changes, but it can be found by searching ASHA's web site with the keyword "telepractice"). New practice policy documents were approved by ASHA in March 2004 on "SLPs Providing Clinical Services via Telepractice" and "Audiologists Providing Clinical Services via Telepractice." These documents are available to members on the ASHA web site and address issues such as client eligibility and outcomes, knowledge and skills for clinicians, ethics, licensure, liability, and reimbursement. *Telepractice* is an umbrella term used to include many clinical and educational activities. ASHA uses the following definition:

> *Telepractice* may be defined as the application of technology to deliver health services at a distance by linking clinician and patient or clinician and clinician to provide any or all of the following: 1) training, counseling, education; 2) assessment—establishing patient status; 3) intervention—treatment/ management, and to provide remote support and training of practitioners. (http://www.asha.org/members/issues/telepractice/tele_background.htm)

Note that ASHA's definition uses the term *technology* rather than *computers*. Computers may or may not be involved in telepractice. For example, a system that provides a video link between a clinician in a hospital and a patient in a remote clinic may not involve users at either end in any computer-based activity. However, many if not all of the uses of the Internet by clinicians for professional purposes could be encompassed by ASHA's definition.

Important related terms include *telehealth* and *telemedicine*. Telemedicine came first and referred strictly to activities of physicians using advanced technology to provide care for patients at a distance. The concept and definition was expanded in the late 1990s with the term telehealth. Telehealth covers the services provided by all health care providers, including speech-language pathologists and audiologists. These terms, in addition to the professional communication and education functions in the definition above, are all subsumed within the larger concept of telepractice (Telepractice and ASHA: Report of the Telepractices Team, December, 2001).

ON-LINE CLINICAL APPLICATIONS
FOR ASSESSMENT AND INTERVENTION

Already, clinical applications for on-line assessment and intervention of speech and language behavior are appearing on the Internet. Parrot Software Company, for example, has offered a wide selection of communication disorders software to clinicians since the early 1980s. Parrot has specialized in producing primarily drill-and-practice software for adults with aphasia or cognitive impairment. Although Parrot sends catalogs to clinicians and exhibits products at some professional conferences, for a few years now they have also marketed software directly to patients/consumers through their web site.

Parrot gives general consumers the opportunity to "subscribe" to their on-line software collection for a monthly fee. The Parrot web site points out that often medical insurance coverage for speech-language therapy is exhausted long before a patient stops benefiting from services. They encourage consumers to plan for this eventuality by consulting with their clinicians about which of their programs to use and then subscribing to Parrot software as a supplement or continuation of therapy services. No clinician input is required, before or after subscribing. Much like a cable television company might, Parrot provides unlimited use of the software by one person or household in return for the monthly fee. In case no clinician is available to make software recommendations, Parrot offers consumers a free, downloadable "Parrot Diagnostic Kit" that presents a few exercise items across four categories (word recall, cognitive reasoning, vocabulary, and memory). After each set of items is answered, a list of recommended Parrot programs is presented.

Obviously, clinicians who are asked by clients to make recommendations regarding unsupervised on-line therapy activities are put in a difficult situation. This difficulty would be compounded if the clinician was also unfamiliar with the general type of application (in this case, CAI) or factors that should be considered when choosing and implementing such applications (as presented for CAI in Section II). Parrot's direct marketing strategy is just the beginning of what is to come in the area of online assessment and intervention.

A glance at the future is provided on the web site of Beyond Speech Therapy, Inc. This company markets a web-based client management, client–clinician communication and clinician–clinician communication package of the sort that is likely to proliferate as telepractice via computer with clients becomes more common. They claim an "innovative," individualized assessment and treatment protocol delivered online for aphasia, apraxia, dysphagia, dysarthria, and head injury. Aphasia treatment examples provided on their web site, however, included name-the-object line drawings and other drill-and-practice tasks similar to the most basic worksheets and software programs for adult CAI. No information or research references regarding the rationale behind the available therapy modules were available on the web site.

This kind of package illustrates perfectly why clinicians need to have 1) excellent clinical skills and 2) underlying clinical computing competencies. Clinicians need this foundation if they are to make appropriate recommendations and choices when it comes to Internet-delivered assessment and intervention activities and services. Clinicians should be standing up to question the efficacy of Internet-based treatment that is offered in the absence of new research, rationale, or historical evidence of efficacy. Poorly conceived drill-and-practice is unlikely to be any more effective delivered over the Internet than it is when delivered by a live clinician or a worksheet. Unfortunately, many clinicians remain unaware of how much more computers can do. Now and in the future, technology may facilitate self-assessment and treatment in the absence of a qualified clinician, or with minimal consultation. If, however, clinicians show themselves to be competent at identifying and recommending appropriate computer-based therapy activities, their expertise is much more likely to be sought after and paid for.

USING TECHNOLOGY TO PROVIDE
CLINICAL SERVICES AND SUPERVISION REMOTELY

Videoconferencing can be accomplished via computers and the Internet, or via cameras and receivers arranged in two or more separate locations, as is commonly done in distance education facilities. In either case, potentially, persons on both ends can see and hear each other in real time, much like a video phone call. The quality and synchronization of the picture and sound that are transmitted and received are affected by multiple variables. Clinicians who are considering designing or implementing a telepractice project for the purpose of providing services to remote clients are strongly urged to seek professional consultation and inform themselves about state-of-the-art equipment, protocols, legal and ethical considerations, and the challenges that have been encountered and overcome by pioneers in this effort. A good starting point for becoming aware of issues and resources is the ASHA web site.

Many clinicians and agencies are implementing some activities that fall under the wide umbrella of telepractice, including e-mail with clients, on-line support groups for clients and families, and various professional education activities. According to the ASHA 2002 Omnibus Survey results, however, there are still relatively few clinicians who report providing services "via telepractice" (ASHA, 2002). Some clinicians may view the notion of "remote" assessment or intervention as a possible violation of the ASHA Code of Ethics. Although the Code of Ethics has recently been revised to accommodate telepractice wherever it is legal, the ethical concerns about telepractice are still many. Some of these issues are raised in Topic 30.

Two pioneering examples that demonstrate some of the positive potential of simultaneous sound and video setups include a remote video-based clinical supervision project at the University of Virginia and the use of a telehealth network to provide fluency therapy in rural northern Canada. At the University of Virginia, two-way video transmission is used to provide clinical supervision for graduate student clinicians working in public schools.

At the beginning of each practicum period, the student is given use of a standalone videoconferencing unit and portable television. The television serves as a monitor and allows viewing between the two locations. Since transmission of the audio-video data occurs over the Internet, it is necessary for students to have Internet access in the room in which they are providing clinical services. With the equipment in place, the supervisor observes the session with full capabilities for adjusting the view and focus of the camera. The supervisor can interact with the student at any time. After the session is complete and the client is no longer present, the supervisor and student discuss the session. (Dudding & Purcell-Robertson, 2003, p. 7)

The administrative advantages of such a system include making a broader range of clinical practicum sites available to students and conserving supervisor time and travel expenses.

The Institute for Stuttering Treatment and Research (ISTAR) at the University of Alberta, Canada, has been working with clients who live in remote areas. There are places in northern Canada where access to speech-language pathology services is extremely limited and distances are too far to seek regular treatment at the ISTAR clinic (Day, 2001). ISTAR uses the university's telehealth network that provides two-way video/audio communication. For example, program director Deborah Kully reported on the successful case of a 10-year-old boy who was seeking help for fluency problems. The ISTAR clinician and boy met regularly via a simultaneous sound and video connection. A parent was present for each session and sometimes a sibling, as direct training in both fluency enhancement and stuttering management was provided. Systems like this make it possible to provide follow-up services as well as ongoing monitoring of client progress, without causing the client the inconvenience, discomfort, or expense of a lengthy trip to a clinic or rehab facility.

Many Internet sites provide materials or activities that clinicians can use directly with clients in several ways. These sites are not intended to substitute for face-to-face intervention, but rather to provide clinicians, teachers, and families with learning materials and activities related to various content areas. For example, there are many excellent sites related to literacy skills for people of all ages. At *Book Adventure* (www .bookadventure.com), for example, site visitors can check the reading level of popular children's books, get tips for helping a child choose a book to read, and obtain lists of children's books by theme/topic and reading level. The National Geographic site for kids (www.nationalgeographic.com/kids/) offers endless activities, experiments, and games related to nature and world cultures. For adolescents and adults, popular TV games' web sites often provide on-line playable versions. Clinicians can make use of such sites to spark new therapy activity ideas or for real-time therapy activities if Internet access is available during therapy.

USING THE INTERNET FOR PROFESSIONAL EDUCATION AND INFORMATION

On-line universities and degree programs are appearing daily, and new techniques for providing continuing education are being developed with Internet resources in mind. ASHA offers Internet-based continuing education opportunities, which are outlined in the professional section of ASHA's web site at www.asha.org. But clinicians' immediate needs for information and resources can be addressed through Internet access in ways that are less structured than a formal course or event. Clinicians use the Internet to look for information or extend their expertise on their own.

On-line library resources and electronic databases for journal publications have become efficient and sophisticated. Clinicians needing a review of the literature on a topic or the latest research findings should consider visiting a local university library and asking a reference librarian for a quick lesson. The extent of resources and full-text articles that are now available on line will astound anyone who has been out of school for more than a couple of years. Typically, more resources are available to users in the library or who have university library privileges. But the general public has amazing access as well. For example, a free searchable ERIC web site is available at http://askeric.org/Eric/. ERIC is a government-sponsored index and repository of education research and related areas (child development, child disorders, special education, educational technology, speech, language, and hearing development and disorders, etc.). ASHA members have access to full-text articles published in ASHA journals through the ASHA web site. For instance, beginning with Volume 8, February 1999, full-text versions of articles published in the *American Journal of Speech-Language Pathology* are available on line.

Searching for current information in books and journals can be overwhelming in part because electronic databases make so many possibilities available. Much of the time, users must sort out the few perfectly matched sources of interest from dozens that are barely relevant or not related at all to communication disorders. The *ComDis Dome* (ContentScan, Inc.) is a commercial attempt to address this challenge and make access to communication disorders resources more specific and efficient for researchers, students, and clinicians. The *Dome* gives users searchable access to books, journal articles, dissertations, authors, institutions, and web resources, all related to communication disorders. Often more detailed information is available than might be found in other databases. For example, for many books listed in the *Dome,* users can review the complete table of contents, topic index, or reference lists. Purchasing a book is also conveniently accomplished through the web site, which is a for-profit, subscription-sponsored service (http://www.comdisdome.com/).

Jumpstations are web sites that are basically collections of links to other sites—they are like network hubs focused on a certain topic. It can save a lot of search time if a jumpstation on the desired topic can be identified (e.g., communication disorders, stuttering), in lieu of searching for one single resource after another. Using a jumpstation is usually a more efficient and sophisticated approach to getting specialized information and identifying resources than typing a keyword into the typical search engine.

Judith Kuster is well-known for her regular column about the Internet for the *Asha Leader*, and hers is by far the best known and most used "jumpstation" for communication disorders (see the URL at the end of this topic). Note that this site is primarily a collection of links to other sites—most of the content doesn't actually live here. For this reason, clinicians should take care when quoting or referencing materials obtained through Kuster's site. Rarely is her site what should be cited, because the jumpstation was just the route taken on the way to obtaining the information, not the true source. The search that began with Kuster's site most likely ended in an entirely different site. Clinicians should look for and cite the actual location or URL for the material they are using. At any given moment, the URL for the active window or site is listed at the top of the web browser, with http: in front of it.

Web resources that clinicians can use to enhance their practice include new research findings, review materials (phonetics, anatomy, grammar, sign language), computer utilities (phonetic alphabet fonts, sign language, or non-English dictionaries), disorders sites, commercial product sites and product reviews. A brief sampling of the kinds of professional information resources available on the web is presented in Table 26.1.

An innovation in web site design is appearing, in which the functions of professional education and research are combined. Researchers Truman Coggins and Lesley Olswang at the University of Washington are the primary authors of a web site about social communication (http://depts.washington.edu/soccomm/). The site includes content such as definitions, assessment guidelines, and characteristics of people exhibiting social communication problems. In addition, there are several questionnaires throughout the site, designed for caregivers or clinicians to complete. The purpose of the questionnaires, according to the web site directions, is to help provide data for further research on social communication problems in school-age children. In this way, caregivers and clinicians have the opportunity to contribute their experiences and observational expertise back into the research effort, at the same time as they and their clients benefit from access to the latest research findings.

A word of warning is appropriate regarding the difference between information obtained from a public web site and information from peer-reviewed research sources (research journals) or sites sponsored by known professional organizations (ASHA, NIH, APA). Anyone can put anything on the Internet. For the most part, no one checks to see if the information people post on web sites is accurate or substantiated. If information from the Internet is being used to guide clinical decisions or professional activities, clinicians should ensure that the source of the information is indeed expert and legitimate.

Table 26.1. Examples of professional information resources available on the web

Topic/Title	URL (Universal resource locator)=web address
Common Diseases of the External and Middle Ear Study Guide	http://www.bcm.tmc.edu/oto/studs/midear.htm
Citing Internet resources using APA style	http://www.bedfordstmartins.com/online/cite6.html
Guide for Writing Research Papers (APA Frequently Asked Questions)	http://webster.commnet.edu/apa/apa_intro.htm
Nervous System Diseases	http://www.mic.ki.se/Diseases/c10.html
Whole Brain Atlas	http://www.med.harvard.edu/AANLIB/home.html
Word Finding Difficulties	http://www.wordfinding.com/materials.html
Voice Grand Rounds	http://www.bcm.tmc.edu/oto/grand/laryngology.html
Dr. Grammar	http://www.drgrammar.org/
Animated Sign Language Dictionary	http://www.masterstech-home.com/ASLDict.html
Peter Ladefoged's Phonetics Course and Resources	http://hctv.humnet.ucla.edu/departments/linguistics/VowelsandConsonants/
International Phonetics Association (IPA)	http://www.arts.gla.ac.uk/IPA/ipa.html

USING THE INTERNET FOR
PROFESSIONAL SUPPORT AND COMMUNICATION

Communication via the Internet may take a variety of forms. The most frequently used include e-mail, listservs, chat, newsgroups, web logs, and web-based forums. Most clinicians use e-mail for private and routine person-to-person communication. However, group interaction via e-mail is also possible using a listserv. People with a shared interest subscribe to a listserv and every question or comment from group members is re-mailed to each person on the list. It is easy to subscribe or unsubscribe to a list, following directions included in first messages from the list. Listservs pre-date web-based discussion groups and make group interactions convenient even for persons who do not have high-speed Internet access. The main disadvantage of listservs is lack of control over how much and when information appears in members' e-mail accounts. It can be overwhelming if list participants are quite active. Over the years, there have been several active listservs with a focus relevant to communication disorders. Listservs are described and linked on Kuster's jumpstation site.

An updated approach to on-line communication occurs in web-based discussion groups. Unlike "chat rooms" where participants type back and forth in "real time," web-based discussion groups represent conversations that take place without the constraints of simultaneous time and place. Some are "public," but most require registration by the users. Usually discussion coordinators post topics or questions and help encourage interaction. Participants log on at any time to read previous comments and add their own. Conversations on popular topics can be archived for future reference by new participants. Table 26.2 lists some examples of online discussion groups that clinicians will find interesting and useful for communication with colleagues who share their interests and clinical challenges.

USING THE INTERNET FOR
CLIENT EDUCATION, COMMUNICATION, AND SUPPORT

The Internet has been a miracle for non-profit organizations and support groups. From parents of children with autism to stroke survivors, suddenly, people world-wide who need services can access them without the barriers of time and space. Clients may need help from clinicians in identifying and accessing organizations and support groups that may be helpful. Many may not realize the extent of online services that are available, including information about medical and developmental disorders, current research, group discussions for family members, spouses, or clients, legal consultation, funding resources, conference and workshop schedules, and sources for specialized equipment, clothing, and other materials.

Many people with communication disorders have already discovered that the Internet is a great "equalizer." With text-based interactions on line, correspondents cannot tell if a person has a hearing loss, painfully slow typing skills, compromised intelligibility, or disfluent speech. Thus, the Internet can become a place where clients feel less judged and more free to be themselves. Some clients will want to work on improving their computer

Table 26.2. Examples of on-line discussion groups for clinicians

On-line discussion group	URL (web address)
Neurology Web Forum	http://www.braintalk.org
Closing the Gap Forums	http://www.closingthegap.com/cgi-bin/ultimatebb.cgi
Phonology Therapy Discussion Group	http://members.tripod.com/Caroline_Bowen/group.htm

access (Section VIII) and written language skills (Section III) especially for the purpose of making their on-line communications more effective and efficient.

SUMMARY

Telepractice has been broadly defined to include technology applications that facilitate remote interaction between clients and clinicians or clinicians and others for the purposes of assessment, treatment, or education. Although telepractice does not necessarily involve computers, many current and future aspects of telepractice are based on the Internet. Already, there are Internet-based tools for assessment and intervention that are available with and without clinician mediation. Clinicians use the Internet for professional education and information, for professional support and communication, for enhancing client support and information, and for on-line intervention activities and materials. Reportedly few clinicians are involved, so far, in "remote" provision of direct services such as assessment and intervention. Ethical issues regarding such services must be considered.

REVIEW FOR TOPIC 26

1. Define and describe the difference between the terms telemedicine, telehealth, and telepractice.
2. Give an example of telepractice that does NOT involve computers.
3. Give at least one specific example for each of the following categories of Internet use: 1) Clinician education, 2) Clinical materials/activities, 3) Professional communication, 4) Client support.

QUESTIONS FOR DISCUSSION

1. Do you have any concerns about the notion of remotely delivered speech-language pathology services? Explain your position.
2. Visit one of the web sites mentioned in this topic. Based on this experience and others, how would you describe the potential value of telepractice for both professionals and consumers?

RESOURCES FOR FURTHER STUDY

American Speech-Language Hearing Association (December, 2001). *Telepractice and ASHA: Report of the Telepractices Team* [Internal report]. Author.

Kuster, J. Jumpstation for communication disorders. Retrieved May 21, 2004 from http://www
.mnsu.edu/dept/comdis/kuster2/welcome.html

McPherson, F. (2002). *How to do everything with your Pocket PC* (2nd ed.). Berkeley, CA:
McGraw-Hill Osborne Media.

Wynne, M.K. (2001, August 7). The shape of things to come and those that are here today. *Asha
Leader.* Retrieved May 21, 2004 from http://www.asha.org/about/publications/leaderonline/
archives/2001/things_to_come.htm

Note: Kuster's site is accessible via several URLs, including links from the ASHA web
site.

Choosing and Using a Hand-Held Computer or Personal Digital Assistant (PDA)

Clinical computing competency #5: The clinician will demonstrate the ability to use computer-assisted data management tools to document and facilitate client improvement.

Clinical computing competency #9: The clinician will demonstrate awareness of resources that provide continuing education, research results, technical support and information about availability, funding, efficacy, and efficiency of new clinical computing products as well as assistive technology devices and services.

Personal digital assistants (PDAs) represent a class of digital devices that will change the way most people manage their lives on a daily basis, at home and at work. These people will include those who have communication disorders and who may benefit from the use of such powerful, portable, relatively inexpensive tools. In addition, clinicians may find that these new technologies allow them to work more efficiently and effectively by assisting with information management and other aspects of clinical practice. Competency with such new technology includes familiarity with its basic functions and awareness of factors that should be considered before purchase.

WHAT IS A PERSONAL DIGITAL ASSISTANT?

The term *personal digital assistant* (PDA) describes a class of computers that are similar in size and weight to a pocket calculator. They remind many people of the communicators used by Star Trek crewmembers. Most are about the size of a 3″× 5″ note card and about ½″ thick. One side consists of a display screen with several control buttons. The screen is touch-sensitive, allowing the user to make choices or input data with a stylus. Many can be attached to a fold-up keyboard. In this text, the terms *PDA* and *handheld computer*

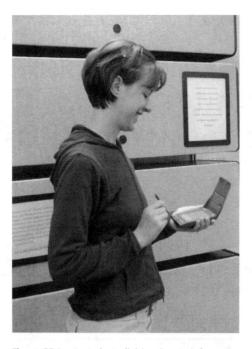

Figure 27.1. A student clinician inputs information into a handheld computer (Courtesy of Truman State University Speech and Hearing Clinic).

are used interchangeably. Handheld computers are powered by batteries and usually weigh from about 4 to 8 ounces.

These small, ultra-portable computers cost between $100 and $600, depending on their features. At this price, they are widely available in office supply stores and discount department stores. Many PDAs are intended to be easily docked to a desktop computer for the purpose of maintaining duplicate files, downloading new applications, or transferring data. This capability is the foundation for one of the chief advantages of a PDA over a traditional paper-based planner. Either wireless transfer or docking to a larger computer allow the user to have a back-up of professional appointment calendars, addresses, and other important information, while still allowing for the convenience of portability (see Figure 27.1). Some agencies, schools, and businesses use a master calendar system so that secretaries can schedule group meetings without having to contact everyone involved. Most central calendar systems now include PDA-compatible modules so that people can frequently synchronize the central calendar with their own personal appointment log.

PDAs have infra-red capability which allows instant transfer of programs or data between users of compatible PDAs. Infra-red can also be used for communicating with other devices for purposes such as printing or TV remote control emulation.

Although handwriting recognition on PDAs is improving, for some clinicians, combining a PDA with a keyboard will be the defining moment in converting from a paper planner to a handheld computer. This combination is ideal for portable access to client data, records, calendars, and notes from meetings and telephone calls. Notes typed during a parent interview or IEP meeting will not have to be re-typed or transcribed in order to be integrated into a case report. A simple press of the synchronization button when the hand-held is connected to a desktop computer will transfer the files and ensure that identical information is present on both systems. If another professional needs the information before the report is ready, notes can be "beamed" via infra-red connection from one PDA to another. Infra-red communication between two devices, such as a PDA and a printer or two hand-helds, requires that the devices be in relatively close proximity and in direct line with each other, just like a TV and an infra-red remote control.

Many handhelds have Internet access and e-mail capability via wireless data transfer, in addition to infra-red functions. Like cell phones, PDAs with such wireless-data features help itinerant professionals to stay connected to other professionals, a central office, or personal contacts.

The definition of PDA continues to undergo changes as this market of miniature digital devices expands. The typical handheld described previously represents the smallest and least costly end of a continuum of products that gradually increase in size, cost, and capabilities. The more expensive, feature-rich devices often include a miniature built-in keyboard or an even smaller keyboard usually accessed by thumbs. Presently these cost $700–$900.

The range of applications available for hand-held computers grows daily. Functions that usually come pre-installed include such basics as a note pad, calculator, to-do list, appointment calendar, and address book. However, of particular interest to clinicians are the hundreds of other applications distributed via the Internet that are available commercially or at no cost or at low cost as shareware. A sampling of low-cost and no-cost downloadable software includes word list generators, billing code tables, timers and alarms, dictionaries, drug reference materials, anatomy study guides, and thousands of games from hangman to sports trivia.

CASE EXAMPLE: *Wordlist*, version 3.0 by Kevin J. Lang

This 51k program for the Palm OS will instantly develop a list of English words to the user's specifications.

Palm display: Enter search pattern.

    Word length   _____
    Pattern   _____
    Anchor left   _____
    Anchor right   _____

(Choosing anchor left or anchor right indicates whether to match by beginning or end of word.)

User: Fills in blanks using stylus as follows:

    Word length   __5__
    Pattern   __st__
    Anchor left   __X__

Palm display: A list of five-letter words beginning with "st" appears immediately. The first of five screens of words includes stack, staff, stage, staid, stain, stair, stake, stale, stalk, stamp, stand, stank.

Wordlist is just one of the many readily available applications for hand-held computers that may be of interest to speech-language pathologists for both personal and professional use.

CHOOSING A PLATFORM TO SUIT INDIVIDUAL NEEDS

How should a clinician go about choosing a handheld computer? First, it is a good idea to do some hands-on investigating. Get the feel of several devices by actually handling them and viewing their screens. For example, the form factor may be especially important to some users. *Form factor* is a term appearing in product reviews which refers to the physical design of the product. Some users will highly value the convenience of a hand-held computer that is the perfect size and shape for slipping into a shirt pocket. For others, the clarity and color of the display or a built-in microphone will be more important.

After a hands-on shopping trip, check the reviews on some of the major technology web sites and trade magazines (e.g., *PC Computing, WINDOWS Magazine, MacWorld*). The newest and most popular products and models will be there, often with more detailed information than is typically available in a retail setting. Do not depend on the advice of the clerk in a discount electronics or office supply store. Instead, ask for advice from friends and colleagues who may already be using a handheld computer. As more information is collected prior to a purchase decision, there are several additional factors to consider that are somewhat unique to this new category of personal tool.

Choosing the platform and model of a handheld computer is comparable to choosing the brand and model of an automobile or a cell phone. The best choice will depend a great deal on personal preferences, budget, and individual needs. The term *platform* refers to the combination of physical features and operating system that results in a uniquely designed product. One platform is likely to meet a person's individual needs better than another, and the fit can be further tailored by choosing the right model.

In the early development of hand-held computers, a clear difference in purpose distinguished the most popular platforms available. Two operating systems came to the forefront, Palm OS and a miniature version of Microsoft Windows (currently called Windows Mobile). On the one hand, the developers of the Palm line of handhelds placed high value on streamlined design and simplicity of operation. These values are still apparent in the products that use the Palm OS (e.g., Handspring, Palm, Sony). On the other hand, developers of Pocket PCs that run a version of Windows (e.g., Casio, Dell, HP, Toshiba) had a different vision. This vision valued consistency with Windows appearance and a larger subset of desktop computer functions. In this way, the hand-held was viewed as an extension of the individual's desktop computer. Applications developed for one or the other of these two operating systems may or may not be available for the other.

Additional platform factors that prospective purchasers may want to consider include market share and compatibility. There will always be more and better applications available for hand-helds that have the largest number of buyers. However, even if it means purchasing a less popular PDA, it makes problem-solving, sharing, and repairing easier when your handheld is compatible with those used by family members or associates at work. Thus some institutions and businesses, such as the University of Virginia Medical School, include specific PDA information and recommendations on their web sites, so that employees and students will make purchases that allow them to take full advantage of specialized applications being widely used in their facilities.

BUILT-IN HAND-HELD FEATURES AND ACCESSORIES

Specific hand-held computers vary somewhat in the quality of display, amount of memory, features, and power consumption that come as part of a standard configuration. For example, the *Cassiopeia* handheld from CASIO was among the first to include a built-in microphone and headphone jack. The *Palm IIIx* from 3Com had a handy page-up/page-down arrow button, but no built-in microphone. New handheld products are coming along so quickly that a feature comparison in a book would be quickly outdated. The best source for such a feature comparisons are current reviews in trade magazines and Internet web sites.

If an owner realizes that a particular function is missing on his handheld computer, there is a good chance that either a software program or an add-on accessory can help fill the need. For example, accessories that add new functions to handheld computers include a digital camera, a pager card, or a storage media card reader such as those used by digital cameras. The *GoType!* portable keyboard can be added to Palm handhelds for silent, rapid text input on-the-fly. Most users will input major text documents or numerical data using their desktop computer and then transmit needed files to their hand-held computer. Users who know they need to do extensive text input in various locations are apt to invest in a notebook computer with a full-size keyboard and larger display. However, some situations in which the hand-held computer is needed, a detachable keyboard may be an excellent way to achieve faster text input away from home base. Paired with an infra-red compatible printer, complete document preparation independence is achieved.

SUMMARY

These small digital devices are just the beginning of a movement toward portable, personal devices that will impact the way people manage their lives, just as cell phones have done. They are changing rapidly in form and features, although at present the two dominant operating systems are Palm OS and Windows Mobile. There are many administrative, personal, and clinical applications for handheld computers, awareness of which may help some clinicians make purchasing decisions. It is suggested that clinicians do some hands-on shopping, read product reviews on line, consult friends and colleagues, and investigate potential clinical applications, prior to making a PDA purchase.

REVIEW FOR TOPIC 27

1. What are some examples of applications that are likely to come pre-installed in a hand-held computer?
2. Why is infra-red capability useful in a PDA?
3. How should clinicians investigate their options prior to purchasing a handheld computer?
4. Explore the listings of available PDA software by visiting a major PDA web site (just search on "personal digital assistant" and "software"). List three programs that might have potential use for clinicians.

QUESTIONS FOR DISCUSSION

1. Based on the information presented in this topic, how do you envision handheld computers being of use to speech-language pathologists?
2. Imagine that you could commission a computer programmer to develop software for your use on a PDA. Describe the program you would request and how you would use it.

RESOURCES FOR FURTHER STUDY

McPherson, F. (2002). *How to do everything with your Pocket PC* (2nd ed.). New York: McGraw-Hill Osborne Media.
Pogue, D. (1998). *PalmPilot: The ultimate guide.* Sebastopol, CA: O'Reilly & Associates.

How Clinicians Use Hand-Held Computers and PDAs

Clinical computing competency #10: The clinician will increase and maintain personal productivity by using a computer for administrative purposes.

Clinical computing competency #5: The clinician will demonstrate the ability to use computer-assisted data management tools to document and facilitate client improvement.

Hand-held computers bridge the gap between administrative and clinical uses for new technology. The same PDA might be used by the competent clinician to record a brief speech sample, calculate a client's fluency rate, document billable time and service codes, take notes at an IEP meeting, time a client's ability to sustain a vowel, and take a digital photo of a client's new AAC device to include in a report. This competency requires clinicians to be familiar with the basic operation of hand-held computers and conversant with some of the many potential clinical and administrative uses for this new portable technology.

Hand-held computers bring into grasp a set of low-cost, portable, flexible tools for speech-language pathologists. Already ubiquitous in many other professional arenas, hand-held computers are being taken for granted like pocket calculators and cell phones. In fact, it is likely that all three of these functions and more will be affordably combined into a single device that some clinicians will purchase.

How could such tools impact the daily professional activities of speech-language pathologists? The basic applications (notepad, address/telephone database, to-do list, calculator, expense record, calendar) discussed in Topic 27 will appeal to many professionals. At present, at least five additional categories of applications are of particular interest to both working clinicians and student clinicians:

- Record keeping and billing
- Diagnostic, intervention, and research tools

- Reference and study tools
- Multimedia capture/play
- Applications for direct use by clients, such as reading activities, AAC, and expert system aids

Examples of all but the last of these categories of applications are discussed here in Topic 28. A discussion of how clients themselves might make use of PDAs and hand-held computers is found in Topic 29.

USING A HAND-HELD COMPUTER TO FACILITATE ADMINISTRATIVE TASKS

Time management and billing applications include utilities that help a user track contact time with clients or patients. Many clinicians work in health care settings that require the use of special billing codes. Look-up tables for most major billing code systems have already been formatted for installation on PDAs. These and the other applications mentioned in this topic can be downloaded from the Internet and readily installed on a hand-held.

Some complete applications are provided free of charge; others are shareware and require registration and a minimal fee before access to all features is available. Some shareware applications are provided in their entirety as soon as they are downloaded, but they expire and cease to function after a few days unless they are registered. In most cases, registration is a simple matter of sending an e-mail message or making a phone call, and providing a credit card number or sending a check. Typical shareware registration fees for hand-held applications cost $15–$25.

Although most users actively seek out free programs or shareware from the Internet, there is also a commercial software market for hand-held computers. Sophisticated and highly specialized applications for particular professions and industries are appearing. In medicine especially, both expensive and inexpensive applications seem to be proliferating. Medical dictionaries, pharmaceutical references, growth charts, recommended immunization schedules, billing codes, medical study and review materials, new research publication subscriptions, and many more applications for doctors, dentists, nurses, and others are widely available.

In his book *PalmPilot: The Ultimate Guide*, David Pogue (1998) described the example of a powerful commercial database program that interfaced with the most popular standard PC database software (Oracle, Lotus Notes, DB2, Microsoft Access). The idea was that custom data-collection forms could be designed for the hand-held. The information was entered into these forms on-site by research associates and then easily transmitted into a central database. For example, interview survey data could be collected and recorded in a variety of public places. The data could be stored in digital format on hand-held computers and then transmitted into a standard PC database without having to be re-coded or typed.

USING A HAND-HELD COMPUTER DURING DIAGNOSTIC AND INTERVENTION ACTIVITIES

The convenience of the management/administrative kinds of applications of hand-held computers for clinicians is obvious and compelling. Perhaps less obvious but equally interesting are applications that have potential to directly impact intervention and evaluation procedures. With the appropriate utilities installed, a single 4-ounce hand-held computer could easily take the place of a pocket calculator, dictionary, stopwatch, digital camera, and pitch pipe. In additon, some PDAs have built-in microphones and can record short speech samples. These applications alone would make many itinerant clinicians consider purchasing such a device. A more complete list of software already readily available for clinical tasks is found in Table 28.1. (Note: Because the details of the web addresses of downloading sites change so frequently, they have not been included in this table, to prevent reader frustration. A brief search on the web will produce several examples of each kind of software described.)

Hand-held computers, however, have clinical potential that goes beyond gadget/device replacement. Information for spur-of-the-moment therapy activities can be at the clinician's fingertips. For example, word lists could be instantly generated to match the specifications of the user (see example in Topic 27: Choosing and Using a Hand-Held Computer or Personal Digital Assistant [PDA]). So a clinician who suddenly needs a list of 10 words that start with /sl/ or 20 words that end with /ts/ could obtain such a list in a matter of seconds, without a major interruption in the session.

What about taking full advantage of those last few minutes of therapy when the planned activities have been completed? An instantly accessible bank of jokes or sports facts or entertainment trivia may be just the right thing. The clinician who has these readily available might give an elderly patient something to talk about for the rest of the day or an adolescent with a recent TBI the feeling that she is still connected with the real world of teenagers outside the rehab facility. A hand-held trivia game could even be the center of a brief group activity in which the clinician serves as game host. The clinician could read the questions aloud and pairs of clients would team up to answer them orally. The clinician could quickly enter answers into the PDA and let teams know the correct answer and the score.

An important role for PDAs in direct service activities involves collecting and storing client performance data for diagnostic or therapeutic purposes. A hand-held computer would seem to be an ideal tool for tracking multiple behaviors (or multiple clients) simultaneously. Envision, for example, a "counter" application that would allow clinicians to tap the screen to tally each correct or incorrect response, save the client file, then transmit the data to a desktop computer or print it in graph form on an infra-red compatible printer.

Clinicians, student clinicians, and researchers all have an interest in discovering convenient uses for PDAs in the area of client information and data management. Itinerant clinicians who work in more than one setting may find the capabilities of a PDA to be especially convenient.

Table 28.1. Examples of free or shareware software for handheld computers that clinicians could use for common diagnostic and intervention activities

General category of clinical application	Examples of existing programs and utilities available on the Internet
Reporting and billing	Time logs
	Mileage and expense trackers
	Billing code databases
	Client databases (contact information, IEP dates, referral sources)
Diagnostic and intervention tools	Mirror and flashlight simulators
	Metronome and tone scales
	Counters, timers, clocks
	Game tools: dice rollers, turn timers
	Word games: hangman, buy-a-vowel games, anagram generators
	Trivia games and collections
	Non-English dictionaries
	Games: Drawing, puzzles, card games
Reference and study tools for clinicians	Medical and other dictionaries, thesaurus, spellcheckers
	Statistics calculators
	Phonetic alphabet reference and practice
	Anatomy & neurology review programs
Multimedia capture/play	Photo display/slideshow utilities
	Speech recording (with capable PDA)
	Music and MP3 players
	Digital camera (built-in, added on, or emulated)

CASE EXAMPLE: Using a PDA in Fluency Research

Following is an excerpt from a recent e-mail correspondence between the author and a new owner of a PDA, a former student beginning her doctoral studies at Vanderbilt University:

Let me tell you! It is soooooo helpful in therapy. This is what I have learned to do on mine in only a few short weeks. In addition to keeping my daily schedule of classes, meetings, and everything else, I developed a spreadsheet today where I can input formulas to calculate speech rate of utterances and disfluency percentages without using a calculator (just like using Excel). My next step is going to be hot syncing that info into my computer and printing it out to include in the report and/or file! Isn't that cool? Dr. Conture actually takes his PDA and his keyboard on home visits and types all the info into the PDA so we can bring it up on the computer back at the clinic. In his office and ours we have cradles hooked to our computers for the PDAs. I also have PowerPoint capabilities and Word which I have been taking notes on from meetings. Dr. Conture showed me a PowerPoint presentation on his and said he uses that when he's traveling to practice (I have an extra memory card that will come in handy when I start doing those things). (Kia Hartfield, personal correspondence, September 10, 2003)

If the clinician's PDA is equipped with the right features and software, she could use a wireless phone as a modem to access the Internet for web-browsing or e-mail. Client data or billing information could be transmitted back to a central system this way, too, without the clinician returning to a particular desktop computer and "hot-syncing" it with her PDA to backup her data. Of course, it would be important to ensure the security and privacy of any method of confidential data transfer. The surprising new convenience of such applications will change the way some clinicians schedule their time and manage their "paperwork." In the same way, hand-held computers are introducing exciting possibilities for direct use by clients themselves, which is considered in Topic 29.

SUMMARY

The applications for hand-held computers that working clinicians and student clinicians might find useful are numerous and increasing by the moment. Individuals are likely to discover new and important functions as they become accustomed to the convenience and efficiency that is possible with continuous access to the power of a computer. Already, clinicians use PDAs for tasks related to recordkeeping and billing; diagnostics and intervention; research, reference, and studying; and multimedia.

REVIEW FOR TOPIC 28

1. List at least three categories of hand-held computer applications of particular interest to students and clinicians in speech-language pathology.
2. Give examples of five specific clinical tasks or functions that could be implemented with the assistance of a hand-held computer.
3. How is most software for hand-held computers acquired by end users?

QUESTIONS FOR DISCUSSION

1. Does a hand-held computer sound like something you could use in your clinical practice? What are the strengths and drawbacks as you see them at this time?
2. If you know someone who is already using a hand-held computer for some personal or professional purpose, interview them about the pros and cons. What new ideas does this additional perspective give you?

RESOURCES FOR FURTHER STUDY

American Academy of Family Physicians. (2003). *Why Get a PDA?* Retrieved September 2003 from http://www.aafp.org/x476.xml
McPherson, F. (2002). *How to do everything with your Pocket PC* (2nd ed.). New York: McGraw-Hill Osborne Media.

How Clients Use Hand-Held Computers and PDAs

Clinical computing competency #9: The clinician will demonstrate awareness of resources that provide continuing education, research results, technical support and information about availability, funding, efficacy, and efficiency of new clinical computing products as well as assistive technology devices and services.

Portable, inexpensive technology has much appeal for clients, not just clinicians. Clinicians may find themselves in the position of consultant as hand-held computers or PDAs are recommended and configured for client use. Competent clinicians will be aware of the variety of special applications available for this computing genre and comfortable exploring and personalizing the use of such technology for their clients.

Many clinicians, teachers, physicians, and students are already using personal digital assistants (PDAs) as personal organization tools. The use of hand-held or pocket computers and other small, portable computing products as assistive technology devices for clients in education and rehabilitation settings is less common. However, this will change as clinicians and clients become more aware of the possibilities and learn to integrate such portable technologies into everyday life. Applications designed for and used by clients can be organized into several categories including augmentative and alternative communication (AAC) tools, expert systems, personal educational assistants, and classroom tools.

HAND-HELD–BASED AUGMENTATIVE AND ALTERNATIVE COMMUNICATION

Portability and flexibility have always been highly valued in AAC devices. Developers have been quick to jump on the potential of hand-held and palm-size computers to provide portable, flexible communication devices. For example, Enkidu Research markets a family of communication devices called the *IMPACT* series. This collection of devices integrates the latest hardware and software technology in lightweight, highly configurable packages that can be tailored to the needs of a wide variety of AAC users. The range of basic devices in the *IMPACT* series includes a Palm PDA, a hand-held computer w/keyboard, two sizes of tablet computers, and a dedicated tablet called an "e-talk." They range in weight from about ½ pound to 5 pounds for the largest device, including a case. As of 2003, all *IMPACT* devices included the full Mayer-Johnson (Boardmaker) symbol set, an expanded 128 MB memory card, and a rechargeable speaker for voice output. Each package costs several thousand dollars.

Additional innovations in using palm-size technology come from Gus Communications, Inc. This company claims to have developed the first "dynamic display" software product for a Windows operating system, releasing *Gus! Multimedia Speech System for Windows* in 1992. "Dynamic display" refers to the way symbols/messages can be stored in layers that change as the user makes choices, so that additional items become visible/available automatically. According to the Gus web site, this original product "was an instant success due, in large part, to the fact that it could convert any Windows based personal computer into a much more powerful and versatile 'communication device' than typical single purpose communication devices" (www.gusinc.com). With this background in converting off-the-shelf computers and Windows for AAC purposes, it was natural for this company to develop AAC applications for Pocket PCs. Several models for several languages are available.

HAND-HELD–BASED EXPERT SYSTEMS

The concept of an "expert system" comes from the early days of artificial intelligence when the potential and limitations of computers were first being envisioned. Even then, innovators were describing the notion that the right computer application might serve as an "expert system" for persons with cognitive deficits (Bull, Cochran, & Snell, 1988; Lent, 1982). An "expert system" helps prompt a user by taking on the role of an expert coach. A human expert considers not only factual information, but also the specific task and context relevant to the situation. Therefore, a computer-based expert system is different than a mere database of information. An expert system is designed to help a novice consider what actions are appropriate under certain conditions. Thus a computer-based expert system for emergency room doctors might step them through a protocol of patient history questions and test results to ensure that key diagnostic possibilities are considered and systematically ruled out, much in the way that an expert ER physician would. A simpler expert system for clients with cognitive disability, TBI, or Alzheimer's disease, might help them take medication on time or correctly sequence a daily living task.

Research has documented the successful use of traditional picture and word cues by persons with cognitive and memory impairments. Such cues can help them remember and complete tasks that increase their independence (see Bull et al., 1998, for a review of some of this literature). Transferring this role to small, portable technologies is a natural step. This function was explored in a study of four individuals by Tackett, Rice, Rice, and Butterbaugh (2001). Their goal was to determine if off-the-shelf PDA equipment (experimental condition) would work better than traditional paper lists (control condition) for helping people with prospective memory loss do two types of tasks. All four subjects experienced both conditions. The tasks were either 1) chosen by the subject or 2) assigned by the experimenters because they required the subject to be attentive to doing things at a certain time. Results suggested better performance when subjects used the PDA, and better performance in the control condition among subjects who experienced the experimental condition first. In other words, the regularity and process of using the PDA seemed to carry over into making traditional reminder strategies more effective. Special software for making the PDA interface easier to use as a memory support system was described by researchers at the University of Colorado (Carmien & Hudak, 2003).

Patricia Wright and colleagues at Cardiff University pursued a line of research regarding similar uses of PDAs with clinical populations. They compared the efficacy of particular styles/feature of PDAs to support memory functions in people who had sustained non-progressive, closed head injury. They reported that most of their subjects (10 of 12) found the use of the PDAs helpful in everyday life (Wright et al., 2001).

Approaching the use of PDAs as expert systems for people with cognitive disabilities has been the particular mission of Ablelink Technologies, Inc. Over a period of several years and in collaboration with several major grant sources, Ablelink has developed an impressive product line based on the Windows Pocket PC operating system. Products are designed to help people with cognitive impairment be more independent and successful in many areas of life, including independent living, money management, transportation, menu planning, schedule maintenance, and supported employment. For example, the *Pocket Coach* is described on the Ablelink web site as "a software/hardware system designed to provide fully customizable, step-by-step audio instructions or reminders to persons with mental retardation in any educational, vocational or residential setting" (www .ablelink.com). The *Pocket Coach* makes use of off-the-shelf consumer technology that is adapted for a special use. In order to simplify operation for someone with limited cognitive skills, for example, the physical "buttons" on a Pocket PC are disabled so only the touchscreen interface works. Instructions are recorded by an assistant and associated with screen buttons. Recording is simple and easy to change, much like a clinician or teacher might record speech messages into any small voice output device or talking switch. Compared to most assistive technologies, the Ablelink products boast an impressively documented research and development record.

Some uses of a PDA for and by clients extend and blur the traditional definition of an expert system. An individual client may use a PDA for multiple purposes, some more clearly in the nature of an "expert system" than others. Gayton and Ferrell (2001) described a series of clients and their use of Palm PDAs. For example, they have used a Palm with a young adult who had suffered viral meningitis. It provided picture memory cues to help him recall family members and his residence as well as diary and to-do list functions. Attached to a portable keyboard, a Palm PDA was used with a bright 7-year-old with cerebral palsy, primarily as a writing assistant. A 60-year-old stroke client was taught to use a Palm PDA to help him succeed in his job as an apartment building manager. He used the Palm as a contact manager, personal scheduler, and maintenance job calendar.

Beyond use as an expert system or AAC device, there seem to be two other notable categories of PDA use by people with special needs at this time: use of PDAs as personal educational assistants, and use of PDAs as classroom tools. The distinction lies primarily in whether the PDA is individually purchased and configured (personal educational assistant) or whether the PDA is being used by most or all of the students in a class as part of the curriculum (classroom tool).

HAND-HELD–BASED EDUCATIONAL ASSISTANTS

Many students of all ages and in all educational settings find the convenience of hand-held computing devices helpful. The standard capabilities, like a calendar, to-do list, and address book are helpful for almost anyone. Students with learning disabilities, ADHD, TBI, or other conditions that may affect organization and memory may particularly benefit from the use of a PDA to help manage their educational responsibilities. Appert (2002) noted that these students may find the use of a PDA especially helpful for

- Tracking assignments
- Important dates like exams
- Note taking in class
- Study tools
- Outlining and concept mapping

Affordable, portable, and inconspicuous alternatives to handwriting class notes on paper are desirable for many students who have special needs. Sometimes a paid or volunteer note taker is the solution of choice. Some students, however would like to achieve this task more independently (see Section VIII for more information about adapting computer access). Although laptop computers are more common than ever in high school and college classrooms, they are still somewhat cumbersome and remain desirable targets for theft compared to their lightweight PDA counterparts. PDAs that fit easily into a pocket or backpack compare favorably in price as well. Very small, collapsible keyboards can be attached to hand-held or pocket PCs if necessary, to make keyboard entry possible. Other input choices include handwriting recognition, speech recognition (with the right software) or the use of a touchscreen keyboard on the display of the PDA. No matter what the input method, notes can be uploaded and printed using a desktop computer and printer or "beamed" to a printer using the PDAs infrared capability. Text such as to-do lists or notes can be spoken to the user for review using a text-to-speech utility such as *PDSay* (Scansoft). *PDSay* also adds speech recognition functions to a PDA, so that it responds to voice commands and dictation (see more about speech recognition in general in Topic 39).

Although accessibility options are limited, there are new developments every day. New larger fonts are available on some PDAs and users who have had difficulty seeing the small displays on PDAs may find the use of a specialized screen magnifier helpful. For example, the Magnifico Portable PDA Screen Magnifier (Office on the Go Go) is economically priced (under $40), compatible with most PDAs, and offers two times the magnification of the display.

Examples of programs and utilities that might be of special interest and value to students using a PDA as a personal educational assistant include:

- Expanded notepad programs
- Clocks and alarms
- Dictionaries
- Handwriting tutorials
- Concept mapping
- Alphabet flashcards
- Make-your-own flashcards
- Memory games and puzzles
- E-book readers (Appert, 2002)

Electronic books (e-books for short) are often available at no cost (as a free download) or at a reduced price compared to hardcopy versions. If a student (or anyone else) is already carrying a PDA almost all of the time, a clear advantage to an e-book is the constant availability of the text, as well as the possibility of having the text read aloud simultaneously and inconspicuously. To other people, it just appears as if the person is listening to MP3 music, when really he or she is getting English literature homework done.

With the right software utilities, all Palm OS and Pocket PC hand-helds can function as e-book readers (Broida, 2003). With additional utilities, such as Audible Player (Audible, Inc.), hand-helds can be used to play books aloud, like music files. "Audible, Inc., is the leading provider of Internet-delivered spoken content for playback on personal computers and Pocket PCs" (McPherson, 2002, p. 354). The sound files are purchased from the Audible web site (www.audible.com). Listening to pre-recorded sound files is like listening to a CD or a book on tape. This is different from the *PDSay* (Scansoft) utility that converts text-to-speech using synthesized speech to "read" whatever the user types into a PDA. The exact procedures for obtaining and installing utilities, sound files, or e-books vary a bit according to platform and e-book source, so the details are not presented here. PDA web sites, how-to books, and popular tech magazines (e.g., *Hand-held Computing*) routinely publish updates on the ins-and-outs of how to use a PDA for such purposes.

HAND-HELD–BASED CLASSROOM TOOLS

School systems all over the country are exploring the use of PDAs and hand-helds in classrooms, as a supplement and alternative to providing each individual student with more expensive but less portable computer capabilities. Students and teachers are using PDAs with a broad range of utilities including mapping applications, databases, counters, drawing and photography tools, field guides, and decision-tree models (Tinker, Staudt, & Walton, 2002). In one study, Palm Pilots were given to 28 sixth-graders, six of whom had special needs. Results indicated that the students preferred using their PDAs over traditional notebooks for recording assignments, accessing spelling lists, and checking math and spelling (Bauer & Ulrich, 2002).

The PDAs, hand-helds, and Pocket PC devices that have been developed for personal and business use are being adopted into educational settings as well. There are some small, inexpensive computing devices, however, that have been especially designed for classroom use. The AlphaSmart company is among the leaders in this area, best known for the *AlphaSmart* and the *Dana* product lines. The *AlphaSmart* and *Dana* devices are portable, inexpensive, self-contained computers that include small built-in displays and full-size keyboards. The *AlphaSmart 3000*, for example, is about $12'' \times 9''$ in size and weighs about 2 pounds. It runs on batteries and is described as a "simple, low-cost computer companion" (www.alphasmart.com). It has infrared capability that allows transfer of data to either Mac or Windows PCs or a variety or printers. The *Dana* is similar except it is designed to operate with the Palm OS, giving it access to the thousands of shareware and public domain applications available for Palm devices. The latest *Dana* devices are available with wireless Internet capability (Wi-Fi) and expansion slots. Larger than PDAs but much lighter and less expensive than laptop computers, these devices have found a market niche in both regular and special education classrooms.

Devices such as these make it possible for schools to provide whole classes with several hours of computer access per day, which otherwise would not be financially feasible. Don Johnston, Inc., markets a utility that will allow *Write: Outloud* (talking word processing) and *Co:Writer* (word prediction) to run on AlphaSmart products, which can be an extremely useful configuration for students needing extra support in acquiring emergent and beginning literacy skills. (Note: These are computers with limited functions that do not include speech recognition or speech output; however, files may be transferred back and forth to desktop computers that have these capabilities.) For further examples and strategies for classroom and lab use of these and similar products with children who have language impairment, see *The Writing Lab Approach to Language Instruction and Intervention* (Nelson, 2004), available from Paul H. Brookes Publishing Co.

ADVANTAGES AND DISADVANTAGES FOR CLIENTS

There are obvious advantages and disadvantages of hand-held/palm-size technology for clients. Leading the list of advantages is extreme portability—pocket-sized technology can truly be with the client at all times, unlike bulkier systems for communication, reminders, or educational support. In addition, because hand-held and palm-size devices are becoming ubiquitous, they do not draw unwanted attention to the user. They are viewed as age-appropriate at all ages, and may even be perceived by the client to be socially "cool." For clients who may be at high risk for losing a device as small as a PDA, the fact that data can be backed up on a larger personal computer may be especially important.

Chief among the disadvantages of hand-held/palm-size devices for clients is that they are small enough to be easily lost or damaged. Even with care, the constant use and risky environments (kitchens, classrooms) that some clients require may cause devices to wear out relatively quickly. It may be difficult to determine cost-effectiveness if the device does indeed meet some client needs, but requires frequent repair or replacement. Other serious limitations include the fact that devices this small can be prohibitive for users with low vision, arthritis, or other fine motor control difficulty such as tremor. Although touch screen or optional keyboard interface is excellent for some users, adapted access options are limited at this time.

SUMMARY

Clients are using PDAs and hand-held computers for as many diverse purposes as everyone else. Some clients, however, have needs that are being addressed in special ways using this technology. Such specialized applications generally fall into four categories: 1) AAC, 2) expert systems, 3) personalized educational assistants, and 4) classroom tools. It is valuable for clinicians to be aware of the range of uses and applications that are available to assist clients in choosing and adopting this kind of assistive technology. Researchers are already exploring the use of these devices with a wide range of clinical populations, including those with developmental/cognitive disabilities, acquired brain injuries, and learning disabilities. Although the price and size are hard to beat, accessibility options are limited as yet, and input is primarily managed via built-in touch screens/stylus or optional portable keyboards. As portable technologies continue to evolve, exciting new possibilities for people with special needs can be expected to unfold.

REVIEW FOR TOPIC 29

1. List at least three categories of hand-held computer applications used by clients.
2. What does the term "expert system" mean?
3. Visit one of the web sites for specialized applications mentioned in this topic. Describe a potential client who might benefit from the use of one of these products.

QUESTIONS FOR DISCUSSION

1. Discuss the advantages and limitations that characterize the use of hand-held/palm-size devices by clients.
2. If you know someone who is already using a hand-held computer for personal or professional purposes, interview them about the pros and cons. What new ideas does an additional perspective give you?

RESOURCES FOR FURTHER STUDY

Broida, R. (June/July, 2003). Book-mobile: The best e-book reader on the planet is already in your pocket. *Hand-held Computing, 6*(2), 47–48.

Pownell, D., & Bailey, G.D. (2002). Are you ready for hand-helds? *Learning and Leading with Technology, 30*(2), 50–57.

Tackett, S.L., Rice, D.A., Rice, J.C., & Butterbaugh, G.J. (2001). Using a Palmtop PDA for reminding in prospective memory deficit. In *Proceedings of the 2001 Convention of the Rehabilitation Engineering and Assistive Technology Society of North America* (pp. 23–25). Arlington, VA: RESNA.

Wright., P, Rogers, N., Hall, C., Wilson, B., Evans, J., Emslie, H., & Bartram, C. (2001). Comparison of pocket-computer memory aids for people with brain injury. *Brain Injury, 15*(9), 787–800.

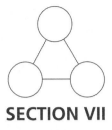

SECTION VII

Using a Computer as a Diagnostic Tool

Introduction to Using a Computer as a Diagnostic Tool

Clinical computing competency #6: The clinician will make appropriate use of computer-based instruments designed to assist in the evaluation or diagnosis of communication disorders.

Specific examples of how clinicians could achieve this competency cross all areas of communication disorders. Clinicians can use computer-assisted speech or language sample analysis, computer-assisted voice analysis, as well as computer-assisted test administration, scoring, or interpretation. Initial personal objectives might include learning how to transcribe and code a speech or language sample for accurate analysis or practicing a computer-based voice evaluation protocol that includes appropriate software settings and microphone placement. Competency in this area includes awareness of both the strengths and weaknesses of computer-based tools used during diagnostic activities.

Since the 1980s, the diagnostic uses of computers in communication disorders have been described in a well-developed body of published research (e.g., see the special theme issue of *Seminars in Speech and Language*, May, 1999, Vol. 20, No. 2). In addition, an extensive array of papers, demonstrations, and workshops at peer-reviewed professional conferences attests to this major aspect of clinical computing. This research, as well as the early availability of interesting software, has affected clinical practice. As early as 1996, school clinicians reported that diagnostics (not including report writing) accounted for an important share of their overall use of computers (13%) (McRay & Fitch, 1996).

Nevertheless, many clinicians, including new graduates, remain unaware of the potential uses of computers in this part of their clinical practice. A 1997 survey of communication disorders program directors suggested that academic and clinical training might be lagging behind the practice of working clinicians in the use of computer-based diagnostic tools (Walz & Cochran, 1997). In response to the survey, only 15 of 88 program directors (17%) indicated that modules or courses in computer applications particular to communication disorders (e.g., computer-assisted language sample analysis) were available in their programs. Even new textbooks on diagnostics in communication disorders often give little attention to this major topic. Because such specialized training would be difficult to find elsewhere, it is unfortunate that it remains rare in ASHA-accredited graduate programs. Pre-service clinicians who do obtain experience with the diagnostic applications of computers are at a definite advantage when they become working clinicians. They are already familiar with state-of-the-art procedures, the technology itself, and important professional concerns that may apply. Clinicians with this background are better able to assess new computer-based tools that will compete for the attention of their colleagues and their clients.

The purpose of the present topic is to provide an overview of how computers can be used by clinicians during clinical assessment activities. A historical perspective of the diagnostic uses of computers is provided, followed by consideration of how computers can assist with each major aspect of assessment: data collection, data analysis, and data interpretation. The potential for "on-line" diagnostics and computer-assisted data interpretation, especially, raise professional concerns that warrant clinicians' attention.

HISTORICAL PERSPECTIVE AND THE NOTION OF "TOOL"

Although clinicians may regard the use of computers in assessment as something new, computers have been utilized this way since the late 1970s. Interest in diagnostic applications blossomed as soon as personal computers became available. Given the limitations of the computers that early innovators were using, they envisioned and implemented an amazing array of applications. Consider the following list of software products already being distributed by 1985: *Frenchay Dysarthria Assessment: Computer Differential Analysis* (Enderby, 1983), an online articulation test; *Computer Managed Articulation Diagnosis* (Fitch, 1984), a computerized step-by-step protocol for testing articulation; *Lingquest 1: Language Sample Analysis* (Mordecai, Palin, & Palmer, 1982), a complex and sophisticated early tool for grammatical analysis of language samples; *Phonological Analysis by Computer* (Weiner, 1984), a simplified tool for phonological process analysis; *Computerized Assessment of Intelligibility of Dysarthric Speech* (Yorkston, Beukelman, & Traynor, 1984), an innovative approach to assessing intelligibility through random selection of test stimuli.

Developing commercially viable products for a relatively small market like speech-language pathology is risky and time-consuming. Even though some early applications worked well even in 1985, rapid changes in microcomputers (e.g., systems, disk formats, memory capacity, printer interfaces) meant that developers had difficulty keeping such products current and providing appropriate technical support to the clinicians who ordered their software—often beginning computer users. Of the software tools for diagnostics that were among those originating in the 1980s, few are still commercially available. *Phonological Analysis by Computer* became *Automatic Articulation Analysis Plus* and then *Automatic Articulation Analysis 2000*, still available from Parrot Software. An updated version of *Computerized Assessment of Intelligibility of Dysarthric Speech* was developed for Windows/Mac and distributed by Tice Technology Services, Inc., under the title *Sentence Intelligibility Test (SIT)*. It remains available, along with other Tice software such as *Pacer/Tally*, from Madonna Rehabilitation Hospital (www.madonna.org). In summary, one of the barriers to wider use of computers for diagnostic purposes has been not just development, but also maintenance of excellent software tools available from dependable sources.

A common expectation is that computers will make work easier and faster. This expectation is difficult to fulfill for the clinician first encountering a complex tool. Another barrier to wider adoption, therefore, may be the perceived difficulty of some diagnostic applications. In an attempt to encourage their fellow professionals, some converts may promise efficiency and accuracy that can seldom be achieved by a novice user. This is a familiar pattern related to the dissemination of innovation (Rogers, 1995). At first, innovation is adopted by a small group of enthusiasts and risk takers. However, when the benefits become known and the tool becomes part of a "standard" approach, then novice users are more willing to adopt the innovation themselves, persisting till they achieve competency. Many of the most exciting diagnostic applications of computers, such as computer-assisted speech and language sample analysis, are in the midst of this transition from novel to standard approach.

Videofluoroscopy is a clinical technology that is well past the "novel" point, providing a useful analogy. Many clinicians are familiar with videofluoroscopy and its role in helping evaluate swallowing disorders and orofacial anomolies. With dysphagia patients, clinicians and radiologists routinely use videofluoroscopy to study the details of the swallowing process. The results are similar to a moving x-ray that can be viewed repeatedly if necessary. This procedure helps clinicians and physicians determine the precise nature of a swallowing problem and how to intervene. For example, it might be revealed that the patient does better with foods or liquids of certain consistencies.

Videofluoroscopy is a diagnostic tool that was once relatively unknown. It requires significant investment in training and experience. Although a tool can accomplish an important purpose in the hands of the right user, a beginning clinician may take longer to obtain the needed sample of behavior during a swallow study or may require repeated viewings of the tape in order to observe what a more experienced clinician would have noticed at once. However, with practice and experience, the beginner becomes more efficient at making good use of the tool (saving time) and more expert at noticing idiosyncrasies that may affect patient care (client benefits). In a similar way, computer-based diagnostic applications for speech, language, and voice can be powerful additions to a clinician's resources. Initially, most of these tools require more than a trivial investment of time and energy. Once the basics have been mastered, time and energy savings become apparent to the clinician and benefits for the client begin to accrue.

USING THE COMPUTER TO ASSIST WITH DIAGNOSTIC DATA COLLECTION

The therapeutic role of computer-based feedback and the acoustic analysis of speech have been described in Section V. Applications that capture and analyze human speech can also be invaluable in the evaluation or diagnosis of a communication disorder.

For example, the *Nasometer* from Kay Elemetrics is a computer-based tool that quantifies the otherwise subjectively judged aspect of speech called *nasality*. In English, nasality is desirable when producing "nasals" like /m/ and /n/. When air escapes through the nose at inappropriate moments, however, too much nasality is perceived and the speaker is judged to be *hypernasal*.

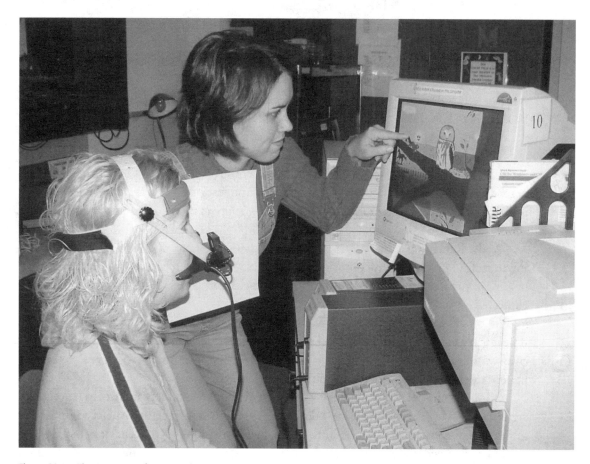

Figure 30.1. The *Nasometer* from Kay Elemetrics helps clinicians quantify nasality during a speech evaluation (Courtesy of Truman State University Speech and Hearing Clinic).

For a clinician, judging hypernasality reliably from moment to moment requires extensive experience, not to mention endurance. The *Nasometer* assists the clinician by measuring physical attributes of speech production that are generally associated with nasality. During data collection, the client wears a headpiece. The headpiece is equipped with microphones situated on either side of a sound separator that rests on the client's upper lip. As the client talks, the computer calculates the relative proportion of nasal to nasal-plus-oral acoustic energy and displays the results on the computer monitor. Clinicians use the *Nasometer* to help quantify the impact of orofacial anomalies (e.g., cleft palate) and neurological impairments that affect speech (see Figure 30.1).

The *Nasometer* illustrates the use of the computer to obtain data directly from a client during an assessment. Other computer-based tools are available for collecting information such as pitch range, habitual pitch during speech, vocal loudness, and other attributes of speech and voice production. Judging the presence or absence of a communication disorder involves consideration of many factors, including the speaker's own opinion, the perceptions of listeners, standardized performance measures, and the informal impressions of an expert clinician. Computer-based tools can help clinicians and researchers assess parameters of speech and voice that otherwise are difficult to objectively measure.

USING THE COMPUTER TO ASSIST WITH DIAGNOSTIC DATA ANALYSIS

One of the most tedious and time-consuming tasks regularly undertaken by clinicians is speech and language sample analysis. When a clinician analyzes a conversational speech or language sample "by hand," several hours may be required to transcribe the conversation from tapes and then analyze it. The sample could be examined for various features such as phonetic or phonological patterns, morphological development, grammatical structures, vocabulary, and/or discourse rules. In practice, clinicians would rarely complete all of these analyses on a single sample, because of time constraints. Instead, they are likely to review the transcript and look for problem areas that seem most in need of detailed examination. They apply their clinical judgment and choose the analyses that they know how to do, and that their limited time permits.

Researchers claim that the use of computer-based speech and language sample analysis not only makes the process of transcription more efficient, but also dramatically improves the speed and reliability of analysis (Evans & Miller, 1999; Long, 1999, 2001; Long & Channell, 2001; Long & Masterson, 1993; Miller, Freiberg, Rolland, & Reeves, 1992). Once the sample is transcribed and coded, analyses such as phonetic inventories, phonological processes, MLU, vocabulary lists, or discourse measures can be obtained almost instantly. Examples of specific software applications that perform such analyses are discussed in Topics 31, 32, and 33.

Analysis of systematically gathered speech and language samples can be an ideal measure of treatment progress, unlike standardized tests. Standardized tests provide a general gauge of an individual's communication skills, but they are not intended for frequent, repeated administrations. Often they do not reflect the gradual improvements that should be considered for effective intervention planning. Speech and language as it is used in a genuine communicative context (versus a testing task) is sought as the best reflection of a person's communication ability. Computer-based tools for language sample analysis have the potential to help clinicians make more regular use of speech and language sampling as clinical measures.

The judgment and experience required for selecting and implementing speech or language analyses by hand should not be abandoned, even if a computer reduces some of the tedium. Most experts in computer-based speech and language sample analysis urge clinicians to hold onto the notion that their clinical expertise is crucial. Long described the computer assisting the clinician as follows:

> Microcomputers can simplify clinical transcription by providing efficient methods for recording and editing responses. They can process large quantities of client data, thereby relieving the clinician from many tasks that are both time-consuming and, because of their repetitiveness, mentally exhausting. Current software can also scan for subtle patterns within the data. Nevertheless, it is the clinician, not the microcomputer, who remains in charge of the assessment process; although technology can get the data to the clinician, only a clinician can derive information from that data. (1991, p. 2)

No matter how clinically useful conversational speech and language samples may be, they will not be used to their potential if they are too time consuming for clinicians to manage.

USING THE COMPUTER TO ASSIST WITH DIAGNOSTIC DATA INTERPRETATION

In 1991, extensive clinical training and expertise were necessary to derive useful information from an assessment. More recent computer applications, however, can automatically compare an individual's speech or language to that of age-matched peers.

Systematic Analysis of Language Transcripts (SALT) has a companion reference database of language sample measures from 252 children ages 3–13 called *PROFILER*. The comparison process results in a profile of language performance in which individual measures can be checked relative to the mean and standard deviation of the reference sample of typical children (Evans & Miller, 1999). A more complete description and discussion of *SALT* and other language sample analysis software is found in Topics 31 and 32.

Test publishers are developing computer tools to assist clinicians with the scoring and interpretation of standardized, norm-referenced instruments administered either traditionally or with computer assistance. Typically, test-scoring programs take individual raw scores, automatically calculate standard scores, and provide norm comparisons. Some applications also offer narrative interpretations and recommendations that are intended for inclusion in assessment reports.

CASE EXAMPLE: Computerized Articulation and Phonology Evaluation System (CAPES)

Computerized Articulation and Phonology Evaluation System (CAPES) can be administered to clients ages 2 through adult. The software includes stimulus items, transcription assistance, and extensive analysis options. Interpretation features include age comparisons, dialect filters, treatment suggestions, and customizable reports. A more complete description and discussion of *CAPES* and other software for speech sample analysis is found in Topic 33.

Some clinicians have qualms about sending or receiving client reports that contain "computer-generated" test interpretations or treatment recommendations. An argument could be made that the reader of a report should, at least, be informed about which parts of the report reflect a clinician's personal assessment of the client and which were generated by a computer, entirely on the basis of test data. Computer-assisted scoring and interpretation are discussed in more detail in Topics 34 and 35.

The Internet provides yet another way that computers will and do affect the interpretation of diagnostic data. The use of the Internet as a means of providing access to large reference databases against which individual performances can be routinely compared is still in its infancy. Used more by researchers than clinicians so far, the CHILDES project offers Internet access to an extensive reference database of child language samples transcribed in many different languages (Evans & Miller, 1999). Ready access to national and international databases of speech, language, and voice samples is likely to increase dramatically, as researchers and developers resolve issues surrounding copyrights and funding. Clinicians and consumers will soon have access to large collections of video, audio, and photographic examples illustrating the physical and behavioral characteristics of speech, language, hearing disorders, genetic syndromes, learning problems, neurological impairments, orofacial anomolies, and major developmental milestones.

"ON-LINE" DIAGNOSIS OF COMMUNICATION DISORDERS

The Internet connects professionals and consumers to on-line medical chat rooms, support groups, and vast amounts of information about communication disorders. ASHA has organized its web site to be more useful to professionals and consumers, and declared that a priority will be making consumer information about communication disorders and service providers easy to obtain. Already, the web is providing a convenient and seemingly confidential way for individuals to consult with all kinds of service providers, from psychic mediums and car mechanics to midwives and veterinarians. Every day, audio and video conferencing over the Internet become more common and convenient. A person can go to the web and take a hearing screening test in complete privacy. How far are we from "on-line" speech and language screening and diagnosis? The beginnings of on-line assessment and treatment (telepractice) are discussed in Section VI.

In his description of the "cyber speech and hearing clinic" of the future, Tanner (2001) predicted that computers will take on much of the collection and analysis of data that clinicians do at present. For example, computers will acoustically analyze a client's speech and compare each phoneme to known norms for intelligibility and precision. Language samples and tests will be entirely computerized, making use of sophisticated new speech recognition technology. Computers will automatically develop a complete profile of a person's voice parameters, detecting not only obvious deviations that a clinician would notice, but also perhaps subtle early signs of neurological diseases such as ALS, MS, or others. For most clinicians, this vision of the future is both enticing and frightening. Like other service professions, we need to prepare for the dramatic changes that new technologies will bring to the everyday clinical experience.

PROFESSIONAL CONCERNS SURROUNDING THE DIAGNOSTIC USES OF COMPUTERS

"Garbage in, garbage out." This phrase, sometimes abbreviated "GIGO," is how computer programmers acknowledge the limitations of computerized data analysis. No matter how well designed and executed a computer program is, the end result can only be as good as the information entered by the user. Thus, if misleading or inaccurate data is the source, misleading and inaccurate results are the inevitable product–thus, garbage in, garbage out. Clinicians and consumers must not give too much credence to an analysis of assessment data merely because a computer was used. Complex printouts and graphs can give the impression of professionalism and expertise that computers on their own do not possess. The analysis can only be as valid as was the original data, and the quality of this raw information still depends heavily on a clinician's assessment skills (Schwartz, 1986).

For example, it is possible to obtain a very impressive printout analyzing a client's voice. In seconds, the computer can report and graph not only basic parameters such as pitch and loudness, but also detailed measures that are more commonly used in research. Imagine the implications of relying on this data if the microphone was inappropriately placed or the speaking task was poorly chosen. In either case, the sample recorded and analyzed by the computer may not be an accurate reflection of the client's vocal behavior. A computer cannot make this judgment.

Mastery of computer-based diagnostic tools requires time and effort. They may produce results that are more accurate, more consistent, or more detailed than are generally available without a computer, but at first such tools are time-consuming. They may even seem more difficult than low-tech alternatives, especially to student clinicians. Students are simultaneously learning not only the computer-based tool, but also the basic assessment procedures and underlying content. A student clinician learning to use computer-assisted language sample analysis, for instance, may struggle with the coding of morphemes in the sample. This may be less a matter of learning to use the computer-based tool than it is just a matter of mastering the basics of morphology. The latter would be necessary whether the student was using traditional or computer-assisted methods of calculating MLU.

So, just like other clinical computing competencies, effective use of computer-assisted diagnostic tools depends less on computer expertise than on clinical expertise. Computers can help clinicians and students acquire or review communication disorders content. The web is a source for professional development and student study aides on many clinical topics. For example, Barbara Fazio at Indiana University has posted a web-based tutorial for learning and practicing the counting of morphemes and the calculation of MLU. Many publishers and instructors have tried to help students and working clinicians overcome some of the barriers to adoption of new computer tools by providing on-line tutorials and demonstration copies of their software at low or no cost. Clinicians and instructors who are interested in improving their general skills or trying computer-based language sample analysis should seek out such support materials.

The professional concerns described thus far focus on the clinician's skills, training, and understanding of the strengths and limitations of computer-based diagnostic tools. What will happen when either the clinician is not present at all, as with "self-diagnosis" tools, or is available only as an "on-line" consultant who never meets face-to-face with the client? It is likely that these situations will give rise to more professional issues and ethical concerns. Certainly clinicians, professional organizations, consumers, and third-party payers, will want to address the following questions at the very least:

1. How will consumers of "on-line" services know that providers have appropriate qualifications and experience?

2. Who will be responsible for misdiagnoses and lack of appropriate follow-up services?

3. How should charges for "on-line" diagnostic and treatment services be determined, and by whom?

4. Who owns the "data" created by thousands of "on-line" evaluations and how will consumers give their consent for their data to be included in online research projects and databases?

5. How will the confidentiality of client data and records be maintained in cyberspace?

Predicting the future with regard to how computer technology will be used is always risky. Many famous mistaken predictions from "experts" amuse computer users today. In 1977, at the World Future Convention, the well-known president, chairman, and founder of Digital Equipment Corporation Kenneth Olson, said "There is no reason for any individual to have a computer in his home." In 1981, about the time that diagnostic uses for computers were first being explored in communication disorders, Bill Gates, founder and chairman of Microsoft, made his now famous statement about computer memory: "640K [1 megabyte] ought to be enough for anybody." Just two decades later, 256 MB of RAM was considered minimal on new computers. The only thing that can be said about the future for sure is that computers will be used in the process of diagnosing speech, language, and hearing disorders, in ways that at present we cannot foresee.

SUMMARY

Since the early 1980s, clinicians and researchers have been exploring the routine clinical use of computers to assist with the evaluation of communication disorders. At present, many successful computer applications are available for assisting clinicians in the collection, analysis, and interpretation of diagnostic information. These applications cross a wide span of disorders. They include applications used directly with clients during an evaluation as well as those employed as analysis tools later by the clinician. Professional concerns that arise from using computers this way include the old adage "garbage-in, garbage-out." The clinician must ensure the quality of the procedures used and the data collected during an evaluation. Clinicians are reminded that computers cannot fully understand and synthesize clinical data and make judgments about the validity of such data.

Online diagnosis of communication disorders in the future is likely to take at least two forms: 1) self-administered instruments provided via the Internet, and 2) online clinical consultation with a distant clinician via video/audio transmission over the Internet. The advent of on-line diagnostic services will bring many new professional and ethical issues to the forefront.

REVIEW FOR TOPIC 30

1. Give an example of how a computer can be used to collect data during a speech or language evaluation.
2. Give an example of how a computer can be used to analyze data during or after a speech or language evaluation.
3. Give an example of how clinicians could use a computer to assist with the interpretation of diagnostic data.
4. Explain the phrase "garbage in, garbage out" as it applies to this topic.

QUESTIONS FOR DISCUSSION

1. Discuss the availability of "on-line experts" with which you are familiar. Have you made use of such services yet for financial planning, obtaining a loan, medical decisions, plan-

ning a trip, or making a major purchase? In your experience, what were the advantages and disadvantages of online consultation?

2. Describe what entices you and what scares you about the idea of a cyber clinic for diagnosing speech, language, and hearing disorders.

3. Re-read and reconsider Long's statement that only clinicians can derive important and useful diagnostic information from assessment data. What do you think about his position, in light of the new tools and new climate brought about by advances in technology?

RESOURCES FOR FURTHER STUDY

Case, J.L. (1999). Technology in the assessment of voice disorders. *Seminars in Speech and Language, 20,* 169–196.

Hallowell, B., & Katz, R.C. (1999). Technological applications in the assessment of acquired neurogenic communication and swallowing disorders in adults. *Seminars in Speech and Language, 20,* 149–167.

Long, S.H. (2001). About time: A comparison of computerised and manual procedures for grammatical and phonological analysis. *Clinical Linguistics and Phonetics, 15*(5), 399–426.

Long, S.H., & Channell, R.W. (2001). Accuracy of four language analysis procedures performed automatically. *American Journal of Speech-Language Pathology, 10,* 180–188.

Masterson, J.J., & Oller, D.K., (1999). Use of technology in phonological assessment: Evaluation of early meaningful speech and prelinguistic vocalizations. *Seminars in Speech and Language, 20,* 133–148.

Using a Computer to Assist with Language Sample Analysis

Transcription and Coding

Clinical computing competency #6: The clinician will make appropriate use of computer-based instruments designed to assist in the evaluation or diagnosis of communication disorders.

Every clinician should become familiar with the pros and cons of computer-assisted language sample analysis. Then, if the clinician sees potential benefits, personal goals can be developed for achieving competency with one or more computer-based analysis tools. Goals could include learning to collect, transcribe, and code the language sample according to the software's specific conventions, then choosing and implementing appropriate analyses. A further goal is learning to correctly interpret the results of computer-assisted language sample analysis.

Topic 31 is designed to get clinicians started on acquiring competency with computer-assisted language sample analysis. It provides an overview of available tools and an introduction that follows the usual first steps in this diagnostic procedure: collecting, transcribing, and coding a language sample. The remaining steps—analyis and interpretation—are discussed in Topic 32, as well as consideration of the advantages and limitations of using computer-based tools for these purposes.

CURRENTLY AVAILABLE TOOLS

Computer-assisted language sample analysis appeared early in the history of the clinical applications of computers. Important progress has been made in the development and dissemination of these tools, from research to clinical settings. Common analyses and measures facilitated by computer software include: the total number of words, number of different words, number of utterances or words per conversational turn, mean-length-utterance in morphemes (MLU), Developmental Sentence Scoring (DSS) (Lee, 1974), and type–token ratio (TTR) (Templin, 1957). Many additional measures and analyses are available, depending on which software is employed. Table 31.1 presents examples of currently available software designed to assist clinicians with the task of language sample analysis.

Table 31.1. Examples of clinical software available to assist clinicians with language sample analysis

Software exemplar	Abbreviation	Program components	Measures available
Child Language Data Exchange System (first developed by MacWhinney & Snow, 1986) (WIN)	CHILDES	A collection of tools including the CHILDES Transcription Editor (CED), CHAT (Codes for Human Analysis of Transcripts), CLAN (Child Language Analysis), and the CHILDES international language sample archive. Includes a parsing module that automatically adds grammatical tags after utterances in transcript; clinician must review these and correct errors before utterances are sorted or tallied.	MLU, DSS, lexical frequency counts, suprasegmentals, speech acts, code switching, signed language, dysfluency, timing, number of words, number of different words, type–token ratio, tally of sentence types, length of conversational turns, additional user-determined codes
Systematic Analysis of Language Transcripts (first developed by Miller & Chapman, 1981; current version 8.0, 2003) (WIN; older versions for MAC). Trial versions can be downloaded and complimentary copies are available.	SALT	Standard, instructional, student, and research versions of SALT are available. A collection of related products including SALT Transcription Tutor CD-ROM, SALT analysis program, and PROFILER for comparing results to a normative reference database of 252 children. Clinicians must individually code structures to be sorted or tallied. SALT analysis is available for English or Spanish.	MLU, lexical frequency counts, words per minute, utterances per minute, % intelligible, number of words, number of different words, type–token ratio, tally of sentence types, length of conversational turns, additional user-determined codes
Computerized Profiling v. 9.5.0 (Long, Fey, & Channell, 1998; 2003) (DOS). Free downloadable.	CP	A collection of separate tools that automatically generate tentative analyses of grammar [MLU, DSS, LARSP, IPSyn], pragmatics [NAP], semantics [APRON, PRISM-L], and/or prosody [PROP]. Profile of phonology module [PROPH, part of Computerized Profiling], profile of prosody [PROP], transcription utility with phonetics font [PROPHecy]. Clinicians must review and correct analysis errors before structures are sorted and tallied.	MLU, DSS, Syntax Complexity Score (SCS), IPSyn, LARSP, Analysis of Propositions (APRON), semantic themes, semantic categories, narrative analysis prosody profile, number of words, number of different words, type–token ratio, tally of sentence types, length of conversational turns
Parrot Easy Language Sample Analysis Plus (Parrot, 1998) (Win)	PELSA	Clinician must enter target forms as well as actual utterances.	Organizes sample according to 26 grammatical forms

Although there is some overlap in the functions of the tools presented in Table 31.1, they are diverse in their specific features and outcomes. For more detailed comparisons of the history and mechanics of these tools, readers should consult Evans and Miller (1999) for CHILDES and SALT, and Long (1999) for Computerized Profiling (CP). PELSA is much more limited than the other programs listed in Table 31.1. It has been dismissed as having "far more weaknesses than strengths" (Baker-Van Den Goorbergh, 1994, p. 335).

COLLECTING AND RECORDING A LANGUAGE SAMPLE

The various approaches that clinicians use to collect language samples from clients reflect how the clinicians were trained, the age and overall functioning level of the clients, and the purposes for which samples are collected. Current best practice encourages collecting samples of language across multiple contexts and tasks. For example, a different perspective on a person's language competence is obtained when the sample consists of a conversation, a personal narrative, a picture description, or the retelling of a story. In addition to the task, factors such as the gender, age, ethnicity, and familiarity of conversational partners may influence the results.

In 1994–1995, Kemp and Klee (1997) surveyed the language sampling practices of ASHA-certified clinicians working with preschoolers in the U.S. Not surprisingly, they found a great deal of variability in the typical length of samples, methods of recording, and analysis procedures. Eighty-five percent of the 253 respondents used language sample analysis to assess preschoolers with language impairments. This suggested to the researchers that clinicians value language sampling as a measure of language performance. Surprisingly, 59% of them reported that their primary method of capturing a sample was to record it by hand in real time without a tape recorder. Only 4% reported transcribing from videotape, while 37% transcribed their samples from audiotape. Obviously, scribbling utterances as a client speaks is efficient, but it leaves no opportunity for re-checking or re-interpreting communication attempts and it captures only one side of the conversation. A great deal of the information that justifies using a language sample for assessment may be lost in this procedure.

At the time of the Kemp–Klee survey, digital tape recorders and other portable digital technologies (e.g., hand-held computers and hand-held digital video cameras) were not options. Today their popularity in the general market makes them accessible for clinicians as well. Although digital recording equipment does not solve all of the problems associated with transcription, it does make it possible to take advantage of some of the transcription aids. In addition to dedicated digital audio recorders and video recorders, clinicians may want to consider using other new technologies for capturing their client's speech and/or language. There is a growing push to equip personal digital devices—such as personal digital assistants (PDAs), cell phones, and MP3 players, to do more and more diverse tasks (see Section VI). For example, a new iPod accessory called *iTalk* (Griffin Technology) turns Apple's popular MP3 music player into a sound recorder with thousands of hours of recording time. The *iTalk* also has a built-in speaker, releasing iPod users from their headphones. Thus a clinician could use an iPod for recording and playing speech or language samples as well as easily uploading the files to a computer. Likewise, audio files (music or speech, such as audio books) are easily downloaded from a web site to a computer to the iPod.

The classic and most commonly recommended length of a language sample is 100 utterances. This length helps ensure that the sample is representative of the person's ability and often allows for comparison to reference data provided by researchers (e.g., Miller, 1981; Weston, Shriberg, & Miller, 1989). However, in practice, clinicians often use shorter samples. The majority of clinicians surveyed by Kemp & Klee (1997) used 50 utterance samples. Research suggests that some valid measures can be obtained from samples as short as 25 utterances in length (Miller, 2000). Clinicians often develop their own favorite methods and materials for collecting language samples from the types and ages of clients they most frequently encounter. It is well known that many variables affect language sampling results—such as materials, tasks, and conversational partners. Developing and perfecting sampling protocols is desirable, so that some consistency in elicitation conditions from one language sample to another can be assured (reliability). However, for the same reason, clinicians should become familiar with the sampling tasks and conditions that were used to establish any norms or guidelines against which they plan to compare the results obtained by their clients. Because convenient comparison to a reference database is one of the frequently cited advantages of computer-assisted language sample analysis, the issue of how to collect a sample warrants extra attention.

Comparing the results of just any language sample to a reference database of samples collected in a particular way is unlikely to yield results that are reliable and valid. Eisenberg, Fersko, and Lundgren (2001) presented clinicians with a cautionary note to this effect, accompanied by a summary of the research showing the effects of variables such as setting, task, and speaking partner on the MLU of preschoolers. Clinicians often use as a guideline for interpreting MLU, the well-known early research of Miller and Chapman (Miller & Chapman, 1981; Miller, 1981). Table 31.2 summarizes the procedures that were used for collecting language samples in this early research (children ages 2–5), as well as the procedures used to collect samples later incorporated into the SALT reference database (children ages 3–13) (Leadholm & Miller, 1992). As one might expect, these procedures vary considerably in order to accommodate children of different ages and samples of different types (e.g., conversational versus narrative).

Computer-assisted tools such as those listed in Table 31.1 can be used to analyze language samples collected from clients of any age. Because of its child reference database, the SALT manual provides suggested tasks and materials for collecting samples from preschool and school-aged children. Specific examples in the manual contrast the elicitation of conversational versus narrative samples (Miller & Chapman, 1988). The examples are similar to the procedures described in Table 31.2. If clinicians follow these suggestions, they can be reasonably confident that the resulting samples can be validly compared to SALT's child reference database.

TRANSCRIBING A LANGUAGE SAMPLE

Transcription is the process of converting a language sample from an oral event to a written document. For the most part, computer-based tools for analyzing a language sample

Table 31.2. Procedures for eliciting language samples that have been used to establish performance expectations for MLU and other language characteristics

Procedure variables	MC	LM/SALT conversation context	LNM/SALT narrative context
Sampling size	50 utterances	100 utterances	100 utterances
Sampling time	• 10–15 minutes (older than age 2) • 20 minutes maximum (for age 2)	• 15 minutes • Provide separate data on 12-minute sampling time	• 15 minutes • Provide separate data on 12-minute sampling time
Setting	Child's home, an experimental play room, or therapy room	Therapy room	Therapy room
Interactant	Parent	Speech-Language Pathologist	Speech-Language Pathologist
Instructions	Mothers instructed to "play with toys as they usually did"	• Provide sample questions and prompts to facilitate child talk • Introduce at least one topic absent from the time and space of the sampling condition	Provide questions and prompts to facilitate child talk
Activity	Play with toys	• Play with clay (young children) • Question about classroom and other activities	• Tell a favorite story • Retell an episode of a TV program • Retell a familiar story
Materials	Set of toys that "varied from study to study, but always included both novel and familiar ones"	Clay (children 3–5 years)	• None • For 3-year-olds, pictures may be used for story retelling

From Eisenberg, S.L., Fersko, T.M., & Lundgren, C. (2001). The use of MLU for identifying language impairment in preschool children: A review. *American Journal of Speech-Language Pathology, 10,* 323–342. Reprinted with permission.

Note: MC=Miller & Chapman (1981); LM=Leadholm & Miller (1992); SALT=Systematic Analysis of Language Transcripts.

come into play after the sample has been collected and transcribed. However, transcription is key to any kind of language sample analysis. Even experienced clinicians dread after-the-fact transcription of a language sample from audio or videotape. Transcribing a 100-utterance tape of interaction with a school-age child reportedly takes experienced clinicians 1.5–2 hours (Miller, Freiberg, Rolland, & Reeves, 1992). This is probably why so many clinicians in the Kemp and Klee (1997) survey reported that they just write what they can at the moment and leave it at that. They would probably agree that transcribing in real time leaves much to be desired, but the realistic alternative may be no language sample at all.

High-tech and low-tech tools—from the business world and from clinical software developers—are available to help clinicians with transcription. From business settings, clinicians might benefit from the special transcription equipment used by secretaries in typing pools. Such tools include relatively inexpensive tape players with foot pedal controls that leave both hands available for typing. There are also computer-based controllers for digital recordings, but they still depend on a person to convert the auditory signal to a text document by typing what is heard. A freeware utility called *Sound Scriber* has been developed by Eric Breck at the University of Michigan; it aides in the transcription of digitalized sound files.

From clinical software developers come transcription editors and tutorials to assist clinicians in the process of preparing a language sample for analysis. For example, the CHILDES transcription editor (CED) displays three windows that give the clinician simultaneous access to a video display, an acoustic waveform of whatever sound is occurring, and a transcript window for typing. The CED requires digitized audio or video as input. The display includes on-screen controls that replace the rewinding and replaying on tape players, the use of which the developers claim "reduces transcription time by almost one-third" (Evans & Miller, 1999, p. 105). *Transcript Builder* (Thinking Publications) is a similar cross-platform (Mac/Windows) utility developed by Moore. It requires digital audio or video files as input, but is designed to make the transcription process faster and easier with onscreen controls and windows. Transcripts developed with *Transcript Builder* can be saved as text files and imported later into conventional word processing programs for clinician analysis or into computerized analysis programs such as SALT or CP.

It is important that the format for a transcript maintain enough coherence that the nature of the original interaction can be gleaned from reading it. In other words, transcription conventions should accommodate human readers, not just computer programs. Toward this end, CHILDES, SALT, and CP developers have attempted to keep the distraction of coding and transcription conventions to a minimum. Figure 31.1 shows a traditional transcription of the first few interactions between a clinician and a client during the elicitation of a language sample. It is easy to get a sense of the interaction from this classic three-column format. This format is convenient for handwritten transcription, however, it can be difficult to squeeze in additional notes or analysis codes such as utterance numbers, discourse errors, or morpheme counts.

Compare Figure 31.1 to a transcript of the same interaction, this time prepared according to SALT conventions (see Table 31.3). Again, it is easy to get a sense of the interaction by scanning the transcript. When SALT prints the transcript, utterance numbers can be automatically added.

Researchers and clinicians appear to be in complete agreement on this point: language sample transcription remains a barrier to more frequent and more effective use of language sampling for diagnostics and for documentation of progress (Evans & Miller, 1999; Kemp & Klee, 1997; Long, 1999). To date, there is no miracle solution to the difficulty of converting an analog speech signal (live or from video or audiotape) to a text document. However, digitizing speech and converting it to text—such as the process used in popular speech recognition systems—is a technology undergoing rapid improvement (see Topic 39 for an explanation of speech recognition). Because transcription of dictation is crucial in many businesses and medical settings, there is economic incentive for making the process of transcription more efficient through the use of technology. International business needs are also driving the pursuit of technological solutions to the challenge of cross-linguistic communication. Future solutions for clinical transcription may therefore also derive from improvements in technology for simultaneous translation of one language into another.

CODING A LANGUAGE SAMPLE

Clinicians who have never prepared a transcript for computer-assisted analysis may be intimidated by the phrase "coding the transcript," because it sounds technical and com-

TRUMAN STATE UNIVERSITY
Speech and Hearing Clinic
Language Sample Transcript Form

Name of Client __Eddie__ Age __7:6__
Type of Situation __Interview, narrative, free play__ Date __1-31-02__
Materials Present __Crayons, paper, cars, car wash__
People Present __Client & Clinician__
Portion of conversation transcribed: BEG _____ MID __✓__ END _____ ALL _____
Length of transcript: __11:53__ minutes __114__ utterances

CLINICIAN	CONTEXT	CLIENT
	Client & Clinician drawing pictures of their families	
		Hey! I'm drawing faster than you!
Yeah, you are. I draw slowly.		
		Actually, I'm going to make that my sister. We'll pretend she she grew um four inches last night.
She grew four inches in one night?		
		Yeah, and she's only three!
She's only three. Is she bigger than you?		
		No, I'm seven.
You're seven. But you're still taller than her.		
		Mmhm.
Wow		
	Client looking at crayon box	

Figure 31.1. A traditional transcription of the first few interactions between a clinician and a client during the elicitation of a language sample.

Table 31.3.   Excerpt from a transcript prepared according to SALT transcription and basic coding conventions

Eddie, Carol (client and clinician; not real names)

CA: 7;6 (chronological age of the client)

MODE: Interview (what kind of interaction is this? narrative? small group?)

DATE OF SAMPLE: 12/22/03

E Hey, I/'m draw/ing fast/er than you!

C Yeh, you are. I draw slow/ly.

E Actually, I/'m go/ing to make that my sister.

E We/'ll pretend she (she) grew (um) four inch/s last night.

C She grew four inch/s in one night?

E Yeh, and she/'s only three.

C She/'s only three.

C Is she big/er than you then?

E No, I/'m seven.

C You/'re seven.

C But you/'re still tall/er than her.

E Mhm.

C Wow.

=E looking at crayon box.

E If you ever want to take out that crayon sharpen/er, just take out all these.

E I/'ll show>

E Cause this thing is slant/ed and if (if) you ever want to pick it up, do that.

C Oh, I see.

C Then you can grab it out.

E Want me to?

C No, that/'s ok.

C We can leave it in.

=E puts finger in sharpener

E Oh, my finger/'s in there!

C Is your finger get/ing sharper?

=both laugh

:

C I need brown.

=E looks at crayons

E These crayon/s look like (in the : :02) they/'re in the wrong: thing.

E (It/'s like) That look/3s like a black and it/'s really brown.

C It almost look/3s gold.

Software: *Systematic Analysis of Language Transcripts* (University of Wisconsin-Madison, Language Analysis Lab).

plex. But "coding" occurs no matter how a transcript will be analyzed, even by hand. Clinicians "code" when they write each utterance on a new line and number the morphemes in each word; every time they underline topic initiations or circle errors in the use of articles or verbs, clinicians are "coding the transcript" according to their own system or conventions. Some examples of SALT coding can be seen with a closer examination of Table 31.3. The $ symbol denotes the speakers' names, the plus sign (+) precedes general information, and equals signs (=) precedes comment lines in the transcript. Slashes (/) are used to help the computer identify grammatical morphemes, and a colon (:) indicates a pause or time marker. This is basically all the coding that is necessary in order for SALT to calculate MLU, the total number of words, the number of different words, distribution of speaker turns by length, and frequency counts of word roots and bound morphemes (i.e., -ing, -ed, -s).

The trade-off seems more than worth it, and these basic transcription conventions are easily mastered. Nevertheless, even this amount of special formatting may seem like a lot to remember at first. Clinicians using computer-assisted analysis are advised to transcribe the client–clinician interaction and comments first, then go back and add formatting or codes that may be required by the computer program. The SALT program includes a transcript error-checking step that ensures that basic SALT formatting requirements, such as punctuation at the end of each utterance, are in place prior to analysis. Since the marking of bound morphemes such as -ing, -s, and -ed, depends entirely on the clinician when using SALT, the same chance of making a coding error occurs as if the clinician were using a non-computer method. However, there is less likelihood of making simple counting and mathematical errors since the SALT program numbers the utterances, tallies and lists the morphemes, and calculates MLU. Advanced coding can include time markers and symbols indicating any kind of structure or behavior (e.g., discourse rules) that the clinician would like to have the computer tally.

On-line training is available to aid clinicians in learning to transcribe and code language samples using Computerized Profiling (CP) version 9.5.0 and SALT version 8.0; a tutorial CD supported previous Windows versions of SALT. The on-line tutorials and training materials for both programs include short video clips and corresponding transcripts that take the user through the steps of transcribing and coding a sample, including some advanced codes and analyses. Examining the effect of the basic training provided by the SALT CD tutorial, researchers claimed that "Early versions of this program that were developed for transcription training have proven to be very efficient, reducing training time from 40 to 50 hours to 5 hours" (Evans & Miller, 1999, p. 107). Topic 32 provides more discussion of the potential time savings, advantages, and limitations of computer-assisted language sample analysis.

SUMMARY

Current software tools can assist clinicians with every aspect of language sample analysis: transcribing, coding, analyzing, and interpreting. Such software tools provide clinicians with a wide range of clinically useful measures and analyses that can be applied to conversational or narrative samples from clients of all ages. Most of the research of the developers of these tools has focused on language samples from children. Even before the language sample is collected, it is important for clinicians to consider whether they intend to use computer-assisted language sample analysis. That way, procedures for collecting, recording, and transcribing the sample can be consistent with the recommendations of the software developers. Elicitation procedures are especially important if the clinician expects to compare the eventual results of the analysis to a reference database.

Researchers and clinicians agree that the transcription step remains a primary barrier to more routine clinical use of language samples. Converting an audio or video signal into a text document remains a cumbersome and time-consuming task. Improvements to this aspect of language sample analysis will result from new technologies developed primarily for business and international communication.

REVIEW FOR TOPIC 31

1. What is the classic and most commonly recommended length for a language sample?
2. Describe a non-computer tool and a computer-based tool for helping clinicians with the process of transcribing a language sample.
3. What does "coding" a language sample mean? Give an example of an informal coding convention that a clinician might invent. Give two examples of SALT coding conventions.
4. Visit the web site of one or more of the software tools described in this topic. Look at examples of transcripts and print one if possible so that you can examine it more closely.

QUESTIONS FOR DISCUSSION

1. How important is it for clinicians to know what procedures were employed to collect the language samples used to develop normative data or to create a reference database? Discuss the factors that can influence the performance of a client during the elicitation of a language sample.
2. There are many possible formats for language sample transcription, and most clinicians have a favorite. What are some of the advantages and disadvantages of transcript formats you are familiar with? What is your preference and why?
3. Based on the information in this topic, what appear to you to be the advantages and disadvantages of computer-assisted language sample analysis?

RESOURCES FOR FURTHER STUDY

Eisenberg, S.L., Fersko, T.M., & Lundgren, C. (2001). The use of MLU for identifying language impairment in preschool children: A review. *American Journal of Speech-Language Pathology, 10,* 323–342.

Evans, J.L., & Miller, J.F. (1999). Language sample anaylsis in the 21st century. *Seminars in Speech and Language, 20*(2), 101–116.

Kemp, K., & Klee, T. (1997). Clinical language sampling practices: Results of a survey of speech-language pathologists in the United States. *Child Language Teaching and Therapy, 13,* 161–176.

Long, S.H. (1999). Technology applications in the assessment of children's language. *Seminars in Speech and Language, 20,* 117–132.

Using a Computer to Assist with Language Sample Analysis

Analysis and Interpretation

Clinical computing competency #6: The clinician will make appropriate use of computer-based instruments designed to assist in the evaluation or diagnosis of communication disorders.

One way that clinicians could approach this competency would be to master the use of one or more computer-based tools for language sample analysis. Personal goals for achieving this could include learning to transcribe and code the language sample according to the software's specific coding conventions, choosing and implementing appropriate analyses, correctly interpreting the results of computer-assisted language sample analysis, and being aware of the strengths and weaknesses of computer-assisted language sample analysis software.

As discussed in Topic 31, several computer-based tools are available to help clinicians with language sample analysis. Collecting, transcribing, and coding the sample are all affected by the decision to use computer-assisted analysis. Table 31.1 provides an overview of the specific software programs discussed here in Topic 32. Here the emphasis is on analysis and interpretation of language samples with the help of computer-based tools. Current research results and future perspectives are also offered.

ANALYZING A LANGUAGE SAMPLE

The software tools most widely used for language analysis by clinicians are of two types: the *data retrieval* type and the *symbiotic* type (Long, 1999). SALT is primarily a data retrieval program, in which words and codes that have been entered by the clinician are retrieved from a data file and tallied. Child Language Analysis (CLAN), which is part of the CHILDES system, and Computerized Profiling (CP) have both data retrieval components and symbiotic components. Long described "symbiotic" analysis as follows:

> The computer attempts to carry out some of the metalinguistic portions of the analysis based on linguistic information and decision-making algorithms pro-

The author thanks Janet Gooch, Steven Long, and Jon Miller for their comments and suggestions regarding the content of this topic.

grammed into it. The computer's analyses are displayed, and clinicians must review and correct them before asking the computer to sort and count the data. (1999, p. 121)

For example, the utterance "Him diving board" [He's on the diving board] might be parsed by a computer as having the following grammatical structure: subject (him) + verb (diving) + object (board), the same as the sentence "Him eating cookie." A clinician, however, would know that "diving" was not something being done to the board. In other words, even though the word "diving" can be a verb, as in "He is diving under the water," "diving" in the first sentence was used instead to describe the board. So, the clinician corrects the computer's interpretation before further grammatical analysis and calculations take place.

The manner in which a program approaches the task of language analysis can have implications. Consider MLU, a measure frequently of interest to clinicians. CLAN and SALT calculate MLU using the data retrieval method, counting and sorting root words and bound morphemes according to how each one has been marked in the transcript by a clinician. By contrast, CP calculates MLU using a symbiotic approach. It parses the sample based on its analysis of each word's syntactic function, and codes bound morphemes accordingly. Clinicians should check this analysis to be sure the parsing is correct. The typical margin of error for CP, even without a clinician's correction, is less than 2% (Long, 1999; Long & Channell, 2001). Additional descriptions of how coding and analysis are managed with CLAN, CP, and SALT can be found in Evan & Miller (1999) and Long (1999) as well as on the web sites associated with each program. These resources provide detailed information about particular analyses and measures produced by each software package (see also Table 31.1).

Researchers are continuing to evaluate and improve automated language sample analysis (e.g., the symbiotic approaches previously mentioned). Some computer tools for this purpose use a "probability" model in which the analysis is based on the probability of combinations of certain words. The grammatical categorization of each word is based on such probabilities. For example, given the sentence "The girl petted the dog with her hand," most English speakers would predict that the last word in the sentence will be a noun, and probably would guess the word *hand*. So, the syntactic and semantic context in this sentence makes "noun" a high probability. Grammatical categorization of this sort is called "tagging." Automated "whole-utterance tagging" means that a computer correctly categorized each word in the utterance. Channell and Johnson (1999) reported an overall accuracy rate of 95% for the automated word-by-word grammatical tagging of 30 naturalistic language samples from typically developing preschoolers. Whole-utterance tagging accuracy was notably lower, at 78%. The researchers concluded that additional improvement is needed "before the tagging is reliable enough to avoid manual postediting of any automated analysis" (p. 731). Automated syntactic, semantic, and pragmatic analysis will become increasingly accurate as artificial intelligence capabilities improve and computers are able to consider more of the contextual features of natural languages.

INTERPRETING THE RESULTS

Whether using traditional or computer-assisted analysis methods, clinicians must effectively interpret the results. There may not even be a demarcation between analysis and interpretation in the minds of some clinicians. Generally, clinicians analyzing and interpreting a language sample do some or all of the following

- Look for patterns surrounding noticeable breakdowns in communication
- Look for evidence of age-appropriate structures and functions
- Compare the actual occurrence of linguistic functions and structures to obligatory contexts where they should have occurred
- Compare numerical results to normative data when appropriate and available

How can computer-assisted language sample analysis help clinicians with these interpretive tasks? Experienced users find that all four of these interpretation activities can be facilitated directly or indirectly by computer-assisted language sample analysis.

Consider the way interpretation starts for most clinicians. The beginning of analysis and interpretation comes with detailed familiarity with the language sample. Miller et al. pointed out "Analysis and interpretation begin long before the 'print' of the transcript is ready" (1992, p. 79). They suggest that "While transcribing the sample, the speech-language pathologist cannot help but begin to form hypotheses about the student's language performance . . . [and] become aware of interactions in the data" (p. 79). As clinicians repeatedly view, hear, and read the interaction, they consider and reconsider the communication and the strengths and weaknesses exhibited by the client. They decide whether the sample is a good reflection of the client's usual language performance. They notice and evaluate their own contributions to the conversation. Just the process of transcribing a language sample, then, contributes to the clinician's understanding of the client and the interpretation of the sample.

After becoming familiar with the sample and the client's communication, the clinician may decide that no further analysis or interpretation is warranted, either because 1) the sample is not a good representation of the client's ability or 2) sufficient evidence of typical development and adequate skills is apparent. These are judgment calls, just like declaring the results of an oral peripheral examination "unremarkable." At present, computers are a long way from being able to certify a language sample as either unusable or unremarkable. Ability to make such judgments and feel confident about them comes with the linguistic expertise of a native speaker and the clinical training and practice of a speech-language pathologist.

Many times, a closer examination and more thorough documentation of linguistic structures and functions are warranted. At this point in analysis, the computer may be extremely useful. In a matter of moments, lists of morphemes, root words, or grammatical structures evident in the sample can be generated, depending on the software chosen. Computer-assisted analysis facilitates looking for patterns of errors or evidence of developmental milestones (e.g., did third-person singular –s occur in this sample? How many WH question words did the client use? What was this client's rate of speaking?). Depending on the software tool in use and the details included in transcription, information about actual occurrence of linguistic structures versus obligatory contexts can be rapidly obtained. For example, SALT analysis of bound morphemes produces a table that presents each morpheme, the number of times it occurred, the number of times it was omitted, and the resulting percent of obligatory contexts in which the morpheme was present.

Thus, rapidly searching the transcript for target structures, vocabulary, or discourse patterns may be the most useful advantage of computer-assisted language sample analysis such as CLAN, CP, and SALT. Beyond helping to document whether a problem is present, such analysis can help a clinician identify and track potential intervention goals. Goals based on a client's actual use (or non-use) of certain aspects of language during conversation or narrative tasks can be supported through this close examination of language samples, regardless of what formal measures are taken. When clinicians fail to make use of the search functions of computer-assisted language sample analysis tools, they miss an important opportunity. "Unless computerized language sample analysis software is used in this way, its function becomes pretty much the same as norm-referenced testing, namely, to identify children in need of language intervention" (Steven Long, personal communication, January 27, 2002).

Finally, clinicians and researchers may want to compare some aspects of an individual's language to that of age-matched peers. As previously noted, it is important to consider the methods, contexts, and tasks used during elicitation of the sample if such comparison is anticipated. Computer-assisted analysis shines when it comes to producing and displaying numerical data and manipulating large databases.

The CHILDES system offers an international archive of samples against which a particular child's language sample can be compared, albeit by hand.

> Researchers can transcribe languages such as Dutch, French, German, Italian, Japanese, Portuguese, and Spanish, and use coding schemes that have been developed for the phonetic features, suprasegmental information, speech acts, code switching between languages or dialects, signed language, written language, dysfluent speech, and even specialized idiosyncratic use of linguistic features . . . The CHILDES system is designed to provide rapid, free, multimedia access to the entire database, via either the Internet or CDs. (Evans & Miller, 1999, p. 109)

SALT provides an automated comparison of an individual child's transcript to a reference database of 252 children ages 3–13 years. The database includes measures such as MLU, number of different words, total number of words, TTR, mean speaking turn length, percent of intelligible utterances, utterances per minute, words per minute, pauses, number of omitted words and bound morphemes, and number of abandoned utterances. In addition, comparative data is available for mazes if they are coded in the transcript by the clinician (mazes are repetitions or revisions of parts of words, words, or phrases). An individual's performance can be compared to the means and standard deviations of the reference sample of typical children. This elevates language sample analysis from a descriptive process to a criterion-referenced assessment procedure.

ADVANTAGES AND LIMITATIONS: WHAT THE RESEARCH SUGGESTS

The question many clinicians ask is, "Can I obtain and interpret the results of a language sample more quickly and more thoroughly by using computer-assisted analysis?" The best answer to this question right now is not "yes" or "no." The best answer is, "probably yes, eventually." This is the best answer because rapid changes in technology will continue to improve how clinicians are aided in this task. However, even with existing technology and tools, "probably yes, eventually" is a good answer. It means, yes, this tool will probably help you save time and get more accurate results. Why say "eventually?" The time required at first will probably be the same or longer than when doing language sample transcription and a common analysis like MLU by hand. The amount of advantage will depend on individual practice with the tool and the actual analyses completed.

In an effort to estimate the time savings that clinicians could expect from computer-assisted language sample analysis, Long and Masterson (1993) gathered data from both trials with students and surveys of working clinicians. Their estimates suggest that time savings increase directly as a function of the amount of analysis that is desired. In other words, the more thoroughly a language sample is examined, the more efficient computer-assisted analysis becomes. This is in part because of the "up front" time invested in transcribing and coding the sample—this takes about the same amount of time, whether manual or computer-assisted analysis is intended. But once the transcript is available, the time involved in completing additional analyses or measures via computer is trivial. To complete additional analyses manually, however, the clinician has to code/count/analyze each utterance again from the start. For example, transcribing a 100-utterance sample and calculating MLU was [very conservatively] estimated to require about 25 minutes by hand and 35 minutes on computer. But then calculating total number of words, number of different words, and a ratio of different words to total words (type-token ratio or TTR) was estimated to take another 25 minutes by hand and only 1 additional minute by computer, for a combined estimated time savings of 20% (Long & Masterson, 1993). Time savings became more dramatic as analysis became more extensive.

Are there disadvantages to having readily available extensive or unusual analyses? One possible problem would be misinterpretation of the results of an analysis the clinician did not thoroughly understand, and would never have generated on her own. Schwartz pointed out, in an early caution about analysis software, that

> While extensive analyses are impressive, they are functional only if the user needs that information. It is possible to be inundated by detail. The individual who encounters difficulties coding samples may also have trouble sorting information in tables and identifying patterns of performance. (1986, p. 5)

Just because an analysis can be done, does not mean that it always should be done, or that the results will be informative. Authors on the topic of computer-assisted speech and language sample analysis almost always reiterate some concern on this point. Computers do not and will not absolve clinicians from needing excellent preparation. For example, Long and Masterson cautioned against the notion that computer-generated analysis could somehow take the place of a clinician's expertise:

> Clinicians bear an equal responsibility for interpreting numbers on a computer printout as they do for numbers on a test score-sheet. They must understand how these numbers are calculated and what factors could make them more or less representative of a client's competence. (1993, p. 41)

However, the clinical usefulness of new measures and analyses only becomes apparent if they are available. Ready access may help a clinician identify and describe the language characteristics of an individual client in a way that otherwise might have been overlooked. More accurate description of behavior may lead to more appropriate treatment strategies. "Language impairment" is a complex term that researchers and clinicians are still defining. Miller et al. (1992) outlined six clinical types of language production disorders, aside from language delay, that experienced speech-language pathologists working in public schools had described. Some of the language parameters that best distinguished these types—such as length and frequency of pauses, rate of utterances and words per minute, repetitions, and vocabulary diversity—are most easily obtained by computer-assisted analysis. Clinicians are more likely to notice such parameters and perceive patterns in them if the information is easily or automatically available for their consideration.

SUMMARY

The software tools most commonly used to assist with clinical language sample analysis are of two types: 1) the data retrieval type and 2) the symbiotic type. Data retrieval programs retrieve and tally codes that have been entered by the clinician, depending heavily on clinician coding accuracy but eliminating much of the tedium of counting and calculations. Symbiotic programs use algorithms to label or "tag" linguistic elements, depending on the clinician to review and correct the inevitable coding errors that occur when the computer does not have the necessary contextual information to interpret each utterance appropriately. Researchers have high expectations for clinically dependable fully automated language sample analysis in the not-too-distant future.

The ease of availability of some measures provided by computer-assisted analysis, such as speaking rate and vocabulary diversity, have increased the attention of clinicians and researchers to those parameters of language development and language impairment. More complete description of language impairment may lead to more accurate diagnosis and more appropriately designed intervention. In general, the efficiency and accuracy that result from computer-assisted language sample analysis is a function of the number of measures obtained. That is, once the sample is transcribed and coded, obtaining more measures and analyses from the computer requires a minimal investment of additional time. Clinicians must be responsible for appropriate interpretation of language sample analysis, whether obtained traditionally or with the assistance of new technologies.

REVIEW FOR TOPIC 32

1. What are the two types of computer programs used most frequently in clinical language analysis and how are they different?
2. What does the phrase "grammatical tagging" mean?
3. The answer is "Probably yes, eventually." What is the question?
4. Have you ever derived the measures "total number of words" and "total number of different words in a language sample" by hand? How about "speaking rate in utterances per minute" and "words per minute"? Explain how you could obtain this information without a computer, and estimate how long it would take you for a 100-utterance sample (assume that the sample is already transcribed).
5. Visit the web site of one or more of the software tools described in this topic. Look at examples of analyses and print one if possible so that you can examine it more closely.

QUESTIONS FOR DISCUSSION

1. Review the description of what clinicians do when they interpret a language sample analysis. Do you agree with these four points? Are there others you would add? Based on the information in this topic, how would you expect computer-assisted analysis to contribute to a clinician's interpretation?

2. There is an implied trade-off in the risk of having too much analysis of a language sample (overwhelming detail) versus the risk of missing important characteristics of a language impairment (insufficient analysis). Discuss this trade-off as an argument for or against computer-assisted language sample analysis.

3. Based on the information in this topic, how has your perception of the advantages and disadvantages of computer-assisted language sample analysis changed?

RESOURCES FOR FURTHER STUDY

Long, S.H. (2001). About time: A comparison of computerised and manual procedures for grammatical and phonological analysis. *Clinical Linguistics and Phonetics, 15*(5), 399–426.

Long, S.H., & Channell, R.W. (2001). Accuracy of four language analysis procedures performed automatically. *American Journal of Speech-Language Pathology, 10,* 180–188.

Miller, J.F., Freiberg, C., Rolland, M.B., & Reeves, M.A. (1992). Implementing computerized language sample analysis in the public school. *Topics in Language Disorders, 12*(2), 69–82.

Using a Computer to Assist with Speech Sample Analysis

Clinical computing competency #6: The clinician will make appropriate use of computer-based instruments designed to assist in the evaluation or diagnosis of communication disorders.

Several tools for computer-assisted speech testing and speech sample analysis are available to clinicians. Clinical competency in the use of such tools includes taking responsibility for eliciting and recording an appropriate sample of the client's speech and transcribing or coding it with a high degree of accuracy. Software tools help with each of these steps. In addition, competent clinicians must be familiar with traditional and computerized analysis options available and how the results should be interpreted.

It is the rare clinician who works in a setting where speech testing is not a routine part of his or her responsibilities. Clinicians frequently administer picture-based articulation tests that have long been the cornerstone of speech assessment. Some clinicians depend more on their own judgments of the spontaneous running speech of their clients than they do on articulation test results. Some clinicians want a detailed index of sounds the client produces correctly or incorrectly, some need phonological process analysis, and some are more interested in estimates of client intelligibility. Most clinicians in training have been encouraged to use phonetic transcription to record the articulation of their clients, so that detailed analysis can be conducted when warranted. Computer applications are available to assist with each of these aspects of speech assessment, in addition to measurement of stuttering behaviors. Table 33.1 describes some examples of speech sample analysis and testing software.

An early example of computer-assisted speech sample analysis resulted from a collaboration that began in the late 1980s between researcher Kim Oller and biomedical engineer Rafael Delgado of Intelligent Hearing Systems. Their work resulted in the *Logical International Phonetic Programs* (LIPP) (Intelligent Hearing Systems), which has contin-

Thanks to Steven Long and Julie Masterson for their helpful comments and suggestions regarding the content of this topic.

ued to be revised and refined over the past two decades. *LIPP* is used in universities and research labs in the United States, Canada, and Europe. Oller described the rationale for computer-assisted speech sample analysis during the initial stages of *LIPP* development, explaining that

> The two major trends of modern child phonology are 1) an ever increasing complexity of symbology to keep pace with discoveries about international phonetic systems as well as special sound types occuring in development and speech disorders, and 2) increasingly sophisticated phonetic/phonological systems of analysis to be applied to transcribed data. While these trends have provided the foundation for vastly more significant insight into processes of phonological development and disorders, they have also created a great need for more convenient, automated means of recording and analyzing data. (1991, p. 57)

Two especially important needs drove some of the early design decisions in the development of *LIPP*: 1) the need for ongoing flexibility so that the tool could be modified to accommodate new discoveries and goals in phonology research, and 2) the need for a way to establish and easily check the reliability of the coding of large amounts of detailed data. These prime directives, clearly related to the state of phonology as a field of study, might not be the same for a software tool that a clinician would design for everyday use. Although other computer-assisted speech sample analysis programs have come and gone, they have not had the same priorities as *LIPP*, possibly making them more vulnerable to changes in both clinical practice and technology.

LIPP is a collection of modules and programming tools. In many ways, *LIPP* embodies the low-threshold and high-ceiling characteristics of learner-based tools described in Topic 13. Although flexible and complex enough to allow experts to create new phonetic symbols and analyses for particular research protocols, *LIPP* is also comprehensible enough that student clinicians can learn the basics relatively quickly. By the end of a semester of practice and exercises, students are proficient at using *LIPP* as a tool for phonetic transcription and standard phonological analysis (Kim Oller, personal communication, June 16, 2003). A shareware version, *THINLIPP* provides phonetic transcription and standard phonological analysis capability.

Like many of the software tools developed for language sample analysis, programs for speech sample analysis have often arisen initially to meet the needs of a particular researcher or research team. This is in contrast to other types of clinical software, more likely to have been developed with working clinicians and a commercial market in mind from the start. Computers excel at data analysis: bring on the tasks that require matching, tallying, and calculating. Speech sample analysis for the purpose of diagnostics, with or without computer assistance, consists largely of exactly these tasks: determining how closely a production matches an ideal model, counting how many times an attribute, sound, or error occurs, and calculating percentages or other statistics. This is not to suggest that diagnosing speech disorders is merely a matter of computation; but the art of diagnosis and the purposes of assessment are often aided by such data. Computer-assisted speech sample analysis is a natural application of technology in communication disorders.

COLLECTING A SPEECH SAMPLE

Collecting a speech sample involves eliciting it and recording it in some fashion. There are at least three available software applications that were especially designed to be used during elicitation of a traditional, confrontational naming speech sample. These include *AAAP*, *CAPES*, and *PROPHet*, which are described in Table 33.1. In all three cases, single-word stimuli are presented in the form of computer graphics or digital photos and the clinician immediately uses the computer program to provide partial or complete transcription of the client's response.

Some clinicians will want to collect a conversational speech sample as an alternative to or in addition to a single-word test. For example, Masterson and Oller (1999) recommend a brief conversational sample of 100 different words (usually about 200 words, total) for an initial speech sound assessment. There are advantages to each format (single-word versus running speech), as has been debated in the literature (Masterson & Oller, 1999; Morrison & Shriberg, 1992; Shriberg, 1993). Computer-assisted analysis, described later in this topic, is available for both single-word elicitation and connected speech samples.

Speech fluency and how to assess it is another area about which there is lack of universal agreement, as illustrated by lack of consensus regarding a definition of stuttering (Bakker, 1999a). Some professionals put less emphasis on the counting or measuring of disfluent speech as part of a differential diagnosis. These clinicians may not be interested in the computer-based tools for assessing disorders of fluency described in Table 33.1. These tools assist the clinician in determining the number and types of dysfluencies occurring in the speech of the client, which for many clinicians is among the most important features considered in fluency assessment (Bakker, 1999a).

DIGITALLY RECORDING A SPEECH SAMPLE

The technology for creating digital recordings of speech or music continues to become more portable, economical, and reliable. Among the computerized speech testing programs to date, only *CAPES* allows for actual capture or digitization of the client's speech during testing. Capturing a client's speech for later listening or analysis can certainly be accomplished without special communication disorders software. Clinicians use digital tape recorders or computers (e.g., desktop, laptop, hand-helds, or personal digital assistants [PDA]) for this purpose. Sound cards/chips have become a standard feature of most personal computers and their smaller cousins.

CASE EXAMPLE: Using a PDA to Capture a Brief Speech Sample from a Client Who Has Just Produced the Target Sound Correctly in a Word

Clinician: Wow! You did it Emil! I heard you make a perfect /l/ in "lake."

Client: [grins]

Clinician: Let's record that so you can hear how good it sounds, and I can keep it to play for your teacher and your mom at our meeting next week. When I point, you say "lake" three times, okay? Ready? (pushes button on her handheld PC and holds it near Emil's mouth; points to him)

Table 33.1. Examples of speech testing and speech sample analysis software

Software exemplar	Program features	Measures available
Automatic Articulation Analysis 2000 (AAAP, Parrot Software, WIN)	72 cartoon-like picture stimuli are used to elicit responses from the client. The phonetics font included is compatible with other Windows applications. Only program stimuli words can be analyzed.	Analysis consists of listing of patterns of misarticulation including: stops for fricatives, nasals, or affricates; glides for fricatives or liquids; vowels for syllabic consonants; fronting of velars and fricatives; prevocalic voicing; initial consonant devoicing; final consonant deletion; cluster reduction.
Computerized Articulation and Phonology Evaluation System (CAPES, Psychological Corporation, WIN)	Photographic and video stimuli, phonemic profile, in depth analysis, connected speech sample analysis, online demo, online transcription assistance, dialect filters for African American English and Spanish-influenced English, customizable parent letter, customizable age comparison guidelines to accommodate state/local guidelines. Only program stimuli are used for phonemic profile or individualized phonological evaluation, but conversational speech sample could include novel vocabulary.	Detailed analysis based on phonemic profile, individualized phonological evaluation, and/or connected speech sample. Extensive collection of detailed reports generated for each level of evaluation completed. Some describe/report client performance, (i.e., list of phonetically transcribed target words and initial position errors), some analyze productions according to theoretical stances such as nonlinear phonology, some provide simplified overview for parents, some provide treatment recommendations for the clinician's use. Summary report showing all target words and client's productions not available.
Computerized Scoring of Stuttering Severity (CSSS, Pro-Ed, DOS-WIN)	The CSSS provides measures that are required in the Stuttering Severity Instrument for Children and Adults–Third Edition (SSI-3) (i.e., percentage of stuttered syllables and duration of the three longest stuttering events). According to the authors, users of the SSI-3 will appreciate how much time can be saved when the longest events are located and measured automatically. Results of CSSS scoring can be displayed as graphs, printed, or stored.	Types of measurement include percentage of stuttered syllables, mean duration of the three longest stuttering events, mean duration of all stuttering events, fluent speaking rate, and length of periods of fluent speech. According to the authors, these data are useful for tracking stuttering severity during treatment or in research over time.
Computerized Profiling v9.5.0: Phonology (PROPH, DOS-WIN)	Optional photographic stimuli database and online response transcription with mulitmedia "rewards" for client (PROPHet), profile of phonology module (PROPH, part of Computerized Profiling), profile of prosody (PROP), transcription utility with phonetics font (PROPHecy), utility that generates phonetic text compatible with Windows applications (PROPHer). Phonetically transcribed target word lists for commonly used word lists/articulation tests are available for download, but tools could be used to analyze any words.	Comprehensive phonological analysis of any spontaneous speech sample or articulation test items; structural statistics variability/homonymy analysis; analysis of word shape, vowel target, consonant target; percentage consonants correct; phonetic inventory; phonological process analysis.

322

Interactive System for Phonological Analysis (ISPA, Psychological Corporation, MAC)	Analysis program for speech samples. Clinician must enter target word plus actual production using phonetic transcription symbols and conventions. Files for target words from frequently used tests can be developed by user so that they do not have to be entered each time. Phonetic font utility for Mac, sample files, and manual with tutorial included. Analysis not limited to any particular stimulus set.	Phonological and phonetic analysis of any speech sample or items from any traditional articulation test. Detailed and summary reports for phonological processes, phonetic inventory.
Phoneme Intelligibility Test (PIT, Tice Technology Services, Inc., WIN)	Database of text-based stimulus words and phrases; new item set randomly generated for each administration (can be printed out). Computer-guided intelligibility data collected by having judge(s) listen to tape of speaker and choose target words on the computer, much like an auditory discrimination test. Computer analyzes listener judgments to determine speaker intelligibility and articulatory breakdowns.	Overall percent accuracy; percent of accurate vowels; percent of accurate consonants; vowel and consonant matrices plot actual target sounds vs. perceived sounds; additional scores for stop consonants, fricatives, affricates, semi-vowels, nasals, and pressure consonants.
Logical International Phonetics Programs (LIPP, Intelligent Hearing Systems of Miami, WIN)	Primarily used by researchers, LIPP is sophisticated phonetic transcription and phonological analysis software that includes tools for creating novel phonetic symbols and analyses. It has been used to study the vocalizations of typically developing infants and toddlers as well as infants with hearing impairment and infants in bilingual homes. A CHILDES database interface is available.	LIPP is an extremely flexible tool that allows the user to define analysis needs and display of results. Modules include a full implementation of Hodson's Phonological Analysis and automatic scoring for Jakielski's Index of Phonetic Complexity, among dozens of other standard analyses and measures.
Stuttering Measurement Module (SMM, WIN)	Aids clinician in ongoing count of stuttered and non-stuttered syllables and speech naturalness ratings as client speaks, or could be used by clinician while listening to a recorded sample. Can be used to inform client of current performance during treatment sessions. Stimuli, topics are not unlimited.	Provides percentage of stuttered syllables, speech rate, speech naturalness ratings in text or graphical form. Also available: mean length of stutter-free intervals in syllables or seconds.

Client: Lake, lake, lake.

Clinician: Lovely! Listen while I play it back for you.
            [presses play button; recording plays immediately]
            You sound awesome!

When the clinician in this case example returns to her "home base" computer, she may transfer this audio file to a more permanent location, to free up her handheld for new recordings. She may just leave it on her hand-held computer for easy transport and reproduction at the upcoming IEP meeting. If this was assessment data, she might listen to it repeatedly, while she transcribes it into a computer-assisted speech analysis program. Note that recording and playback quality varies considerably among small portable devices, and that some articulation errors, such as fricative distortions, may be difficult to discriminate. Good headphones will improve the playback of speech or music, assuming the hand-held has an earphone jack.

Clinicians who want to use a computer to capture speech samples need three things: 1) a sound input device (e.g., microphone), 2) a sound digitizer (e.g., a *SoundBlaster* card in Windows machines), and 3) software to record, stop, play, and save. External speakers or good quality headphones are desirable if the speech sample is to be phonetically transcribed. All of the required recording components are often included in desktop and hand-held PCs and can be added to some PDAs. An add-on device from Griffin Technologies, Inc., called *iTalk* adds recording and speaker playback capability to Apple's popular MP3 player, the iPod.

Although speech recording capability and a microphone were automatically included with Macintosh desktop and laptop computers for many years, some recent models have eliminated audio input capability as a standard feature. Presumably, this is so that consumers can choose (and pay for) the quality and type of audio input desired. For a very reasonable price, clinicians can add stereo input and output to any Mac or PC that has a USB port with an *iMic* USB audio interface from Griffin Technologies, Inc. A microphone is also required, which will plug into the *iMic* interface. The manufacturer claims a resulting quality of sound recording that exceeds the performance of built-in audio (e.g., the iMac's built-in microphone).

Speech samples in digital format have advantages similar to the advantages that DVDs have over analog videotapes and that music CDs have over cassette tapes. Analog audio or videotape requires the user to fast-forward and rewind repeatedly to find the desired segment, in a linear fashion. Digital video and audio, in contrast, offer immediate access to any point in the recording. In addition, storage of digital files is easy, inexpensive, and space-saving. Repeated playing does not cause a digital recording to deteriorate, as it does analog media. Clinicians could even store audio files of special or unique clients permanently by making a compact disc (see Section IV for a discussion of multimedia tools). Client files of all types (text, audio, video) can be permanently stored on CD-ROM today, and other digital media in the future.

TRANSCRIBING (CODING) THE SPEECH SAMPLE

Similar to tools for computer-assisted language sample analysis, most computer-assisted speech analysis comes into play after the sample has been elicited and recorded, either with analog or digital methods. Unlike language samples, speech samples are generally transcribed and coded in one process: phonetically transcribing the client's productions, using the International Phonetic Alphabet (IPA). Some computer-based speech testing and analysis software offers assistance with this phase.

For example, *CAPES, LIPP*, and *PROPH* have a "phonetic dictionary" utility. To use a phonetic dictionary, the user types in target utterances in traditional orthography. Then the phonetic dictionary software automatically translates the words into phonetic symbols. Clinicians only need to make special transcriptions when the client's production includes errors or the target word isn't in the phonetic dictionary database (Masterson & Oller, 1999). Theoretically, this could include words in other languages, as long as the clinician enters both the target and the production, using the IPA.

The *Interactive System for Phonological Analysis* (ISPA) (Masterson & Pagan, 1993) was a Macintosh platform tool for speech sample analysis available until recently. One of the strengths of *ISPA* was the fact that it could be used to analyze any speech sample. Clinicians could enter a connected speech sample (one word at a time), a collection of single word utterances, or a wordlist associated with a major articulation test. In contrast to the phonetic dictionary approach, however, clinicians using *ISPA* used a phonetic font to enter all target words and client productions. Much time was saved if the target words were predictable (as in a standardized articulation test). Clinicians could create, save, and share template files of frequently used word lists in advance. These files could be edited to indicate client error productions, rather than entering all targets and productions from scratch for each analysis. Now *LIPP* and *PROPH* offer similar capabilities.

Whether using computer-assisted speech sample analysis or not, many clinicians will find it useful to have a phonetics font available. A phonetics font allows for printing correct transcription of sounds in IEPs and reports, rather than hand-writing special symbols onto the hardcopy. New fonts and shareware utilities are developed each time a major upgrade of system software occurs. The best way to find these fonts and utilities is to search for them on the Internet. Many are free and downloadable. One example is the *SIL Encore IPA Fonts*, a free downloadable Mac/Win font collection from International Publishing Services. These IPA fonts are automatically installed with *Computerized Profiling* (i.e., *PROPH*), a collection of programs that can be downloaded from the *CP* web site (see Table 33.1). Alternatively, clinicians can purchase a phonetics font, such as *Phonetic Font Plus* (Parrot Software).

Neither a phonetic dictionary nor a phonetic font actually helps a clinician decide on a correct phonetic transcription of a target that is produced in error. Clinicians are assisted with speeding up transcription of errors in *PROPH* and *PROPHet* (Long et al., 2003) and *CAPES* (Masterson & Bernhardt, 2001). These programs present a correct phonetic transcription for each target word as well as several common error productions for the clinician to choose from. The clinician also has the opportunity to add unique phonetic transcriptions for each target. This support helps clinicians listen to and consider each error production more carefully, perhaps, although there is also the risk that the clinician's perception will be influenced by available transcriptions.

Obviously, in order to provide the phonetically transcribed alternatives, the targets must be known in advance. So, *CAPES* has its own target word set that is individualized for the client at the deep testing level, as determined by the software based on errors produced during the initial 46 items. This is the traditional articulation test model, in which clinicians do not choose the target words. *PROPHet* is more tool-like, leaving the clinician to choose targets from a library of approximately 400 digital images (some duplicates) and 3–4 accompanying phonetic transcriptions per item (see Figure 33.1). Pictures for the wordlists from popular traditional articulation tests are available, but a clinician could also create his own "deep test," for example, using items weighted with fricatives or liquids and glides. The responses collected and coded with *PROPHet* are then analyzed using the *PROPH* module of *Computerized Profiling*. Both *CAPES* and *PROPH* can also be used to analyze connected speech samples, as discussed further below.

CAPES: THREE LEVELS OF ASSESSMENT

CAPES is intended to be a complete, start-to-finish computerized speech assessment tool, for use with clients ages 2 and up. It provides single-word photo stimuli, video and text prompts for eliciting connected speech, preliminary analyses and detailed analyses of single-word productions, analysis of connected speech, and a variety of interpretation and report options. Initially, a basic set of 46 words is elicited from the client in response to digital photos; responses are digitally recorded for later transcription, or transcribed online immediately by the clinician. To facilitate this process, likely errors are phonetically transcribed on the screen in a multiple-choice format. Clinicians may click on one of the suggested transcriptions, or transcribe the entire response on the screen themselves. At the clinician's choosing, the client's production can be flagged for later consideration (see Figure 33.2).

After the phonemic profile (initial 46 items) is complete, the assessment could stop, although that would not be recommended unless no speech problems are observed. At this point, a phonemic profile summary (initial, medial, final phonemes produced) and/or a parent report could be generated. The parent report indicates sounds that are advanced for the child's age as well as the sounds with which the child "is having difficulty." If the clinician has indicated that the client uses African-American English or Spanish-Influenced English, mismatches between targets and productions that might be dialectal do not appear in reports. So, based on fewer than 50 words, clinicians can obtain a quick idea of how the client compares to norms and consider whether a larger sample and more detailed analysis is warranted. Clinicians choose the criteria by which developmental errors are determined. The "standard" used by the program are the *Iowa-Nebraska Articulation Norms* (Smit, Hand, Freilinger, Bernthal, & Bird, 1990). If clinicians want to use local or state guidelines instead, those are entered in the Preferences section of *CAPES*.

An Individualized Phonological Evaluation (IPE) is completed at the clinician's discretion, by eliciting 20–100 words that are selected by *CAPES*. The number and phonetic content of the stimuli used for the IPE depend on the developmental level of the client and the errors transcribed during the Phonemic Profile. According to program developers, there are four IPE levels:

- **IPE Level 1** is for clients at the earliest stages of development who have several deletions in the Profile responses; it checks simple word shapes with early developing consonants.

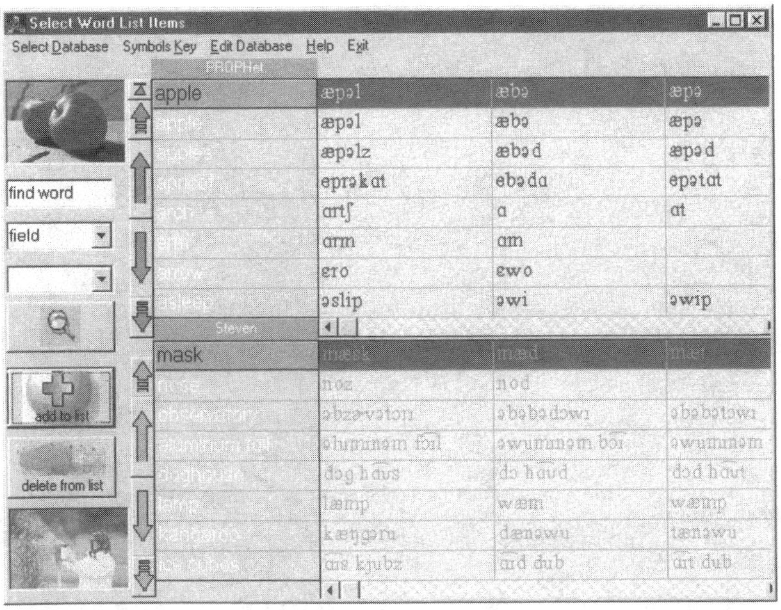

Figure 33.1. Screen shot from *PROPHet* showing the utility that the clinician uses to choose which target words/images will be presented to the client during speech sample elicitation. Common error productions are pre-transcribed, but clinicians can add unique transcriptions as needed (Courtesy of Steven H. Long).

- **IPE Level 2** is for clients who have few deletions (maybe cluster reduction), but several substitutions. Every possible target is elicited at least three times in each position.

- **IPE Level 3** is for clients who have three or four sounds in error. It functions as a "deep test" with multiple opportunities to produce each sound in each position.

- **IPE Level 4** is for clients who had few errors, if any, on the initial Profile. It consists of complex multi-syllabic words with a variety of stress patterns.

CAPES developers consider the IPE levels one of its outstanding features. Stimuli items are tailored to the client, unlike traditional tests that use the same words to sample the speech of every client (Julie Masterson, personal communication, July 2003). When elicitation and transcription of all IPE items is complete, a wide range of analyses and reports are available. The reports/analyses consist primarily of tables that are not generally interpretable by anyone unfamiliar with clinical phonetics. In some reports, treatment suggestions are available.

The third level of assessment facilitated by *CAPES* is sampling and analyzing brief samples of connected speech. This assessment can be done with or without the other assessment components. Brief video segments can be used to elicit connected speech if desired, or the clinician can type in any brief sample. A phonetic dictionary is used to match as many words as possible, with others being phonetically transcribed by the clinician. Then error productions are coded and the entire sample is available in 1) orthographic form, 2) target phonetic transcription, and 3) actual production in phonetic transcription (see Figure 33.3). Connected speech analysis options are similar to those available in the IPE.

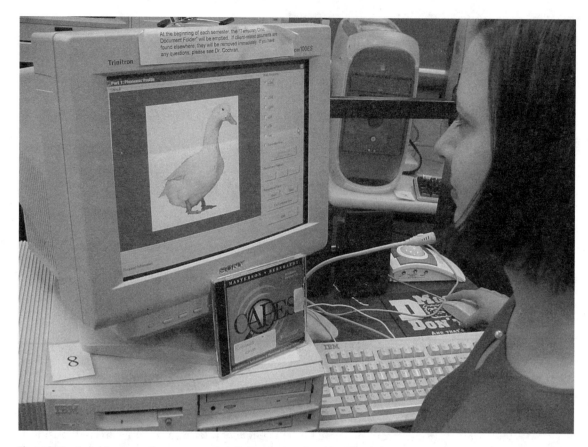

Figure 33.2. A clinician transcribes a pre-recorded client response using CAPES (Psychological Corporation; Courtesy of Truman State University Speech and Hearing Clinic).

ANALYZING A SPEECH SAMPLE

Clinicians analyze speech samples for a variety of purposes. For some, this has become so automatic that they may not even think about the kinds of information they are gathering or the various audiences that it may have. In some evaluations, the speech sample serves to document that articulation and phonology are not problematic for the client. Analysis in such cases is likely to be limited to reporting a simple articulation test score, or providing a clinical judgment of the client's functional speech (e.g., "Sharon's intelligibility is good even when the topic of conversation is unknown, and she is developing speech sounds as expected for her age").

In other cases, speech sample analysis may be used to 1) qualify the client for services, 2) help determine appropriate intervention goals, 3) document progress resulting from intervention, or 4) provide data for studying normal or disordered speech development. Computer-based tools for speech and language sample analysis have often begun as research tools that may or may not eventually become clinical tools. Some of the programs described in Table 33.1 reflect such a history. Thus, some of the analyses that they are capable of may strike some clinicians as obscure or unnecessary, depending on their habits and training. Other users may find such measures to be useful and enlightening in part because they have never routinely calculated them before.

> The bear is eating carrots.
>
> ₃ðə ₁bɛɾ ₁ɪz ₁i₃ɾɪŋ ₁kʰɛ₃ɾɪts
>
> ₃ðə ₁bɛʊ ₁ɪz ₁i₃ɾɪŋ ₁kʰɛ₃wɪts
>
> They are fighting.
>
> ₁ðɛ ₁ɑr ₁faɪ₃ɾɪŋ
>
> ₁ðɛ ₁ɑ ₁faɪ₃ɾɪŋ
>
> The bear sat down.
>
> ₃ðə ₁bɛɾ ₁sæt ₁daʊn
>
> ₃ðə ₁bɛʊ ₁sæt ₁daʊn

Figure 33.3. Connected speech sample elicited in response to a brief video clip showing panda bears. The clinician typed in the sample line by line (first line of text). The software provided a target phonetic transcription from a phonetic dictionary (first line of phonetic transcription under text). The clinician edited the targets to reflect actual client production (second phonetic line). Lines of phonetic text are color-coded on the computer monitor, as viewed in *CAPES*.

For example, most clinicians do not regularly tally the instances of every consonant in each position (initial, medial, final) that occurred in a sample. This is an analysis instantly available from *CAPES* and *PROPH*. Using computer-assisted analysis shifts the focus away from the tedium of tallying and analyzing the sample. Instead, the challenge becomes answering questions such as: "What does this information tell me?" or "How can I use this information to benefit my client?" Recall that computer-assisted language sample analysis has brought attention to measures such as rate, total number of words, and total number of different words. These measures, previously rarely calculated by clinicians, are now helping them to distinguish between clinical types of language impairment (Evans & Miller, 1999; Miller, Freiberg, Rolland, & Reeves, 1992).

Very possibly, some measures calculated routinely in computer-assisted speech sample analysis will eventually yield similar clinical insights. According to Long (personal communication, June, 2003), certain speech analyses have been developed and recommended for clinical use, but were rarely implemented by clinicians until computer-assisted methods of analysis were available. In *PROPH*, such analyses include homonym analysis, syllable structure level, and Phonological Mean Length of Utterance (Ingram & Ingram, 2001).

The articulation and phonological process analyses clinicians use most often are available from *CAPES, PROPH*, and to a lesser extent, *AAAP* (see Table 33.1). *CAPES* and *PROPH* also offer word shape analysis (e.g., CV, CVC), vowel analysis, and in the case of *CAPES*, analysis using a nonlinear theory of phonology. Percent of vowels correct and percent consonants correct (PPC) (Shriberg & Kwiatkowski, 1982) are available from *PROPH*.

The number of different possible reports/analyses generated by *CAPES* may be intimidating at first. To date, there is no hard copy manual in which examples of various report formats could be examined. On-line help emphasizes how to generate the reports more than why a particular report or comparison might be of clinical value. In many reports, the context of the client's production is not evident, or only the client's productions (not the target words) are printed out. For a client with many phonological processes it can be difficult for a reader to reconstruct the attempted word. The lack of printed target words and the number and variety of report formats may make it difficult to get an overall view of the client's performance for a beginning *CAPES* user. For example, although thorough information about phonological processes is available, clinicians must request a separate report for each place and manner of articulation in order to get the whole picture. *CAPES* reports can be printed or saved as RTF (Rich Text Format) files for later viewing or cutting and pasting into clinic reports.

INTERPRETING THE RESULTS

In a narrow sense, interpretation of test results usually involves a score and possibly normative comparisons. This would be a typical outcome of traditional articulation testing or phonological analysis. In a broader sense, interpretation involves deciding how well the assessment matches the client's typical performance, how the client's performance compares to expectations or to the performance of peers, whether the client's performance is consistent with the presence of a problem that warrants intervention, whether the results are consistent with other assessment data and observations, and whether the assessment information provides suggestions for possible intervention.

Computer-assisted speech sample analysis can contribute to both types of results interpretation. A *PROPH* profile, for example, automatically includes several well-known normative measures including a Severity Adjective rating (Shriberg & Kwiatkowski, 1982), an Articulation Competence Index score (Shriberg, 1993), Phonological Mean Length of Utterance (Ingram & Ingram, 2001), and Proportion of Whole Word Proximity (Ingram & Ingram, 2001). In the latest version (9.5.0) automatic comparison to the data from the Iowa-Nebraska Articulation Norms Project (Smit et al., 1990) is available. Clinicians are at liberty to use or report and explain all or none of these alternatives.

In contrast, the approach to interpretation taken by *CAPES* could be viewed as either simpler or more complex. The only direct normative information/age comparison is presented in the parent report or initial phonemic profile. A chart shows sounds that would be expected versus sounds the child is actually producing. This seems simple. Other interpretive information, based on combined responses during the Phonemic Profile and the more in-depth Individualized Phonological Evaluation, is presented in customized treatment suggestions that are generated in report format and directed at the clinician.

CAPES treatment suggestion reports review both the strengths and weaknesses identified by the assessments. Specific goals are divided into two categories: word shape goals and segmental or feature goals. Major goals are accompanied by suggestions for possible intervention, such as a minimal pairs approach. Treatment suggestions make a distinction in the kind of therapy procedures to be considered for a phoneme that is inconsistently produced versus one that is entirely absent from the client's phonetic inventory. Treatment options are given for speech elements (sounds, features, processes) that were produced with less than 60% accuracy (Julie Masterson, personal communication, July, 2003). With all of this information provided, why would this interpretation be considered complex? Because the process by which these goals and suggestions were arrived at is not transparent. The computer somewhat mysteriously provides this interpretation, but there is no way to know exactly how or why, and therefore no way to confirm or check it. In some ways, *CAPES*' treatment recommendations are like advice from an expert to a beginning clinician. The advice may be reasonable, but the clinician may or may not understand the rationale behind it. A broader discussion of the issues surrounding computer-assisted test interpretation is found in Topic 35.

A somewhat different approach to lending clinicians expert advice at interpreting assessment data was used in the development of *Childhood Stuttering: A Second Opinion* (ASO) (Bahill Intelligent Computer Systems) (Bahill, Bharathan, & Curlee, 1995; Conture & Yaruss, 1993). *ASO* was developed to serve as an expert system that clinicians could consult after collecting diagnostic information from young clients experiencing dysfluency. The decision matrix in the software is based on the diagnostic opinions and logic of a panel of distinguished experts on childhood stuttering. After the clinician enters requested diagnostic data, the software indicates one of five levels of concern regarding the young client's risk of stuttering (for a more detailed description and critique, see Bakker, 1999a). *ASO* is an early exemplar of "expert system" software for clinicians, which *CAPES* seems to take one step further.

ADVANTAGES AND LIMITATIONS: WHAT THE RESEARCH SUGGESTS

In their early examination of articulation testing via computer, Shriberg, Kwiatkowski, and Snyder (1986) looked at issues such as how presenting test stimuli via computer affected children's performance compared to traditional booklet administration. They found that children "seemed to feel that the computer required that they finish the task," but that it did not make a significant difference in the number or type of articulation errors that they produced (p. 318). They observed that children responded positively to an on-screen progress marker, giving them an idea of how much more had to be done. These are observations that developers of current and new computer-based instruments should keep in mind. The capabilities of off-the-shelf computer systems have come a long way since Shriberg, et al. were testing software on Apple II computers with 128k of memory. Now, computer-based visual materials are extremely high quality, the speed of loading images is instant, the number of responses/records that can be stored is virtually unlimited, the client's productions can be captured and stored digitally, and many interesting and useful tools are available for downloading from the Internet, a dissemination system that was non-existent a few short years ago.

What difference has all this technological progress made? We would hope that such progress would affect at least two parameters of computer-based speech sample analysis: it should be faster, and it should be better (more accurate, more informative). There is evidence that these advantages are occurring, accompanied by the same caveats that exist for computer-assisted language sample analysis. These include the truism that as clinicians become more experienced with the tools, the benefits become greater in time savings and in valid interpretation of the information produced.

Like computer-assisted language sample analysis, computer-assisted speech sample analysis becomes increasingly time-efficient with the number of analyses or measures that are required. Once the sample is transcribed, the time-consuming part is complete when a computer is performing the analyses, but just beginning if analysis is done traditionally. In a study involving 256 students and practicing clinicians, Long (2001) examined the issue of time savings more closely. Participants had been at least minimally trained to use both traditional methods and computerized methods of speech and language sample analysis. They were asked to complete ten common speech sound analyses (PCC, vowel inventory, consonant inventory, phonological processes, and so forth) on speech samples from three different children, by hand and by computer, keeping close track of the time spent on each. Although accuracy was not a focus of the study, the analyses were checked for accuracy as well. The results indicated that "without exception, computerized analyses were completed faster and with equal or better accuracy than manual analyses" (Long, 2001, p. 399). And the time differences weren't small—they were statistically significant at the $p<0.0001$ level, and seemed to be influenced by the type and length of the sample. For one speech sample, subjects completed the computerized analyses an average of 35 times faster than manual analyses (9 minutes versus 274 minutes).

Despite these impressive results, most clinicians and software developers would quickly admit that computer-assisted speech sample analysis still has a long way to go before it meets everyone's expectations. The issues of training and experience are not insignificant, even though developers are clearly making efforts. A collection of brief instructional videos can be downloaded from the *Computerized Profiling/PROPH* web site as needed. The *CAPES* software comes with an on-line demonstration/tutorial. Nevertheless, clinicians will need time and incentive to learn to use these and other computer-based tools to their full advantage.

The transcription feature of *CAPES* demonstrates a trade-off between flexibility (*CAPES* stimuli must be used) and ease of use (likely target errors are pre-transcribed). *LIPP* software demonstrates the same trade-off in reverse; the software is so flexible that clinicians can even design and define their own phonetic symbols (flexibility), but considerable effort is necessary to master *LIPP's* analysis design options (complexity). Software designers make many choices that revolve around this dilemma. Perhaps the software should have a high degree of flexibility and many options for the user, like most of the programs suggested for computer-as-context therapy in Section III. Generally, more orientation and practice are required to make full use of software tools that place a high premium on flexibility. Alternatively, the software could have fewer options, more like the CAI discussed in Section II or the *AAAP* program described in Table 33.1. By severely limiting stimuli and transcription options, *AAAP* keeps the process of analyzing a speech sample fairly simple. However, the price of simplicity is loss of a great deal of information about the client's productions that many clinicians would consider to be essential for grasping and documenting the client's phonological system. Software that locks the user into a more restricted set of activities and options is generally easier to master. What clinicians (and everyone else) find difficult is knowing in advance whether taking the time to master a flexible (and possibly complex) software tool will be worth the investment.

Of course, most clinicians and developers of software for communication disorders assessment are seeking a balance. The perfect software provides enough options to fulfill its purpose, and enough structure for new users to quickly succeed. Sometimes this notion of a trade-off is a helpful way to consider and compare various software tools on the market. Researchers may have resources and needs that make a more flexible, more complex software tool ideal for their assessment purposes. However, the time constraints and limited technical assistance available to clinicians may push them toward software that is less thorough or adaptable, but more comprehensible and efficient.

SUMMARY

Computers are good at matching, tallying, and calculating—processes that are necessary in speech sample analysis. Several products are available to assist clinicians in the task of analyzing speech samples for parameters such as length and type of disfluencies, phonological processes, phonetic indexes, and normative comparisons for speech sound development. Although preliminary research suggests that computer-based tools for speech analysis may yield faster and more accurate results when used by trained clinicians, the issue of training and experience is still important. Some programs have moved past tallying and calculating to offering expert advice intended to help clinicians interpret testing results. Currently available software programs have both strengths and weaknesses, often sharing the history of beginning as research tools that developed into clinical tools. The issue of flexibility versus complexity in software design remains a challenge for software developers and clinicians.

REVIEW FOR TOPIC 33

1. Give an example of one clinical software tool that analyzes any speech sample the clinician enters into the program.
2. Give an example of one clinical program that offers clinicians a choice of most likely error transcriptions for entering a client's response.
3. What is required in order to make a digital recording using a computer?
4. What are the practical advantages and disadvantages of recording speech samples in analog versus digital format?
5. How can a clinician obtain a phonetics font for her computer, and why would she want one?
6. Give three examples of the measures/analyses available from computer-assisted speech sample analysis.

QUESTIONS FOR DISCUSSION

1. Identify a software program that you like and use for any clinical purpose. How does this software illustrate the notion of a "trade-off" between flexibility and ease-of-use?
2. Continuing with the software discussed in Question 1, what features or functions do you wish it had that it does not? What do you think the "trade-off" might be to include those features or functions?
3. Based on the information in this topic, what would you tell other clinicians about the advantages and disadvantages of computer-assisted speech testing and speech sample analysis?

RESOURCES FOR FURTHER STUDY

Bakker, K. (1999). Technical solutions for quantitative and qualitative assessments of speech fluency. *Seminars in Speech and Language, 20,* 185–196.

Long, S.H. (2001). About time: A comparison of computerized and manual procedures for grammatical and phonological analysis. *Clinical Linguistics and Phonetics, 15*(5), 399–426.

Masterson, Long, S., & Buder, E. (1998). Instrumentation in clinical phonology. In Bernthal, J., & Bankson, N. (Eds.) *Articulation and phonological disorders* (4th ed., pp. 378-406).

Masterson, J.J., & Oller, D.K. (1999). Use of technology in phonological assessment: Evaluation of early meaningful speech and prelinguistic vocalizations. *Seminars in Speech and Language, 20*(2), 133–148

Shriberg, L.D., Kwiatkowski, J., & Snyder, T. (1986). Articulation testing by microcomputer. *Journal of Speech and Hearing Disorders, 51,* 309–324.

Using a Computer to Assist with Test Administration and Scoring

Clinical computing competency #6: The clinician will make appropriate use of computer-based instruments designed to assist in the evaluation or diagnosis of communication disorders.

Many examples of computer-assisted test administration and scoring for speech and language disorders already exist, and more are undoubtedly on the way. Clinicians may find themselves attracted to the prospect of saving time and energy this way. Competency with this use of computers should include awareness of the strengths and weaknesses of computer-assisted testing. Competent clinicians will also understand and correctly interpret results obtained by computer-assisted test scoring.

The rationale behind computerized or computer-assisted testing and scoring in most fields emphasizes efficiency in time and therefore reduced costs. It seems easy to argue the case for the cost-effectiveness of computerizing the presentation and scoring of a large number of tests simultaneously administered. We can imagine at least some of the administrative advantages of the computerized version of national tests such as the Graduate Record Examination (GRE). In communication disorders, however, tests are rarely administered simultaneously to large numbers of people. Is it cost-effective to invest in computerized versions of tests designed to assess an individual's communication skills?

Many tests for which computer-assisted scoring software is available are still administered in a traditional face-to-face manner. Most people have had some contact with the idea of computerized scoring via the well known "bubble sheets" they have carefully filled out with a #2 pencil. Computer-assisted scoring, however, goes well beyond scanning bubble sheets these days. Some of the benefits of computer-assisted scoring include

- Fast conversion of raw scores

- Accurate calculation of score conversions such as percentiles or standard scores

- Instant graphical presentation of results

- Easy integration of test results into computer-generated reports.

Computerized testing, by contrast, remains less common in communication disorders than computer-assisted scoring. For the purposes of this discussion, a computerized test is one in which the test taker responds directly to items presented by the computer, usually by typing a response on the keyboard. Computerized testing and scoring of instruments designed to evaluate speech and language began in the early 1980s and continues to be refined. The benefits of computerized testing in communication disorders go well beyond possible cost-effectiveness or time saving for clinicians.

The potential advantages of computerized testing in communication disorders include

- Accessibility for persons with physical or sensory impairments

- Consistency of stimulus presentation

- Adaptation of the test to match individual strengths and weaknesses

- The unique formats and features that computerized testing makes available including the possibility of remote, on-line administration

Currently available software as well as pioneer efforts at computerized testing and scoring will be used to illustrate these features and advantages.

EARLY IMPLEMENTORS

The idea of using a computer to assist with test administration and scoring in communication disorders came along with the very first clinical applications of computers. Among the best-selling early clinical software programs offered by Communication Skill Builders was the series by Fitch, including *Computer Managed Articulation Diagnosis* (1984). This program for Apple II computers provided prompts for 46 single sounds and blends, which the client read aloud from the computer screen or imitated after the clinician. The clinician had the option of using the computer to track responses and calculate a score.

A second program from this era took better advantage of the computer. Also designed for Apple II computers, the *Computerized Assessment of Intelligibility of Dysarthric Speech* by Yorkston, Beukelman, and Traynor (1984) allowed the clinician to calculate speaking rate or quantify the client's intelligibility for single words or sentences. The usual pitfall of having clinicians judge familiar and predictable target sentences was avoided by having the computer randomly choose test items from a database of several hundred. The client could read the stimulus items from the screen or from a printout, but the clinician need not know what each target was until his or her assessment was complete. This sort of "objective" intelligibility testing remains desirable two decades later; a Windows/Mac version this software called the *Sentence Intelligibilty Test* (SIT) is available from the Madonna Rehabilitation Hospital in Lincoln, Nebraska (www.madonna.org).

COMPARING ON-LINE VERSUS OFF-COMPUTER TESTING

Some researchers have attempted to compare traditional test administration to closely matched computer versions of speech and language evaluation instruments. Results to date are mixed. For example, Haaf, Duncan, Skarakis-Doyle, Carew, and Kapitan (1999) found that comparing traditional and computerized versions of the *Peabody Picture Vocabulary Test-Revised* yielded no differences across response conditions. Other research suggests that subtle differences between on and off-computer tasks may be present and that careful evaluation is necessary (Shriberg, Kwiatkowski, & Snyder, 1986; Wiig, Jones, & Wiig, 1996).

Wiig et al., (1996) administered the traditional and experimental computer versions of the *Test of Word Knowledge—Level 2* (TOWK-2) to 30 teens with learning disabilities (LD), some of whom also had attention deficit disorders (ADD/ADHD). When asked about their preferences, the majority expressed a preference for the computer version. Teens with both LD and ADD/ADHD were especially likely to prefer the computer version, and their teachers observed longer than usual attention-to-task. Subjects who self-reported reading slowly, problems with writing and spelling, or difficulties sounding out words, generally preferred standard face-to-face administration. Interestingly, expressed test mode preferences were not necessarily matched by performance advantages. In other words, the teens participating in the study did not necessarily perform best on the test format they said they preferred. The authors report impressive time saving with the computer-based version, providing that available computer facilities permit multiple simultaneous administrations. It is not clear under what circumstances other than for research that someone would need to administer the *TOWK-2* or any other diagnostic language test simultaneously to large numbers of students.

CURRENTLY AVAILABLE COMPUTERIZED TESTING SOFTWARE

Rather than matching a computer-based task to an existing off-computer evaluation instrument, some software developers have designed evaluation instruments with only computer-based administration in mind. Three currently available examples of such software include *Computerized Articulation and Phonology Evaluation System* (CAPES; Masterson & Berhnardt, 2001), *Speech Assessment and Interactive Learning System* (SAILS) (Rvachew, 1994; AVAAZ Innovation, Inc.) and *Automatic Articulation Analysis 2000* (AAAP; Parrot Software). The procedures for administering *CAPES* were described previously in Topic 33.

Designed for children ages 3 through 9, *SAILS* assists with the assessment and treatment of phonemic perception. "The program was specifically designed to treat errors that were characterized by problems in phonemic identification, or the failure to establish appropriate phonemic boundaries" (Masterson & Rvachew, 1999, p. 238). Prior to beginning treatment, *SAILS* can be used to obtain baseline information about a child's ability to receptively distinguish a correct target word (e.g., *rat*) from common misarticulated foils (e.g., [wæt] or [jæt]). Foils and targets included in the software have been recorded by child and adult speakers and are presented via computer. This way of handling stimuli is especially appropriate because it is the specific purpose of this test to see whether a child hears the difference between correct and incorrect productions. Human examiners vary in their ability to produce deliberately misarticulated foils, whereas the computer can replay them reliably and accurately.

CASE EXAMPLE: Child is completing a computerized test of phonemic identification, and is working on an item that tests perception of /r/ as in *rat.*

Software: *SAILS*

Computer display: A picture of a rat, which is the target word, beside a box containing an X, which always represents the negative or "not" the target.

Computer speaker: "[wæt]"

        Child: (clicks on the X box because what she heard was not the target word *rat*)

Computer speaker: "[jæt]"

        Child: (clicks on the X box)

Computer speaker: "[ræt]"

        Child: (clicks on the picture of the rat)

During assessment, such tasks help the clinician understand how phonemic perception may be affecting a child's phonological development. During intervention, similar tasks may help the child learn the significance of sound contrasts.

Automatic Articulation Analysis 2000 (AAAP) can be used with children and adolescents according to the publisher. The program includes 72 picture stimuli showing a cartoon character named Uncle Fred in a variety of situations. Responses are elicited to each picture and the speech-language pathologist records those responses by clicking phonetic symbols displayed on the screen to represent individual omissions, substitutions, and distortions. In other words, the clinician indicates a phonetic symbol to represent an error occuring in either the initial or final position of the target word, but the child's entire production is not transcribed. When the test is finished, an analysis is immediately available that includes a listing of occurrences of common phonological processes. Although results can be saved and printed out, it should be noted that this program is quite different from the other speech testing and analysis tools discussed in Topic 33. In the case of *AAAP*, the computer is used for item administration and coding in real time; no complete transcription or recording of speech (words or sentences) is maintained for later reference. The final product is in many ways similar to a picture naming articulation test form on which errors were marked, but without reference to transcriptions of complete responses, multiple attempts, or running speech.

LOOKING AHEAD AT
COMPUTERIZED SPEECH AND LANGUAGE TESTING

There is growing interest in the development of assessment instruments that truly capitalize on the strengths of available technology. Researchers are excited about the possibilities that computerized test administration holds for precise tracking of response latency and other behaviors that are difficult for a clinician to simultaneously monitor (Hallowell & Katz, 1999). Hallowell and Katz reviewed developments that have promising implications for patients with severe neurological impairments. "New developments in monitoring bioelectric signals from the brain (i.e., electroencephalography or EEG), muscles (i.e., electromyography), or EMG), and skin surfaces (e.g., galvanic skin [response] or GSR) have promising implications for patients' control of a wide range of electronic devices which allow them to respond to a variety of test procedures during diagnostic evaluations" (1991, p. 151). Software would process these signals and respond by implementing certain actions on a computer. Such systems are still in development, but have the potential to provide persons with severe motor impairments with a response mode previously unavailable (Metz & Hoffman, 1997).

Looking at the potential of computerized testing in yet another way, the research team developing *KIDTALK* is focused on increasing accuracy and reducing cultural and linguistic bias in standardized language testing (Jacobs, 2001). *KIDTALK* (Kidtalk Interactive Dynamic Test of Aptitude for Language Knowledge) was designed as a screening test to identify children with language learning impairments, and has recently been adapted for use with preschoolers in a research setting. Through computerized presentation of an invented language based on Swahili, children's potential to learn new linguistic information is assessed. The assumption is that because the content is not based on previous cultural or linguistic knowledge, bias is reduced. Because the test is computerized, items consisting of video segments illustrate target language structures. A dynamic assessment approach adjusts the test to individual children's needs (e.g., number of practice items). In the future, computerized testing will move beyond the boundaries of traditional language testing and make it possible to assess different abilities using unique tasks and response modes.

COMPUTER-ASSISTED TEST SCORING

Computer-assisted test scoring occurs when the results of a test are entered into a computer for analysis. For example, a client's demographic information and raw scores may be input by a clinician after which the computer provides standard scores, standard deviations, age and/or grade equivalencies, percentile ranks, or other statistics. This procedure may not only save the clinician time, but also may result in fewer scoring errors created by hasty misreading of tables in the back of the test manual. The growing number of off-computer standardized tests for which scoring software is available include the *Clinical Evaluation of Language Fundamentals* (CELF; Psychological Corporation), the *Peabody Picture Vocabulary Test III* (PPVT-III; American Guidance Service, 1997), and the *Woodcock Language Proficiency Battery–Revised* (Woodcock, 1998).

Clinicians can expect computer-assisted scoring software to be available for popular norm-referenced diagnostic tests. For example, tests that include several subtests that have separate tables of norms are especially good candidates for computer-assisted scoring. *Scanware for SCAN* and *Scanware for SCAN-A* from Parrot Software are examples of computer-assisted scoring software currently available for clinical purposes. This pair of software programs provides scoring and interpretation assistance for the widely used *SCAN* screening tests for central auditory processing, published by Psychological Corporation. The software provides a complete analysis of all subtest scores and composite scores for each test. In addition, advertising for the software claims that it provides a "complete and accurate analysis of findings in report form . . . for distribution to referral sources." In other words, this software goes beyond scoring to include optional test interpretation.

A product from Psychological Corporation offers clinicians assistance with scoring and interpreting the widely used *CELF–3* (Psychological Corporation). This extensive language test for school-age children provides information about both expressive and receptive language skills. The companion software, *CELF–3 Clinical Assistant*, generates norm-referenced scores, tables, graphs, and confidence intervals for all subtests and composite scores. Additional software features include indications of strengths and weaknesses in subtest performance, recommendations for further testing, and a summary with recommendations. Clearly, this package also goes beyond computer-assisted scoring by providing recommendations regarding how the scores should be used; this is test interpretation.

Some professionals would argue that the most valuable information gained by the administration of a standardized, norm-referenced test is found in the clinician's interpretation and synthesis of the results. Ideally, interpretation is grounded in experience with many other clients of similar age and ability, and by specific observations of the individual client during testing. Many clinicians, therefore, are uncomfortable with the notion of computer-assisted test interpretation. The professional issues surrounding computer-assisted test interpretation are discussed in Topic 35.

SUMMARY

Clinical tools for computer-assisted test administration and scoring have long been available to professionals specializing in communication disorders. Although cost-effectiveness might be easy to document with large scale testing projects, the more common individual testing situation encountered by speech-language pathologists requires a different justification. "Equivalent forms" of traditional off-computer tests have met with mixed results, and do not generally take full advantage of new technology. One currently available example, *SAILS*, and one previously developed example, *Computerized Assessment of Intelligibility of Dysarthric Speech,* are described here because they have capitalized on the unique capabilities and advantages of computer-assisted test administration. Such capabilities include dynamic adjustment of items corresponding to the user's performance and consistency of auditory and visual stimulus presentation. Additional assessment instruments designed for computerized administration are anticipated.

In some instances, computer-assisted scoring saves time and improves the accuracy and illustration of test results. Clinicians can quickly obtain information that helps in their interpretation of individual test scores. Computer-assisted test scoring also increases scoring reliability by reducing human errors occurring during conversions of raw scores.

Clinicians with clinical computing competency will understand the difference between computer-assisted scoring and computer-assisted interpretation of test performance. Computers can assist clinicians in the organization of data and the completion of repetitive and time-consuming sorting and counting tasks. Computers cannot, however, make judgments about the adequacy of a person's communication behaviors or explain why a person responded in a certain way. It is essential for clinicians to recognize the ethical issues associated with computer-assisted test interpretation. Competent clinicians will develop and use their own professional judgments for the interpretation of test results, and consult computer-generated test interpretations with extreme care.

REVIEW FOR TOPIC 34

1. Give an example of an early effort to develop a computerized test in communication disorders.
2. List the advantages of computerized testing in communication disorders.
3. List two advantages of computer-assisted test scoring.
4. Look through a current materials catalog from a major publisher and find an example of software designed to assist the clinician with test administration, scoring, and/or interpretation. Which advantages does the publisher stress?

QUESTIONS FOR DISCUSSION

1. If it were up to you, what kind of computer-assisted test would you develop? Try to envision a testing task or design that has an advantage over common face-to-face testing methods. What will you name your test and which of its virtues will you emphasize in your marketing campaign?
2. Should there be any restrictions on who can purchase or use computer-assisted testing, scoring, and interpretation software? Why or why not?

RESOURCES FOR FURTHER STUDY

Haaf, R., Duncan B., Skarakis-Doyle, E., Carew, M. , & Kapitan, P. (1999). Computer-based language assessment software: The effects of presentation and response format. *Language, Speech, and Hearing Services in Schools, 30,* 68–74.

Hallowell, B., & Katz, R.C. (1999). Technology applications in the assessment of acquired neurogenic communication and swallowing disorders in adults. *Seminars in Speech and Language, 20*(2), 149–167.

Jacobs, E.L. (2001). The effects of adding dynamic assessment components to a computerized preschool language screening test. *Communication Disorders Quarterly, 22,* 217–226.

Using Computer-Assisted Test Interpretation

Clinical computing competency #8: The clinician will demonstrate familiarity with legal and ethical considerations that apply to assistive technology and the use of computers in the management of communication disorders and will adhere to appropriate standards.

Competent users of computer-assisted test interpretation should ensure that test responses are obtained through appropriate procedures, correctly entered into the computer, and stored with the same care for confidentiality that is afforded to client records on paper. Clinicians should be aware of the concerns voiced by some professionals regarding the potential misuse of computerized test interpretation. Competent clinicians will not allow computer-generated interpretations to unduly sway their own professional judgments.

Many clinicians find the task of administering, scoring, and interpreting communication tests daunting. The fact that so many different standardized, norm-referenced tests are in common use in communication disorders further complicates what is already a challenge. Depending on the work setting and caseload, a clinician may find himself administering and interpreting a large number of tests, tapping various areas of communication. Or, a clinician may give just one or two tests so frequently that it remains a challenge to stay attentive and interested in each client's performance. In either case, computer-assisted scoring and interpretation may appear to be a long-awaited solution.

Although there are some genuine benefits to computer-assisted test scoring and interpretation, there are also potential abuses and misuses. Among the pitfalls clinicians should avoid are

1. Failing to take adequate measures to ensure the confidentiality of client information

2. Failing to corroborate a client's test performance with other information or observations

3. Basing intervention goals solely on standardized test items missed

4.   Representing computer-generated test interpretation summaries or recommendations as if they were the professional opinion of the qualified clinician who administered the test

5.   Acting on computer-generated recommendations without due consideration

Nowhere in the clinical process is the clinician's judgment more crucial than in the interpretation of test data. It is the clinician's ethical responsibility to obtain and use test data in an appropriate fashion. This topic focuses on the ethical considerations involved in the use of computer-assisted test scoring and interpretation.

WHAT IS THE PURPOSE OF TEST INTERPRETATION?

There are many purposes for assessment activities, including diagnosis and documentation of treatment progress. Many assessment activities involve comparing an individual's performance to the performance of a large sample of same-age peers. Such norm-referenced testing provides documentation of a person's level of functioning compared to other clinical groups. Often, standardized, norm-referenced testing is administered for the purposes of "qualifying" a person for particular services or benefits. Other testing is done for the purpose of evaluating a person's ability to perform certain tasks, which are deemed to be important. This testing is often used as a guideline for future performance objectives.

The purposes of test interpretation are closely aligned with the purposes of tests themselves. There is little value in the raw score of a norm-referenced test without the perspective provided by descriptive statistics. Clinicians make frequent use of test manuals to obtain such a perspective. When computer software is used to generate this information, it is considered "computer-assisted scoring," as discussed in Topic 34.

Most clinicians would agree, however, that test interpretation goes well beyond scoring individual responses and looking up descriptive statistics. The purpose of test interpretation is to understand and explain what the results mean. Ideally, a test's interpretation should be adapted to a particular target audience, such as fellow researchers, an education team, a client, a spouse, an insurance company, or the client's parents. Each of these target audiences will have slightly different interests and priorities when it comes to assessment results.

A clinician's interpretation is supported by background information, description of the test environment, and examples of behaviors that confirm or contradict the scores obtained. Was this person's performance on this test in good agreement with the results of other assessment activities? If not, what other information should be taken into account? Did this person's test performance give the examiner insights into how this person communicates or learns or approaches novel tasks? Does the examiner believe that this test score reflects the person's typical performance level? What are the clinical implications of the test results? These are the kinds of questions that thorough test interpretation addresses.

HOW COMPUTER-ASSISTED TEST INTERPRETATION WORKS

Computer-assisted test scoring packages often include extra features that include test interpretation. Clinicians may be attracted to the fast and efficient process, such as the one promised in the following excerpt from a materials catalog:

The test's companion software, *XXX*, will generate norm-referenced scores and a narrative report, which can be attached to an IEP. The entire process takes 30 minutes or less.

According to this catalog, the companion software for this popular language test will provide "narrative interpretations of score levels, subtest strengths and weaknesses, recommendations for further testing, a summary, and recommendations."

In order to generate all of this information, the clinician merely enters into the computer the raw scores for each subtest as well as basic demographic information about the client, such as age and gender. This is where the concern for confidentiality arises. Traditional client files and folders are generally stored within locked cabinets and access is limited in most settings. Clinicians must take care that identifying information and test scores entered into special computer-assisted test scoring software is protected as carefully as the information on paper test forms. This means deleting client records or limiting access to the computer/software when not in use by the clinician. Clinicians who share computers or office space or who do test interpretation work at home should take appropriate precautions. Passwords and access codes should be the locked doors that prevent easy access to sensitive and confidential information (Wynne & Hurst, 1995).

Using the raw scores and personal data entered by the clinician, the computer generates a report based on "templates" that have been preprogrammed by the software designers. Such "boiler plate" text is likely to sound something like the following hypothetical example of computer-generated test interpretation:

Lee missed 5 out of 10 items on Subtest #3, *Morphological Endings*. This score is 1.5 standard deviations below the mean score achieved by children this age. A percentile rank of 35 was obtained. These results suggest that morphology may be a weak area of language compared to other subtests completed by Lee.

LIMITATIONS OF COMPUTER-ASSISTED TEST INTERPRETATION

What is missing from this hypothetical interpretation? First of all, it would be good to have some examples of the errors Lee made on the test. Were these errors of morphology, or merely wrong answers? Recently a first grader was observed during administration of a well-known expressive vocabulary test, which includes a section on morphology. When the clinician said, "A person who paints a barn is called a _____," this child said "farmer" instead of "painter." Later his mother confirmed that they had recently seen a farmer painting his barn near their house. The answer was counted wrong by standardized scoring rules, even though the target construction "-er" was correctly used in the word "farmer." This child went on to give several unconventional answers to questions in this subtest, none of which necessarily indicated a problem with morphology. Perhaps something similar happened when hypothetical Lee took the test.

The conclusion that morphology is a comparatively weak area of language for Lee is premature if it is based only on a score; it should be supported by examples that help explain the nature of Lee's errors. But some inexperienced or ill-informed clinicians may be swayed by the "interpretation" provided by test software. The sheer convenience of computer-generated narrative increases the chance that potentially misleading text will inadvertently slip into clinical reports or intervention plans. Credibility is yet another concern. Readers of clinical reports are entitled to know whether the conclusions and recommendations are those of a certified professional who was present for the testing, or whether they are merely the standard boilerplate text provided by a computer program in response to a particular score or pattern of scores.

Most clinicians know that it is inappropriate to base intervention goals solely on the items that a client missed on a standardized, norm-referenced test. Such tests are designed to compare a person's ability to a large peer group, not to identify individual communication needs. Items on such tests are designed to produce a wide range of scores and even clients with average skills or better are unlikely to perform all items correctly. In addition, items are often missed in the artificial context of testing that would be no problem in a genuine communication situation. However, if a computer-generated report suggests the presence of problems and gives recommendations based on an item analysis, an inexperienced clinician or less-informed reader might be inclined to agree.

Thus, the hypothetical interpretation presented in the example above fails to put Lee's score in a context that makes it useful for most readers of the report. As is, it merely repeats the norm-referenced scores in sentence form, and proposes a comparison between this and other subtests. Imagine Lee's parents or teachers, for example, trying to understand the significance of this computer-generated paragraph. There is no clue here that would tell them what "morphology" is, what Lee did or did not do with morphology, or whether difficulty with morphology is actually interfering with communication or academics.

USING REAL COMMUNICATION AS A PERFORMANCE STANDARD

How can clinicians ensure that computer-assisted test administration, scoring, and/or interpretation are implemented appropriately? One protection against misuse or abuse of an isolated test score or interpretation is to ensure that a multi-factored assessment has occurred. The use of multiple measures or procedures to document the presence of a particular problem is good practice regardless of setting. For both children and adults, a component of the assessment should be a sample of real communication. Conversation with clinicians or peers; telling a story; group interaction in the classroom, dining hall, or playground; or explanations to a spouse—all of these constitute genuine communication tasks. Using informal assessment tasks to put test scores in proper perspective is crucial to appropriate test score interpretation.

Clinicians who make use of computer-assisted test interpretation should vigilantly edit and modify computer-generated report narratives to match their own professional observations of the client. Performance on any particular measure should be compared for consistency to other performance indicators, and examples of problematic behaviors should be included. Computer-assisted test scoring and interpretation should never be used as a rationale for turning report writing over to non-certified personnel.

SUMMARY

Clinicians are urged to use informed skepticism with regard to computer-generated test interpretation. Computer-generated text should be edited and refined aggressively to ensure that it does not say anything that the clinician cannot corroborate through independent assessment observations. Client information entered into test interpretation software should be guarded with the same rigor as are other kinds of confidential client records.

REVIEW FOR TOPIC 35

1. What kind of information can a clinician expect from computer-assisted scoring and interpretation software?

2. Describe three potential misuses or limitations of computer-assisted test interpretation.

3. Find an example of computer-assisted test interpretation software in a clinical materials catalog and analyze the marketing strategy. How and why are clinicians being encouraged to purchase this software?

QUESTIONS FOR DISCUSSION

1. The specter of computer-assisted test interpretation disturbs many professionals specializing in communication disorders. Explain why this topic can be considered a "professional issue."

2. In your view, what would constitute "unethical" conduct with regard to computer-assisted test scoring and interpretation?

RESOURCES FOR FURTHER STUDY

Wynne, M.K., & Hurst, D.S. (1995). Legal issues and computer use by school-based audiologists and speech-language pathologists. *Language, Speech, and Hearing Services in Schools, 26,* 251–259.

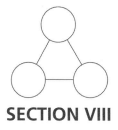

Adapted Access to Computers: Assistive Technology

Introduction to Adapted Access to Computers

with Christine L. Appert

Clinical computing competency #7: The clinician will demonstrate the ability to complete basic computer operations, troubleshoot common problems, and use various assistive technology options to provide adapted computer access.

Clinicians should be aware of common adaptive access solutions for clients of all ages and various special needs. Many clients will require adapted access to computers, at least on a temporary basis. Clinicians should be comfortable with a range of assistive technologies, devices, and software utilities that provide an alternative to regular keyboard input and mouse control. Such clinical computing competency may also be useful in the provision of augmentative and alternative communication services, although it has a different objective and focus.

THE NOTION OF ASSISTIVE TECHNOLOGY

Most of us do not take enough time to reflect on the important things in our lives. What is most important in your life? Your family? Your studies? Your friends? Your work? Financial success, physical fitness, or spiritual growth? In western cultures, most people value control over their environment and self-sufficiency. We require communication with others and seek stimulating surroundings. We use tools, express our creativity, manipulate complex symbols for learning, and pass our knowledge on to others. Many of us resort to destructive or violent behavior when we lack social connectedness or purposeful activities.

The point is, humans have complex needs and expectations. For some people, meeting these needs and expectations in conventional ways is more challenging because of cognitive, sensory, or physical impairments. It is often difficult for bright, successful, physically intact professionals to understand that the presence of an impairment in a person's life does not necessarily mean that their needs or expectations are different than anyone else's. People with impairments still need, and expect, to do and have what other human beings do and have. Sometimes, technology can be used to help them accomplish this. Such a use of technology can be called "assistive technology" (legal and technical definitions of this term are considered in later topics).

It is valuable for speech-language pathologists to have an overview of the ways in which access to a computer can be modified to accommodate a wide range of special needs. That is the primary goal of Section VIII. By most definitions, such accommodation would be considered just one fairly narrow aspect of "assistive technology." Several U.S. laws have a bearing on what persons with special needs are entitled to with regard to both their civil rights and their rights to a free and appropriate public education (FAPE). In addition to technical information, clinicians need to have a basic understanding of these laws and regulations as they relate to technology and the services provided by schools and other agencies. Clinicians must also be aware of funding options, ethical issues, and barriers to implementing assistive technology.

HOW ASSISTIVE TECHNOLOGY DIFFERS FROM AUGMENTATIVE AND ALTERNATIVE COMMUNICATION

Augmentative and alternative communication (AAC) has been defined as an area of clinical practice that attempts to compensate (either temporarily or permanently) for the impairment and disability patterns of individuals with severe expressive communication disorders (ASHA AAC Committee, 1989). Individuals with severe communication disorders are those for whom gestural, speech, and/or written communication is temporarily or permanently inadequate to meet all of their communication needs. For these individuals, hearing impairment is not the primary cause for the communication impairment. Although some of these individuals may be able to produce a limited amount of speech, it is inadequate to meet their various communication needs. Terms that are no longer generally used to identify such individuals include speechless, nonoral, nonvocal, nonverbal, and aphonic (ASHA Report on AAC, 1991).

Within the area of AAC, it is quite useful to know as much as possible about adapted access to computers as well as the broader uses of assistive technology. There is clearly an overlap between assistive technology and AAC in terms of the professionals involved, the technical expertise required, and the clientele who benefit. However, even the most rudimentary coverage of the basic concerns in AAC would go well beyond the scope of this book. Those concerns include motor and communication assessment, selection of symbol systems, vocabulary selection, development of communication strategies, which may or may not include a dedicated device, training communication partners, and long-term AAC follow-up.

Several outstanding resources are available to help clinicians develop an academic understanding of these issues (see Resources at the end of this topic). Readers may wish to contact the International Society for Augmentative and Alternative Communication (ISAAC). We strongly recommend *Augmentative and Alternative Communication: Management of Severe Communication Disorders in Children and Adults, Second Edition* by Beukelman and Mirenda (1998) now in its second edition, and *Augmentative Communication News*, a newsletter written and published by Sarah Blackstone. For gaining clinical expertise in AAC, we recommend seeking out the opportunity to work with an experienced AAC team during assessment, recommendations, and follow-up services.

WHAT IS ADAPTED ACCESS TO COMPUTERS?

Many persons have cognitive, sensory, or motoric impairments such that their control over a computer by conventional methods (e.g., keyboard and mouse) is not adequate (see Figure 36.1). Usually, the way in which the computer is controlled can be successfully modified or "adapted" for a user who has special needs. Adapted access to a computer may have a variety of purposes. Sometimes, such access allows the person with an impairment to participate more fully in prescribed educational or rehabilitative activities. Interim adapted access offers an immediate solution without the intention of establishing either long-term computer use or access in a variety of contexts.

In some instances, a touch screen serves as such a short-term modification. Young children may benefit from using a touch screen to choose animals and actions in *Old Mac-Donald's Farm Deluxe* (SoftTouch) software or other programs commonly used in clinics and early childhood education settings. A touch screen is a transparent, touch-sensitive

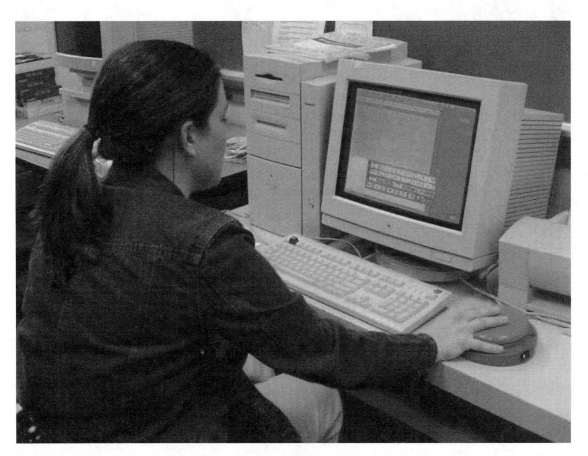

Figure 36.1. Accessing a computer via the Discover Switch (Madentec, Ltd.) (Courtesy of Truman State University Speech and Hearing Clinic).

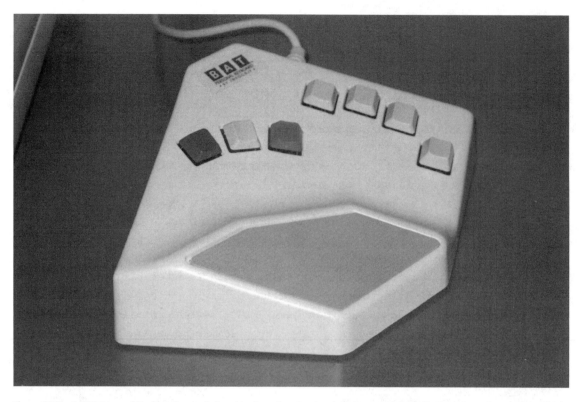

Figure 36.2. A BAT Personal Keyboard, a single-hand keyboard, makes touch typing speed available to typists using one hand (right and left-handed versions are available from Infogrip, Inc.).

membrane that can be temporarily or permanently mounted to cover the regular computer display (see Figure 8.1.). A child can simply touch her choice on the screen, instead of having to point and click with a mouse. Touching the screen is more intuitive than navigating the screen cursor with a mouse. As the child matures, physically and cognitively, she will probably be able to perform the same task without the touch screen by using a mouse or other pointing tool.

The same modification may be desirable to simplify the act of choosing for an adult with mental retardation or acquired brain injury. In these instances, clinicians use short-term adapted access to simplify the cognitive task of controlling the computer, not just to make physical requirements more suited to client abilities.

Technology that plays a part in an education or rehabilitation plan is termed *educational* or *rehabilitative* technology respectively, according to Cook and Hussey in their seminal text on assistive technology. Use of adapted access and computer activities during speech-language therapy would be an example of rehabilitative technology.

In contrast to short-term adaptation for a particular activity, sometimes adapted access is intended to fulfill long-term needs in a variety of contexts. An example of this kind of adapted access could involve a BAT Personal Keyboard (Infogrip, Inc.). A BAT Personal Keyboard attaches to a computer like a regular keyboard, except that it is especially designed to facilitate touch-typing with only one hand (left- or right-hand models are available, see Figure 36.2.). This is accomplished by assigning each alphabet letter a code, which is entered by pressing a combination of the seven keys (a "chord") on the BAT.

Consider an adolescent who has hemiplegia and requires adapted computer access for completing a majority of school assignments at school and at home. A BAT Personal keyboard combined with word processing application and word prediction software (e.g., *Co:Writer 4000* from Don Johnston) may be all that is required in order to make regular classroom participation successful. This adolescent may continue to use the computer in this way during a transition to a community college setting. The adaptive technology is clearly helping the student accomplish a functional activity (writing). Technology that helps an individual to carry out a functional activity is termed *assistive technology*. Cook and Hussey (2001) noted that considered from this perspective, *assistive technology* is a complex term involving a broad range of devices, services, strategies, and practices applied to improve an individual's functional capabilities.

For most clinicians, it is not important to make fine distinctions between educational, rehabilitative, and assistive technology. We raise the issue of various shades of meaning in order to alert clinicians to the overlapping uses of these terms rather than to attempt mutually exclusive categorization. It is important to be aware of the terminology used by various professional groups (educators, rehabilitation specialists, and medical personnel) and various public policy initiatives (insurance and health care regulations, local school policies, state and federal laws).

Clinicians who regularly use computers with their clients will develop an interest in how to make computer access more convenient and effective for them. When clinicians develop this interest and expertise, they probably will not stop to think about which theoretical application of technology (educational, rehabilitative, assistive) they are implementing. What will matter more is improving the communication efficacy of their clients and helping those clients to satisfy needs and expectations. Funding sources, however, may take a stricter stand on the importance of definitions. When it comes to helping clients acquire special technologies for their personal, long-term use, it will be especially important for clinicians to understand the "buzz words" and use them to advantage. The legal definitions and discussion in following topics are intended to help in this regard.

SUMMARY

Assistive technology can help an individual with a temporary or permanent physical, cognitive, or sensory challenge or limitation to perform a functional activity such as walking, listening or writing. Adaptive hardware, software, and strategies can facilitate an individual's access to computers and enhance educational or rehabilitation outcomes. Clinicians interested in acquiring expertise related to adapted computer access should be aware that the field of AAC shares many analogous issues. It is important to note that AAC has distinctive concerns and skills that require familiarity with other references and background knowledge. The topics that follow in Section VIII will provide an overview of technical and clinical considerations related to adapted computer access, educational/vocational programming, public policy, funding, and legal implications.

REVIEW FOR TOPIC 36

1. Based on the information presented in this chapter, how would you explain the notion of assistive technology (AT) to the parent of one of your clients? How would you explain this notion to a colleague?

2. List three functional activities that might involve assistive technology on the part of a client.

QUESTIONS FOR DISCUSSION

1. Think about ways in which technology helps you with the functions of daily life. Make a list of the 10 technologies that are most important to you on a daily, weekly, or monthly basis (keep this list for group discussion). Now, pretend you had to choose only five—eliminate the technologies you are most willing to live without (Your car? The phone? The microwave? Can you live without TV?). If you only had one of the five remaining technologies in your life, which one would it be? What are your reasons for making this choice?

2. If you can recall a time when you did not use a computer, describe ways that computer access has changed your life as a student or as a professional.

RESOURCES FOR FURTHER STUDY ABOUT ASSISTIVE TECHNOLOGY AND ADAPTED ACCESS TO COMPUTERS

Cook, A. & Hussey, S. (2001). *Assistive technologies: Principles and practices* (2nd ed.). St. Louis, MO: Elsevier Science.

Rehabilitation Engineering Society of North America. (2000). *Fundamentals in assistive technology* (3rd ed.). Washington DC: Author.

The Alliance for Technology Access (ATA)

ATA is a network of community-based resource centers. The organization is dedicated to providing information and support services to children and adults with disabilities, and increasing their use of standard, assistive, and information technologies. Web-based materials include a listing of resource centers; book, computer, and web resources for people with disabilities; and a library of resources and links. (www.ataccess.org).

Closing the Gap (CTG)

CTG, Inc., focuses on computer technology for people with special needs. Through publication of a newspaper, presentation of an annual conference, and on-line service "Solutions", CTG provides practical, up-to-date information on assistive technology products, procedures, and best practices.

Closing the Gap, Inc., 526 Main Street • Post Office Box 68 • Henderson, Minnesota 56044 • Telephone: (507) 248-3294 • www.closingthegap.com

Wisconsin Assistive Technology Initiative (WATI)

WATI is a statewide project established to help all school districts develop or improve their assistive technology services. The web site's resources and print materials available from WATI are easy to access and understand for consumers and professionals. (www.wati.org).

RESOURCES FOR FURTHER STUDY ABOUT
AUGMENTATIVE AND ALTERNATIVE COMMUNICATION

Beukelman, D.R., & Mirenda, P. (1998). *Augmentative and alternative communication: Management of severe communication disorders in children and adults* (2nd ed.). Baltimore: Paul H. Brookes Publishing Co.

Augmentative Communication News

A quarterly newsletter focusing on current issues and innovations in AAC; ASHA CEU credits available.

One Surf Way • Suite 215 • Monterey, CA 93940

International Society for Augmentative and Alternative Communication (ISAAC)

This organization sponsors an annual conference and publishes *The ISAAC Bulletin*.

Post Office Box 1762 • Station R • Toronto, Ontario M4G 4AC • Canada

Federal Legislation and Public Policy Related to Assistive Technology

with Christine L. Appert

Clinical computing competency #8: The clinician will demonstrate familiarity with legal and ethical considerations that apply to assistive technology and the use of computers in the management of communication disorders and will adhere to appropriate standards.

Clinicians in every work setting are likely to encounter clients who require assistive technology of some sort. Even when computers are not involved, clinicians may lend their expertise to identifying assistive technology that may help clients develop better communication, achieve educational goals, meet vocational objectives, or accomplish the tasks of daily living. Familiarity with legislation and public policy issues related to assistive technology arms a clinician to help clients and families advocate for provision of appropriate devices and services. This information also contributes to professionals' understanding of their own ethical and legal obligations.

Does the law entitle third-grader Jennifer to take a school-owned computer home with her to do her homework just because she has a learning disability? Does the law say that the employer of your client with a recent traumatic brain injury must provide any equipment he wants in order for him to return to work? Who is responsible for providing funding for the computer-based augmentative communication system needed by the high-school student on your caseload? What rights do clients have, and what responsibilities do clinicians have? Knowing how to find information about the law and where to tap into appropriate resources is critical to keeping abreast of changes and current developments.

An extensive body of statutes, regulations, and court decisions govern rehabilitation and special education in the United States. Historically, the development of laws and policies has reflected the politics, economics, and social sentiments of the times. In the past 30 years, legislation impacting the provision and delivery of assistive technology has emerged along with laws intended to recognize and address the barriers encountered by a growing population of individuals with disabilities. The legislation highlighted in this topic provides an overview of the major statutes associated with the legal basis for assistive technology.

LEGAL DEFINITIONS RELATED TO ASSISTIVE TECHNOLOGY

The definitions of *assistive technology devices and services* are included in the Technology Related Assistance Act (1988, PL 100-407, 29 U.S.C. §§ 2201 *et seq.*). These definitions are widely used and accepted as standard definitions in other laws.

1. An *assistive technology device* is any item, piece of equipment, or product system whether acquired commercially or off the shelf, modified, or customized that is used to increase or improve functional capabilities of individuals with disabilities.

2. An *assistive technology service* is any service that directly assists an individual with a disability in the selection, acquisition, or use of an assistive technology device. This term includes:

   - The evaluation of the needs of the individual with a disability including a functional evaluation of the individual in the individual's customary environment.

   - Purchasing, leasing, or otherwise providing for the acquisition of assistive technology devices by individuals with disabilities.

   - Selecting, designing, fitting, customizing, adapting, applying, retaining, repairing, or replacing of assistive technology devices.

   - Coordinating and using other therapies, interventions, or services with assistive technology devices such as those associated with existing education and rehabilitation plans and programs.

   - Training or technical assistance for an individual with disabilities or when appropriate, the family of an individual with disabilities.

   - Training or technical assistance for professionals (including individuals providing education or rehabilitative services), employers, or other individuals who provide services to, employ, or are otherwise substantially involved in the major life functions of individuals with disabilities. (29 U.S.C. § 2202)

The term *auxiliary aids and services* is another way that assistive technology may be referenced in the law. As defined in the Americans with Disabilities Act, auxiliary aids and services include:

- Qualified interpreters, note takers, transcription services, written materials, telephone hand set amplifiers, assistive listening devices, open and closed captioning, telecommunication devices for deaf persons, videotext displays, or other effective methods of making aurally delivered materials available to individuals with hearing impairments.

- Qualified readers, taped texts, audio recordings, Braille materials, large print materials, or other effective methods of making visually delivered materials available to individuals with visual impairments.

- Acquisition or modification of equipment or devices.

- Other similar services and actions. (42 U.S.C. § 35.104)

For children receiving special education services under the *Individuals with Disabilities Education Act, related services* and *supplementary aids and services* may involve assistive technology. The term *related services* means transportation and such developmental, corrective, and other supportive services as are required to assist a child with a disability to benefit from special education, and includes speech-language pathology and audiology services, psychological services, physical and occupational therapy, recreation (including therapeutic recreation), early identification and assessment of disabilities in children, counseling services (including rehabilitation counseling), orientation and mobility services, and medical services for diagnostic or evaluation purposes. The term also includes school health services, social work services in schools, and parent counseling and training. (20 U.S.C. §1401.22)

The term *supplementary aids and services* means, aids, services, and other supports that are provided in regular education classes or other education-related settings to enable children with disabilities to be educated with nondisabled children to the maximum extent appropriate. (20 U.S.C. §1401.29) For instance, a related service could involve individual training in the use of a speech recognition system. A speech-language pathologist might work directly with the student who will use the system to complete assignments in the special education resource room. A supplementary aid is essentially the same as an auxiliary aid and could include a device such as an amplification system or tape recorder for the student's use in the general classroom.

CIVIL RIGHTS LEGISLATION RELATED TO ASSISTIVE TECHNOLOGY

Several laws are primarily concerned with expanding the constitutional guarantee of equal protection under the Fourteenth Amendment of the U.S. Constitution. The central points of these laws involve equal access to educational programs, transportation, services, and telecommunications, and protection of individuals with disabilities in the workplace.

The Rehabilitation Act of 1973–Section 504

Superceding previous legislation pertinent to disability rights and services, the Rehabilitation Act of 1973 (PL 93-112, 29 U.S.C. §§ 701 *et seq.*) granted a comprehensive plan for providing rehabilitation services to all eligible individuals regardless of their disability and its severity. Over the years, the law has been refined and delineated through the passage of amendments and regulations. Section 504 has endured as an important civil rights statute protecting the rights of individuals with disabilities.

The tenets of Section 504 apply to adults, postsecondary students, and children with disabilities in programs receiving federal financial assistance. Individuals protected under Section 504 must have a physical or mental impairment that substantially limits a major life function, a record of such impairment, or be regarded as having such an impairment (Section 504, 29 U.S.C. §706[7][b]). According to the regulations, a *qualified* individual with a disability meets the academic and technical standards required for admission or participation in a program (Rehabilitation Act Regulations, §104.3[k][3]). Although there are no funds available under Section 504, institutions receiving federal funds must be in compliance or face the possible termination of all federal funding.

Institutions, such as public schools and colleges, are required to be accessible and provide reasonable accommodations and academic adjustments for those who qualify under Section 504's broad definition of disability. Some examples of accommodations might include availability of a height adjustable computer workstation for an individual in a wheelchair, preferential seating for someone with hearing loss, or provision of a laptop computer for a student with severely limited fine motor abilities. Modification of test format, reduced or altered assignments, and use of a tape recorder to tape lectures represent common academic adjustments.

The services designed to meet the needs of students with disabilities must do so as adequately as services designed to meet the needs of students without disabilities. Essentially, equal opportunity must be afforded to students, but an institution is not obligated to provide accommodations or services that produce the same level of achievement or identical results as those attained by students without disabilities.

CASE EXAMPLE: Low-Tech Services that Provide Equal Opportunity

A student in a community college has documented auditory processing difficulties and other learning disabilities. The Disability Services Office at her institution has agreed to provide various accommodations and services that include test administration in a separate, quiet area and having all oral instructions for tests read to her individually. When it is time for an exam in a Western Civilizations course, the student meets with a teaching assistant in a special room. The teaching assistant reads the instructions aloud and shows the student how to complete the response booklet. With these accommodations, the student is expected to meet the same standards of performance as the rest of the class. Even if she fails the test, she is not entitled to exceptions or a chance to re-take the test, unless other students have the same opportunity.

Rehabilitation Act of 1973, Amendments of 1986 (PL 99-506) and 1992 (PL 102-569)–Section 508

When the Rehabilitation Act was re-authorized in 1986, the "computer revolution" was firmly entrenched. Section 508 of the amendments, known as the "electronic curb cuts" legislation, mandated that computers and electronic office equipment used in any federally funded program must be accessible. The major intent of Section 508 was to ensure that persons with disabilities had equal access to telecommunications, databases, and other applications. In 1992, the law was further amended to include collaboration between federal administration agencies and the information and electronic technology industry. An important result of this legislation was the development of guidelines for federal agencies ensuring that electronic and information technology (all media) is usable and available to people with disabilities. Issues related to web-based communication and information delivery were specifically addressed in 1998. Standards were developed to detail the criteria for accessible web page development. Section 508 has also had a significant impact on accessible design features in computer manufacturing.

CASE EXAMPLE: Design Modifications that Enhance Computer Accessibility

- On/off switches near front of machine rather than rear or sides
- Operating system software that includes free utilities for screen enlargement and some keyboard modifications
- Auditory as well as visual alert/error messages

Americans with Disabilities Act of 1990 (PL 101-336)

The Americans with Disabilities Act (ADA) is described as a "sweeping" piece of civil rights legislation. Its primary intent is protecting individuals with disabilities from discrimination in higher education, the workplace, and the community. Provisions of the ADA extend beyond federally funded institutions to all of realms of society in mandating equal access to public services and accommodations, transportation, and telecommunications. In addition, public institutions, such as schools and colleges, have an obligation to consider access to hardware equipment and software in making selections and purchases.

Assistive technology plays a major role in the requirements of ADA to provide individuals with disabilities an equal chance to live independently. The ADA attempts to mandate the elimination of the barriers that exclude anyone from mainstream American life and reduce the incidences of retro-fitting to accommodate people with disabilities. Toward this end, the ADA has prompted changes in building codes to include ramps and other access features that reduce the incidences of physical barriers. In addition, court cases related to ADA requirements have specified that public institutions, such as schools and colleges, have an obligation to consider access in selecting and purchasing hardware and software.

CASE EXAMPLE: Changes in Community Resources as a Result of the American with Disabilities Act

- Public transportation vehicles equipped with wheelchair lifts, tie downs to secure wheelchairs, and auditory stop announcements
- Classroom or meeting facilities equipped with audio amplification systems, Braille signage, and multi-modality emergency alerts
- Assistive technologies, such as screen magnification systems, in public libraries

As described, the ADA includes the terms auxiliary aids and services rather than defining assistive technology. It is not specific about the types of technology, assistive devices, or equipment applied to situations in educational, community, and work environments, rather, decisions are to be made on a case-by-case basis. An underlying issue in determining if an auxiliary aid or service is reasonable and appropriate lies in the concept that the device or service does not have to produce a performance level matched to those without disabilities. It must be effective in providing the individual with an equal opportunity to gain the same benefit or level of achievement as someone without a disability.

Telecommunications Act of 1996, PL 104-652—Section 255

The Telecommunications Act follows the tenets of the ADA. Section 255 requires manufacturers of telephones, fax machines, and other telecommunication devices or services to make products accessible to people with disabilities whenever it is "readily achievable." The Federal Communications Commission (FCC) is responsible for enforcing the Telecommunications Act. The FCC issued regulations and guidelines addressing products and equipment, including input, output, operating controls, and mechanisms, along with product information and documentation.

CASE EXAMPLE: Designing a Cross-Disability Accessible Cell Phone

A cell phone could be designed to incorporate a variety of features that reduce access barriers including

- Visual and reading challenges: auditory and tactile cues for keys and major functions and large print
- Hearing challenges (including a noisy mall!): wide volume range, a stereo phone jack to allow direct audio or electromagnetic coupling to hearing aids, cochlear implants, headsets and other audio enhancement devices, and digital text messaging
- Physical challenges: "touch-and-confirm" and delayed activation key options that reduce unwanted keypresses

FUNDED LEGISLATION RELATED TO ASSISTIVE TECHNOLOGY

The unfunded civil rights legislation forms a backdrop for other laws that do grant funding. Federal monies are intended to supplement state spending for education, vocational rehabilitation, and assistive technology. Funding appropriated under these laws supports specialized educational and vocational programming.

Individuals with Disabilities Education Act of 1990 (PL 101-476)

The Individuals with Disabilities Education Act (IDEA) was originally passed by Congress in 1975 as the Education for All Handicapped Children Act. This legislation introduced landmark changes in the way public schools included and educated students with disabilities. Guided by the "zero-reject" principle, the law mandated that eligible children, irrespective of the nature or severity of their disability, were entitled to a free appropriate public education (FAPE) in the least restrictive environment possible. Essentially, the Education for All Handicapped Chlidren Act combined an educational bill of rights with provisions for funding (Yell, 1998).

Reauthorization of the law and the Amendments of 1990 gave the law a new name, IDEA. The Amendments of 1997 added a number of significant provisions and restructured the format. Definitions of assistive technology devices and services are included. The law states that assistive technology devices and services must be available if they are educationally relevant and it is determined that they are needed to provide the student with a FAPE.

The heart of the law is the child's individualized education program (IEP) (Bateman, 1998). IDEA provides extensive procedural and substantive guidelines for developing and implementing the child's education plan. The IEP is a written statement of the child's education program providing specially designed instruction based on the child's unique needs. According to the 1997 amendments, the IEP team must specifically consider the child's assistive technology needs in formulating and implementing the IEP. Assistive technology in the IEP may be included as part of the child's special education, related services, supplementary aids and services, program modifications, or as support for school personnel who are providing assistive technology services.

For students 16 years and older, a transition plan must be a component of the IEP. The purpose of including transition services is to infuse a long-range perspective into the educational planning process. As with other components of the IEP, assistive technology should also be considered in developing the transition plan.

To address the needs of children younger than three years of age, Part C of IDEA authorizes incentive grants to states in support of comprehensive family-centered early intervention programs for infants and toddlers with disabilities. Assistive technology must also be considered in formulating early intervention plans or an individualized family service plan (IFSP). For instance, very young children often benefit from early opportunities to play with adapted toys or simple voice output devices.

Issues associated with considering assistive technology in the IEP or IFSP include evaluation of the student's technology-related needs, delegation of the individuals involved in the decision making process, and determination of the educational relevance and necessity of the devices and services to be considered. Subsequent topics in Section VIII will deal specifically with funding, training, and implementation of assistive technology.

Technology-Related Assistance for Individuals with Disabilities Act of 1988 (PL 100-407, 29 U.S.C. §§ 2201 *et seq.*)

A primary purpose of the Technology-Related Assistance Act, the "Tech Act," was to provide funds to states to improve assistive technology systems and to develop services for individuals across all age groups. States that applied for funding under the Tech Act were charged with the responsibility of developing consumer responsive assistive technology services, increasing the availability and provision of flexible funding mechanisms, and increasing awareness of the benefits of assistive technology for individuals with disabilities and their families. The emphasis was on fostering interagency cooperation and meeting the assistive technology needs of children and adults with disabilities. Examples of services provided by state projects included information and referral services, equipment libraries, equipment recycling, loan-financing programs, and protective and advocacy assistance. In the absence of continued federal funding, many individual states have continued to support some of their program initiatives.

SUMMARY

The legal definitions of assistive technology devices and services from the Technology-Related Assistance Act are widely used in legislation and policy. Both education and civil rights legislation have provided key laws intended to protect the rights of individuals with disabilities and provide funding to support assistive technology in special educational and vocational programs. Sections 504 and 508 of the Rehabilitation Act of 1975 and the Americans with Disabilities Act are Civil Rights statutes emphasizing the equal rights of individuals with disabilities to be involved in educational, vocational, and community environments. Auxiliary aids and services that include technology are often used to help individuals overcome barriers and support participation. The Individuals with Disabilities Act requires school-based teams to consider and provide for assistive technology in educational programming. Later topics in Section VIII re-visit funding and policy issues and present further description of the devices and services that can facilitate independence and improve an individual's functional potential.

REVIEW FOR TOPIC 37

1. Using the definitions and illustrations discussed in this topic, give examples of two assistive technology devices and two services not specifically identified in Topic 37. For each item, explain how each example might increase or improve the functional capabilities of an individual with a disability.
2. What law first introduced the notion of providing accommodations, such as extended time to take a test or preferential seating for a student with attention difficulties? Why is this law considered a civil rights statute and how does it protect the rights of individuals with disabilities?
3. Describe how assistive technology is included in programming for special education services. Identify the individuals involved in decision making in your response.
4. Explain the key issues involved in deciding if a college student with a documented hearing impairment has made a reasonable and appropriate request when asking for an amplification system to use in a large lecture class.

QUESTION FOR DISCUSSION

1. A school system provides a personal laptop computer with word processing and specialized word prediction program for a student who receives special education services. After the student graduates from high school and enters a community college the family is unable to convince the institution to provide similar equipment. Do you think this is fair? What laws apply to this situation?

RESOURCES FOR FURTHER STUDY

Bateman, B.D., & Linden, M.A. (1998). *Better IEPs: How to develop legally correct and educationally useful programs.* (3rd ed.). Longmont, CA: Sopris West.

Turnbull, A., Turnbull, R., Shank, M., & Leal, D. (1999). *Exceptional lives: Special education in today's schools* (2nd ed.). Upper Saddle River, NJ: Prentice-Hall.

Yell, M.L. (1998). *The law and special education.* Upper Saddle River, NJ: Prentice-Hall.

Standard Computer Access Options

with Christine L. Appert

Clinical computing competency #7: The clinician will demonstrate the ability to complete basic computer operations, troubleshoot common problems, and use various assistive technology options to provide adapted computer access.

Achieving this competency implies that the clinician is familiar with basic computer operations. Clinicians should understand and use a full range of regular access options such as standard keyboards, mouse devices, and speech recognition. They are able to adjust standard system software utilities that are included with computers in order to enhance accessibility. Competent clinicians will be familiar with the application of ergonomic principles, as well as settings and options that can make computers safer and more comfortable for any user.

THE NOTION OF UNIVERSAL DESIGN

Preceding topics in Section VIII introduced the notion of assistive technology and adapted computer access. Topic 38 provides an overview of features that are readily available to all computer users because they are standard options for portable and desktop computers. They are standard features, in part, because of the notion of *universal design*.

The increasing prevalence of survivors of disability and public awareness of issues related to aging and chronic health conditions has prompted innovations in flexible design features that are accessible and available to anyone. The idea that environments and products should be intended for use by as many diverse individuals as possible is referred to as "universal design." Initially, concepts of "universal design" emanated from the legal and social concerns generated by passage of the Americans with Disabilities Act (ADA) and corresponding social initiatives. Flexible architectural models were proposed to accommodate the widest range of capabilities and needs. Cost-effective, front-end access solutions avoided expensive "band-aid" adaptations of bathrooms and other facilities after buildings were complete (Steinfield, 1994). For example, building codes for public structures were revised to include widened doorways and ramps or stair alternatives, thus benefiting parents with strollers, individuals in wheelchairs, and people just too out-of-shape to climb up the stairs. Walkers, scooter-riders, and roller-bladers were able to take advantage of sidewalk curb cuts as they became a norm for pedestrian thoroughfares.

The equivalent of "electronic curb cuts" were subsequently applied to computers (Vanderheiden, 1990). Options to increase access to computers were included in operating system control panels and accessories. New built-in features, such as a selection of cursors and display configurations, enhanced computer functionality for users with and without disabilities. Universal design principles have influenced the development of standards for creating web pages, digital media, and instructional materials. The Center for Applied Special Technology (CAST) has been in the forefront with Universal Design for Learning (UDL), a new paradigm for teaching, learning, and assessment. A central premise of UDL is that curriculum should include alternatives to make it accessible and appropriate for individuals with different backgrounds, learning styles, abilities, and disabilities in widely varied learning contexts (Rose & Meyer, 2002). Technology plays a significant role in applying the principles of UDL by offering flexibility and appealing to the broadest possible range of learners' capabilities.

Topic 38 presents typical aspects of computer access corresponding to universal design principles. Acknowledging that it is impossible to accommodate the needs of everyone all the time, the identification of relatively simple and available technology modifications presented here will be followed by later topics that consider a continuum of more specialized adaptive devices and associated service delivery issues.

THE STANDARD KEYBOARD

Typically, computer users control computers through the use of a keyboard. Whether the user is an accomplished touch typist or devoted to the hunt-and-peck method, the keyboard is just that—a "key" point of entry into the cause-and-effect system, which a computer and a user comprise. Because it is so important, one would assume that much effort has gone into perfecting the efficiency of the standard keyboard. Herein lies one of the most frequently retold stories in computer lore, even though most of it takes place long before the invention of the microchip.

The story of the "QWERTY" keyboard explains the standard arrangement of the keys on typewriters and keyboards designed for writing in English. "Q-W-E-R-T-Y" are the first six letters of the first row on the standard keyboard, and is the name given to this keyboard arrangement. This particular arrangement of keys dates from 1873, shortly after the advent of the mechanical typewriter. The first mechanical typewriter was a huge success and people were quickly becoming accomplished typists. If a typist was too fast, however, the keys on the typewriter would jam. So, one manufacturer scientifically designed a key arrangement that would place frequently used keys on the left and make frequently needed key combinations difficult to access. The result was that typists slowed down and keys didn't jam; typing schools flourished. Many aspects of typewriter design improved and soon the problem of jamming keys was designed away, but meanwhile the QWERTY keyboard had become the standard. Over the years, several attempts have been made to encourage the use of a more efficient keyboard arrangement (notably the Dvorak keyboard developed in the 1930s), but without widespread success. The story of the QWERTY keyboard—deliberately designed to make typing more difficult—is often cited as a classic example of the importance that social and cultural phenomenon play in the diffusion (or lack of diffusion) of technological innovation (Rogers, 1995).

Using the standard keyboard to access a computer efficiently can be accomplished even if the typist uses a hunt-and-peck method and only a few fingers. Minor keyboard modifications (which will be discussed later) can even further expand the range of users for whom a regular keyboard is the access method of choice.

AVOIDING REPETITIVE STRESS INJURY

Use of a keyboard and other computer components for several hours a day can contribute to a painful and debilitating condition called a Cumulative Trauma Disorder or more commonly a *repetitive stress injury* (RSI). *RSI* is an umbrella term used to refer to a family of injuries that occur due to trauma caused by repeating the same movements repeatedly over a lengthy period of time. According to the Cumulative Trauma Resource Network, "initial symptoms may include tightness, general soreness, dull ache, throbbing, sharp pain, numbness, tingling, burning, swelling, and loss of strength in your upper extremities (hands, arms, shoulders, and neck)" (Cumulative Trauma Resource Network, 2002). These problems can occur when there is mismatch between the physical demands of a job and the physical capacity of the human body.

A repetitive stress injury called *carpal tunnel syndrome* results when a bone conduit (carpal tunnel) through which the medial nerve must pass becomes constricted in the same strained position while one action is repeated for a lengthy duration. Typical symptoms include hand numbness, pain, and tingling, which frequently occur at night. When computers replaced typewriters, incidence of carpal tunnel syndrome increased. Using a typewriter was less of a problem due to the frequency with which the typist was required to change positions to insert a new sheet of paper, to correct mistakes, or to push a manual carriage return. Computer keyboards, however, are often awkwardly positioned with regard to height and tilt, and can be used without interruption for hours.

Computer users can take steps to minimize their risk of *RSI* by attention to ergonomic issues (Pascarelli, 1994; Stevenson & Kenny, 2003). *Ergonomics* is the science of adapting the job, tools, and environment to fit the physical and mental abilities and limitations of people (Stevenson & Kenny, 2003). An initial priority for computer users is proper seating. Users who spend appreciable time at a computer should have an adjustable chair that provides firm, comfortable support. The chair should adjust so that the user's thighs are horizontal to the floor and feet are either flat on the floor or on a footrest. The height of the desk or computer table/keyboard rest is also critical. The set up should be arranged low enough so that accessing the keyboard promotes a straight line from elbow to fingertips and does not necessitate bending the wrists back. Shoulder asymmetry can be avoided by ensuring that the keyboard and mouse are on the same level. Correct monitor placement slightly below eye level and away from glare is also important. In some settings, a height-adjustable table will accommodate a variety of users including those in wheelchairs.

Alternatives to typing and cursor movement with the mouse may also be considered. By reducing keyboard entry, speech recognition can serve as a preventative measure and relief strategy. For some users, speech recognition may be a primary adapted access solution. Speech recognition is introduced at the conclusion of this topic and discussed in-depth in Topic 39. Mouse clicks can be minimized through the use of macros (little programs that complete a series of actions as a result of a single click or keypress). Pointing tool options that replace the standard mouse are considered below.

THE MOUSE AND OTHER "CLICKABLE" DEVICES

Since the advent of graphical user interfaces (pull-down menus and icons), the "mouse" has been an integral part of the standard computer control system. With a mouse, users can "point and click" rather than typing in commands to accomplish routine file management and program functions. The "point and click" user interface is one of the most basic differences between the older DOS and newer Macintosh and Windows operating systems.

It is important to realize the connection between the presence of a graphical user interface (GUI) and the use of a mouse to control the computer. The powerful idea behind a mouse is that it permits the user to directly locate and select an item or function anywhere on a computer display. Icons and pull-down menus make the range of available options visible to the user. Basically, the user looks around the screen, finds what he or she wants, and picks it by pointing and clicking on it. This way of making things happen is so intuitive that even preschoolers with normal vision and motor skill development, usually master mouse control quickly (sometimes more efficiently than adults!). This direct select interface was a major change away from a command-based operating system (DOS, Pro-DOS), which required users to remember or look up arcane commands and then type them perfectly in order to do things like format a disk or copy a file.

For most people, the mouse was a fortuitous improvement because it made computer use seem easier. For others, changing over to a graphical user interface has had some distinct disadvantages. Use of a mouse requires sufficient visual acuity and visual scanning abilities to find and change the location of the cursor on the computer display. Individual users vary somewhat in their preferences with regard to mouse "tracking" speed, the relative timing of clicks, and the optimal size of items on the display. Many computer users are unaware of how easily such interface characteristics can be adjusted to suit them. These variables (mouse speed, click speed, cursor size, and icon size or display magnification) can be modified through utilities and options that are included as standard control panel features of major operating systems. Table 38.1 illustrates modifications for keyboard and mouse operations available through system control panels.

For some computer users, moving their hands away from the keyboard to control a mouse is an annoying interruption. To this day there are curmudgeonly DOS users who developed faster-than-lightening touch typing skills decades ago, and still resent the fact that to use Windows they have to move away from the home row and "fool around" pointing and clicking to make things happen. More seriously, mouse control is complicated for users with limited arm/hand movement or those who have difficulty shifting visual attention from keyboard to mouse to computer screen.

Several relatively inexpensive (under $100) variations on a mouse have been developed for general consumers. Trackballs, trackpads, and "super mice" are easily available through local office supply centers and mail-order outlets. These pointing tools may fea-

Table 38.1. Examples of regular access adjustments and modifications available in computer system software, control panels, and utilities

System software modification examples	Function	Result
Standard keyboard		
Keyboard Repeat Function	Key repeat function can be slowed down or turned off	Reduces incidences of repeated character when user does not release key immediately
SlowKeys (Macintosh FilterKeys (Windows)	Requires that a key is held down for a moment before it is activated	Reduces accidental key activation
StickyKeys	Allows key combinations to be typed one key at a time	Single key entry of modifier and function keys requiring simultaneous keypresses
Pointing		
MouseKeys	Allows the user to move the pointer using the keyboard	Moves the pointer on the screen without the use of a mouse
Mouse Speed	Adjusts the speed/lag time of the pointer as user moves it on the computer display	A slow moving pointer may be easier for the user to control with a trackpad or other mouse alternative
Cursor Size /Mouse Tracks	Changes the size and shape of the cursor or displays a trail as the screen cursor is moved	Makes arrow or I-beam easier to see and locate on the screen
Screen display		
SoundSentry, ShowSounds (Windows)	Provides visual alerts/messages or captions whenever a sound or speech is typically generated by a program	Informs hearing impaired or deaf user of sound alerts or program sounds
CloseView (Mac), Magnifier (Windows)	Enlarges screen display	Displays a magnified screen image
Screen Display	Options for changing the colors, icons, and cursor appearance of the screen display	Displays high-contrast colors and the size of screen objects to increase visibility

ture multiple programmable buttons, locking buttons, and an ergonomic design to enhance control and hand/thumb/finger positioning.

JOYSTICKS AND GAME CONTROLLERS

Joysticks and other game controllers constitute a popular method of accessing and controlling computers. Computer-based video games are a big business. New games are predominantly CD-ROM based and typically range in price from $40–$60. To date, males make up the majority of the game market and the sci-fi/war themes of the best-selling games reflect their interests. Adventure games such as *Myst*, sports simulations, and history/culture simulations such as *Civilization*, *Caesar III*, or *The Sims* are notable successful exceptions.

Joysticks and other game controllers are especially designed for efficient game-playing. They facilitate rapid cursor movement and selection (clicking) and increase the "realism" of the user-computer interface. Such rapid control is desirable for many games where pointing the cursor is comparable to aiming a weapon, and clicking a button is comparable to firing it. Game controllers are relatively inexpensive and easy to install. On a Mac they plug into the USB or mouse port and some can function as a mouse alternative in non-game software. Thus on a Mac, at least, some game controllers have potential in the arena of "adapted access."

Although some Windows programs and games allow use of a joystick, the joystick cannot by itself move the mouse cursor, or point and click within Windows. A generic game joystick is not designed to control discrete cursor movements. To use one like a mouse, you need a programmable joystick that goes into a game port. Joystick-To-Mouse software (Innovation Management Group, Inc.) is designed to use with any PC compatible joystick for mouse emulation within the Windows environment. The SAM Joystick (R.J. Cooper and Assoc.) and the Penny & Giles Joystick (Don Johnston, Inc.) with accompanying software drivers are specialized joysticks which offer more control and extra features for individuals with physical challenges (i.e., separate "locking" buttons for drag and click).

VOICE COMMANDS

A computer user who is controlling a computer via spoken commands is said to be using "speech recognition" or "voice recognition." Although these terms are often used interchangeably, "speech recognition" is a more accurate label for what the computer is actually doing. Speech recognition permits a computer to rapidly recognize what a person says, then act on that information by typing a word or doing a command. Ideally, with experience, the user becomes more skilled at dictating in a way that the computer can understand, and the computer becomes increasingly more accurate at recognizing what the user says. Dramatic advances have occurred in speech recognition technology over the past few years.

Speech recognition has become an affordable alternative to keyboard entry and screen navigation. Due to popular demand, technical improvements, and affordability, speech recognition capability is now a built-in feature on new computers with the current MAC OS and Windows operating systems. Software developers have started to include voice commands and dictation capabilities in mainstream programs such as MS Word and other MS Office applications. Although this easily accessed feature is product specific, it offers the user a choice for program navigation and text generation. Specialized commercial software, such as *QPointer Premium* (Commodo) allows automated, hands-free, computer control and dictation into any Windows application.

Successful speech recognition requires a set of skills that are as demanding in their way as the skills required for keyboarding. An overview of speech recognition and the important role which speech-language pathologists can play in assisting potential users are presented Topic 39.

SUMMARY

Universal design models are founded on concepts of flexible planning that makes environments and products available and accessible to the broadest possible range of individuals with and without disabilities. A variety of "built-in" or readily obtainable computer access essentials have been developed for use by the typical personal, educational, and business computer user. These include hardware and software options for the keyboard, the mouse or other pointing tools, and speech recognition. Controlling a computer using these input methods requires particular skills and abilities that clients may not demonstrate. Sometimes, minor modifications applied with "regular" access options are all that is necessary to provide someone with independent computer access. Issues related to overcoming access barriers with adaptive equipment will be discussed in the topics that follow.

REVIEW FOR TOPIC 38

1. Discuss why flexibility is a key element in planning environments and products that follow a universal design model.
2. What are three "standard" ways that a user can input information into a computer?
3. Explain why accessibility control panel options, MouseKeys, and the option for voice commands and dictation with MS Word XP are examples of Universal Design.
4. What does the term "ergonomics" mean?
5. Based on information in this topic, describe three ways that keyboard entry can be modified to accommodate a user who is physically challenged by keyboard access.

QUESTIONS FOR DISCUSSION

1. How can people change their work habits or environment to prevent RSI?
2. Explore some of the features available for altering input and output through the Windows or Macintosh control panels (utilities that come with the operating system software). Try adjusting items in the Sound, Display/Appearances, Mouse, and Keyboard control panels. What happens when you adjust the mouse tracking speed? Sound volume? Screen colors? Cursor size and shape? Experiment with sound alerts and magnification? Do you discover settings that you might prefer? If you are using a computer in a public lab, be sure to note the settings of the control panels before you start making changes and return to the original setups when you are done.

RESOURCES FOR FURTHER STUDY

Cook, A., & Hussey, S. (2001). *Assistive technologies: Principles and practices* (2nd ed). St. Louis, MO: Elsevier Science.

Rose, D., & Meyer, A. (2002) *Teaching every student in the digital age: Universal Design for Learning.* Alexandria; Association for Supervision and Curriculum Development.

Stevenson, D.K. & Kenny, K. (2002). Ergonomics: It's not just for your clients. *Closing the Gap Technology Newsletter, 21*(3), 1, 16–17.

Speech Recognition

with Christine L. Appert

Clinical computing competency #7: The clinician will demonstrate the ability to complete basic computer operations, troubleshoot common problems, and use various assistive technology options to provide adapted computer access.

Speech recognition has become a standard access option, in addition to a keyboard and mouse, employed by computer users in many settings. Clinicians will be keenly interested in this interface between oral communication and technology. Because of their expertise in articulation, respiration for speech, and prevention of vocal abuse, clinicians can play a unique role in helping to identify persons for whom this technology might be supported or counter-indicated as a potential alternative to keyboard access. This clinical computing competency, therefore, requires both familiarity with speech recognition technology and expertise in speech and voice production.

WHAT IS SPEECH RECOGNITION?

Speech recognition technology designed to provide "hands-free" control over computers has been evolving for many years. Anyone who has seen *Star Trek* has seen an enactment of the ultimate in speech recognition systems. In a firm voice, Captain Kirk says, "Computer!" to start the system. The computer promptly replies, "Computer ready!" and the Captain proceeds to dictate his requests as he walks around the command deck. In this fantasy system, there is no keyboard, no mouse, no typing. Using QWERTY keyboards, even excellent typists can only achieve a rate (50–60 wpm), which is a fraction of the number of words per minute that most people speak (150–200 wpm). There is no speech recognition system available at present to rival Captain Kirk's, but dramatically improved products have recently come within the financial reach of users who desire them.

Products such as *Dragon NaturallySpeaking* (ScanSoft, Inc.) and *Via Voice* (IBM) and *EasyVoice* (E-Press, Corp.) allow users to speak with a natural rhythm into a microphone and have their words appear in an application program on the computer. This is called "continuous speech" mode, which is a fairly recent advance in the technology. In a review of *NaturallySpeaking Preferred v.3.5*, the author claimed a corrected text input rate of 50.4 wpm, which was better than his usual typing score of 42 wpm corrected (Linderholm, *WINDOWS Magazine*, August 1999, p. 38). Researchers have examined how speech recognition accuracy changes with experience and the use of particular strategies on the part of the speaker. An "out-of-the-box" accuracy rate of between 85% and 93% was documented for three systems available in 2000 (Koester, 2001). Generally, out-of-the-box recognition accuracy has improved with each generation of products, so it could be expected to be at least as good with currently available software. Earlier speech recognition systems were significantly more costly and required speakers to pause after each word spoken (discrete speech), resulting in a much slower rate of message transmission and low accuracy rates for many users.

For these reasons and others, speech recognition products have found a new level of acceptance by average computer users who may not have physical impairments, but who need or desire some relief from keyboarding (see "Avoiding Repetitive Stress Injuries" in Topic 38). It is this large market of typical business users who are driving the development of better and cheaper speech recognition products. Speech recognition products are already available for languages other than English (e.g., *NaturallySpeaking* in versions for French, Spanish, Dutch, German, Italian, Japanese). Ongoing improvements in this technology will eventually make the prospect of real-time language sample transcription and digital foreign language translation a reality.

Although the term *voice recognition* is sometimes used interchangeably with *speech recognition*, the latter is more accurate. The computer does not recognize a particular person's voice; the computer compares a speech signal produced by the speaker to a previously programmed model and seeks a match. Topic 39 focuses on considerations and issues related to speech recognition and special populations. Assistive technology experts caution that all such systems have important pros and cons when being considered for use by a person with special needs or anyone for whom regular keyboard and mouse control is limited.

WHAT ARE THE COMPONENTS OF A SPEECH RECOGNITION SYSTEM?

Speech recognition used as an alternative method for controlling a computer requires a combination of hardware and software elements. When speech recognition software is purchased, it generally includes a microphone, the software utility itself, an "enrollment" or product training procedure, and sometimes a tutorial. "Enrollment" is a term that may be used for training the computer to correctly recognize the speech of a particular user. The user speaks into a microphone and the computer converts the speaker's words into text displayed on the computer monitor. The programs for which the user wants to use the speech recognition capability (e.g., word processing or e-mail) must be purchased separately.

Speech recognition makes intensive use of a computer's resources, so it is an example of an application in which a more powerful (faster) computer actually makes a difference. In general, the latest computers get optimal performance from the latest versions of speech recognition software. Most products are Windows-based in keeping with the business environment for which they were designed. At present, MacSpeech's *iListen* and IBM's *Via Voice* are also marketed for the Macintosh operating system. It is recommended that Macintosh users investigating speech recognition consult vendors' web sites carefully for information about OS and microphone compatibility.

In addition to a powerful CPU, speech capability, speakers, and a high-quality microphone are the other hardware components that are essential for good speech recognition. In PCs, speech capability is achieved through the addition of an internal sound card. The quality and compatibility of the sound card directly affects the performance of speech recognition software. It is the sound card (or chip) that is responsible for actually converting the spoken word into digits, which the computer can store and then process (digitizing sound is discussed in Sections IV and V). *SoundBlaster* compatible sound cards are generally considered the industry standard. Prospective purchasers must ensure that they have the recommended hardware configuration for the speech recognition system that they plan to buy.

Just as in any speech recording situation, the features and the placement of the microphone are crucial. No matter how good the software may be, success depends entirely on getting the clearest and most consistent signal possible from the person speaking into the computer. Improvements in moderate to low-cost microphone design have taken place in order to optimize speech recognition. Desirable microphone features include

- Noise cancellation
- Easy and comfortable positioning, such as collar style worn around the neck
- A mute button for quickly turning off input to the mic
- A clip allowing easy detachment if the user wants to get up and move away from the computer
- Combination headphone/microphone headsets for reducing environmental noise
- Good quality cables and strain relief
- USB interface bypassing the speech card—best choice for laptops because it reduces computer noise interference

Ironically, because competitive pricing among speech recognition products is so keen, lower quality microphones often come bundled in with the software. Users may find that a modest investment in a better microphone may yield much improved performance.

HOW DOES SPEECH RECOGNITION WORK?

Although much progress has been made in recent years, successful use of speech recognition to control a computer and produce written documents remains a challenging skill for most people who try it. After software installation, the user is required to run through an audio setup wizard intended to help set up audio playback and the microphone; setup is followed by initial training. Training exercises help the speech recognition program match the specific acoustic characteristics of the user's speech with the program's acoustic model. The length of initial training exercises has been dramatically reduced in recent products, and now often takes less than 20 minutes. During this time, the user is asked to read passages as the program establishes a speech file for that user. In most cases, when the computer does not recognize an utterance, the user must repeat it until recognition occurs.

Some tips to keep in mind regarding training with a speech recognition program include:

1. The clinician and user should be prepared for a continuous session (usually at least 20 minutes).

2. The speech recognition software program includes a selection of text passages for the user to read during the initial training. The book excerpts or reading material are usually targeted for literate adult skills and interests, although some products include more variety. For example, passages more appropriately geared for adolescents are included with current versions of *Dragon NaturallySpeaking*. Clinicians should check the reading level in advance, however, because the difficulty level may still be too challenging for clients with limited reading skills.

3. Some practitioners have successfully piloted users with limited reading skills through initial training by reading the text aloud and having the individual repeat each screen of text, line-by-line (requires microphone with mute button).

4. Sometimes, a user is unable to obtain enough accurate speech recognition from the computer to get through the initial training exercise. If this happens, the individual may be encouraged to try again on a different day or different products may be explored.

Following successful initial training, the user can begin to use the speech recognition program with a word processor to dictate written documents or fulfill some other purpose. This constitutes an additional training phase. The individual's spoken words become part of the "active vocabulary" and linguistic sets used by the program to improve recognition accuracy. Concurrently, the user learns how to make better use of the program by applying voice commands and making corrections when a word or phrase is misrecognized.

Making spoken corrections is crucial because the system continues to "learn" and adjust to the individual's speaking characteristics. If corrections are typed instead of spoken, the recognition system assumes that no recognition error was made, and it is even more likely that the same mistake will recur. The user should confirm the correction procedures suggested by the software publisher before using keyboard corrections.

CASE EXAMPLE: Speech Recognition Correction Sequence

User speaks into microphone: Frank is an ice man, period.

Computer displays: Frank is a nice man.

User speaks into microphone: Select 'a nice.' Correct that.

The correction dialogue box pops up on the screen with the word *nice* displayed on the top line. Two possibilities appear: 1) a mice 2) arise. Because neither of the choices is right, the user says "Spell that a - n - space- i-c–e." "An ice" replace "a nice" in the correction box. The user says "OK" and the corrections box closes with the replacement text inserted into the text. After making the correction, it is likely that if the user produced this sentence again in the next paragraph, the program would not make the same mistake and would recognize the whole sentence accurately.

The ongoing process of dictating and correcting text can be tedious and frustrating at first, for any user. For younger clients or adults who have limited attention, low threshold for frustration, or limited reading and spelling ability, this process can seem overwhelming. Over time, the system becomes more attuned and better able to recognize the speech of a particular speaker. Some experts say that it takes about 20 hours of use before a new user with good speech abilities becomes proficient with program use and establishes a satisfactory accuracy rate. It is important for clinicians and others who may be making assistive technology recommendations to realize the investment required to make speech recognition convenient for a client's routine computer use. Although this technology has improved dramatically, the user must still develop skills and learn effective techniques for success.

Portable speech digitizing devices, reminiscent of vintage "dictaphones," are a recent innovation for improving the convenience of speech recognition. An early example was *NaturallyMobile* from Dragon Systems, which included a handheld digital recorder called the *VoiceIt*. Now several companies are developing and distributing portable devices that a person can dictate into anytime, anywhere it is convenient (including personal digital assistants). These portable digitizers dock with a laptop or desktop machine for conversion of the dictation into a text document. Once the document is converted to text by the speech recognition software, the user must to go back and make corrections for all dictated text.

ENHANCING SPEECH RECOGNITION ACCURACY

New users have high expectations, but most will require significant practice to establish their own expertise with a speech recognition program. Even before a new user becomes an expert, however, there are several ways to enhance speech recognition accuracy. The options and directions will vary somewhat from product to product. Here is a brief list of suggestions for quickly increasing speech recognition accuracy:

- Use the audio wizard before each session to be sure the microphone is correctly placed and calibrated for the environment.

- Train/learn commands for making verbal corrections (e.g., "scratch that," "correct that").

- Use the vocabulary builder or expansion procedures if available. This generally involves providing text files of typical writing by the user, so that the system has a better database from which to match words the user probably said.

- Improve the user's individual speech file by practicing/training frequently used or special vocabulary.

New users of speech recognition technology are urged to consult the help files, on-line tips, and documentation that accompany their software. These strategies and suggestions really do make a difference.

FACTORS THAT INFLUENCE THE SUCCESS OF SPEECH RECOGNITION

Many factors influence whether or not a particular speech recognition system can be effectively employed as a sole, primary input method for a client. Such factors include the user's cognitive abilities, speech consistency, persistence, literacy skills, self-monitoring, and vocal stamina, as well as the system's sensitivity, complexity, and flexibility. Speech recognition products vary in features such as degree of hands-free control, software applications compatibility, initial training procedures, and visual display features (Tam & Stoddart, 1997). Speech recognition technology is "hot" right now, and changing rapidly. Clinicians with a special interest in this topic should consult vendors and Internet resources for current technical specifications and capabilities.

The choice of speech recognition software depends primarily on compatibility with hardware specifications, the personal characteristics of the user, and specific features desired by the user. The degree to which the system provides "hands free" control over computer functions other than text entry will be a priority for some users who need an alternative to regular keyboard access. A speech recognition product line from Commodio, Inc. called *Qpointer* has been developed with special consideration for users with special needs, and with particular emphasis on hands-free control of computer functions.

Most speech recognition products were initially designed for business use, and performed optimally with voices like that of a typical adult male. Adult males usually have voices that are lower in pitch (120 Hz) than children or adult women (200–300 Hz). This difference may affect the performance of some speech recognition products. For this reason, young men, boys, and females may have greater success with a product that has flexible settings, such as *Dragon NaturallySpeaking*.

A frequently asked question about using speech recognition with clients who have communication disorders is whether perfect, Standard American English articulation is required. Speech recognition systems depend on consistency of input. So, persons with mild articulation problems or accents are likely to have success, so long as their speech is consistent. Misrecognitions due to intelligibility can be corrected fairly easily and will occur less and less as the system learns how to better predict and match what a speaker says.

Dysarthria is a speech disorder characterized by inconsistency. In a single-subject study, Manasse, Hux, and Rankin-Erickson (2000) investigated the use of speech recognition for generating written language by a traumatic brain injury (TBI) survivor who had mild dysarthria and mild motor impairment of the arms. They used *Dragon NaturallySpeaking v.1*, a continuous speech recognition system, with their 19-year-old client. The subject had been an excellent student prior to her TBI, but post-injury demonstrated some cognitive and academic deficits that were particularly troublesome in the area of written expression. Motor deficits made manual writing painful and difficult. Typing with her non-dominant left hand, her speed was 10 words per minute. The subject was instructed in the use of speech recognition and some techniques for enhancing accuracy rate. Results indicated that after initial training (reading five passages) the subject obtained a recognition accuracy rate of about 65%. This is lower than predicted for persons without dysarthria (closer to 90%). After a second training activity (learning to make corrections) accuracy rose to average 75%–85%. This level of accuracy is still well within the frustration range for most users (because error correction must be done so frequently). In timed trials, the subject produced longer writing samples without speech recognition than with it. The researchers point out that they did not use all of the available accuracy enhancement strategies that might have helped the subject. In addition, they are quick to point out two important caveats: 1) success with other TBI survivors or dysarthric speakers cannot be predicted based on this single case and 2) even with low output rate and less than stellar accuracy, speech recognition may be regarded as a valuable alternative for individuals whose quality of life has been impacted by limitations in written expression.

Early speech recognition systems used a "discrete speech" model, in which the user was forced to pause after each word. This was taxing for some users and resulted in low recognition accuracy rates because linguistic context information was minimal. Therefore, the "discrete speech" technique is no longer supported by new versions of current speech recognition products, which have embraced the "continuous speech" alternative. Continuous speech systems perform best when the user is able to produce strings of words in at a natural, conversational rate, with few unpredictable pauses. (Of course, the user can always pause the system to stop and think.) It is easy to imagine that users with a variety of speech or language difficulties might have more success with a word-by-word approach.

Indeed, much anecdotal evidence and eventually empirical research confirmed that for at least some users with special needs, "discrete speech" systems had advantages. Having more time to compose a sentence word by word is better for some authors and possibly results in fewer mistakes to correct. Also, the specific procedures required to make corrections in discrete speech systems may be better for users who have relatively weak spelling and phonological awareness skills.

In a study of children with learning disabilities, Higgins and Raskind (2000) compared the effects of continuous speech (*Dragon NaturallySpeaking*, v.1.0) versus discrete speech recognition (*DragonDictate*) use on reading and spelling. Both approaches had clear benefits to the users, but results indicated that discrete speech made significantly more impact on students' spelling and phonological deletion abilities. Most striking, however, was the difference in subject attrition. In the discrete speech group, 19 of 21 students learned to use the system efficiently and liked it enough to complete the study. The two who dropped out were already efficient touch typists and found the process of correcting speech recognition errors tedious. In addition, the discrete speech group included three students with articulation difficulties and two with mild motor difficulties, all of whom were able to use the discrete speech system effectively. In the continous speech group, 4 of 17 students were unable to use the system due to poor recognition accuracy. None of this group who were able to complete the initial training had speech or motor difficulties. The four students who discontinued participation were young (9–11) and had relatively high-pitched voices. Some of them were later able to use the discrete speech system (Higgins & Raskind, 2000). It may be that discrete speech will return as an option in future products. It is also important to note, though, that all the students in the Higgins and Raskind study might have had good success with one of the newer continuous speech recognition products.

VOCAL HYGIENE AND SPEECH RECOGNITION

Too often, the role of vocal habits, respiration, and stamina in the long-term success of speech recognition are overlooked. No experimental research data on this topic are available to date. But common sense and experience tell us that we should be on the lookout for problems. Poor ergonomic design of work stations, inadequate postural support, and unhealthy work habits are known to contribute to problems with carpal tunnel syndrome. Similarly, work station design, personal speech characteristics, and vocal habits may contribute positively or negatively to success with speech recognition. It would be unfortunate if a person's solution to reducing typing fatigue or achieving independent computer access came at the price of vocal abuse.

Most people have had the experience of temporary hoarseness resulting from yelling at a ball game or coughing during a cold. Many teachers, lawyers, sales persons and others know that routine use of their voices at work all day sometimes results in vocal strain. It is important to consider the real possibility of vocal damage if talking suddenly increases by several hours a day. This is especially true if the person speaks in a tense or conscientious manner, as is likely when beginning to use speech recognition. Obviously this may be less of a problem if computer use is intermittent and if other potential vocal abuse behaviors are minimized.

Behaviors that sometimes contribute to vocal abuse (and may result in vocal pathology) include frequent throat clearing, coughing, yelling, and using hard glottal attacks during speech. Smoking and alcohol consumption are also negative factors. Allergies and side effects of some medications may put some speakers at risk. Positive vocal hygiene includes drinking plenty of non-caffeine fluids, using appropriate pitch and loudness, managing or avoiding personal stress, using adequate breath support, and avoiding vocal strain. With these issues in mind, users of speech recognition systems may need to gradually develop their vocal stamina, and plan to alternate between traditional keyboard access and speech recognition for optimal health. For some speech recognition users in schools, having water available to drink during breaks may require a modification of computer lab rules.

For some potential users of speech recognition, traditional keyboard access is not an option. They need an alternative access method and would like to use speech recognition exclusively. In such a case, it is valuable to consider whether or not the person's speech consistency, breath support, and vocal stamina are adequate to sustain frequent and long-term use of a speech recognition system. Muttered, inconsistent, and slurred articulation and syllable deletion are likely to result in high error rates. Discrete speech systems are somewhat more forgiving in this regard. Also, continuous speech systems require the user to produce words in chunks or phrases—the longer the better—with consistent pronunciation of each word in the sequence.

It can be a challenge to predict whether this method of access will serve the person's best interests over several months or years, such that the investment in learning how to use the system pays off. The potential user and the team providing consultation about alternative access possibilities should consider these questions.

THE ROLE OF THE SPEECH-LANGUAGE PATHOLOGIST

In many cases, one of the members of the team who recommends or discourages the pursuit of speech recognition as an alternative access method should be a speech-language pathologist. Unfortunately, this may not happen as often as it should for two reasons: 1) assistive technology teams may not know enough about speech and voice assessment to realize when they need an expert opinion, and 2) speech-language pathologists may not know enough about speech recognition technology to realize that they could be helpful in identifying people who will be able to use it. It is extremely useful for speech-language pathologists to have the personal experience of using speech recognition in order to better appreciate the process and skills required.

Common sense and routine precautions will suffice for most users of speech recognition. However, when medical conditions or other special needs are present, a speech and voice evaluation by a speech-language pathologist may be critical. The kind of information such an assessment should yield includes:

- Does the speaker use adequate breath support to sustain clear phonation?

- Can the speaker produce speech with adequate loudness for a microphone to "hear" in normal background noise?

- Is the speaker able to articulate consistently?

- Could the speaker benefit from therapy aimed at increasing breath support and consistency of phonation and/or articulation?

- Does the speaker tire easily from making the effort to speak?

- Does the speaker produce phrases and sentences with adequate fluency for the system under consideration?

- Does the speaker have a history of vocal abuse or vocal pathology?

In addition to assessing the speech and voice of a potential candidate for speech recognition technology, a speech-language pathologist may be useful in patient education. Thus, even someone who meets all criteria for potential success with speech recognition technology should be advised of reasonable precautions and the positive vocal hygiene behaviors described previously.

SUMMARY

Speech recognition occurs when a user speaks into a microphone attached to a computer, and the computer responds. This response is most often the creation of a text message on the screen, but it could also involve completion of various commands and system functions. Speech recognition is being used by many people as an alternative or supplement to manual typing on a keyboard. Exciting new developments in speech recognition, cost, accuracy, and reliability have made it a feasible alternative to a keyboard and mouse for many people who use computers in business, home, and school settings. Therefore, improvements and innovations in speech recognition are of keen interest to the general public as well as to assistive technology professionals and people with special needs.

Implementation factors that impact speech recognition accuracy rates at present include quality and placement of the microphone, sound card quality, and environmental noise. User characteristics that influence speech recognition accuracy include consistency of articulation and phonation, audibility of speech, speech fluency, and use of correction strategies for fixing misrecognized words or sentences. Speech recognition success requires a relatively high level of cognitive skills, literacy skills, persistence, vocal stamina, and respiratory control.

Speech-language pathologists have an important role to play in helping an assistive technology team consider speech recognition as an access alternative for a client. The client's speech intelligibility, breathing, and voice should be assessed before speech recognition is recommended, and new users should be informed of good vocal hygiene habits to prevent vocal abuse.

REVIEW FOR TOPIC 39

1. Identify the essential components of a speech recognition system and describe special considerations for each.
2. What personal speech or voice characteristics could inhibit successful use of speech recognition?
3. Discuss the "training" steps that can increase and improve speech recognition accuracy.
4. What are the recommendations for vocal hygiene for users of speech recognition products?

QUESTIONS FOR DISCUSSION

1. What role should a speech-language pathologist play in helping an assistive technology team recommend speech recognition?
2. Have you ever had a client for whom, looking back, speech recognition might have been a viable computer access solution? Describe this client and a client for whom speech recognition probably would not be successful.

RESOURCES FOR FURTHER STUDY

Berliss-Vincent, J., & Whitford, G. (2002). Talking speech input. *Communication Disorders Quarterly, 23*(3), 155–157.

De La Plaz, S. (1999). Composing via dictation and speech recognition systems: Compensatory strategies for students with learning disabilities. *Learning Disability Quarterly, 22*(3), 173–182.

Fulton, S. (2002). Be a slack-jaw: Advice for voice. Retrieved October 25, 2003 from http://www
.out-loud.com/

Higgins, E.L., & Raskind, M.H. (2000). Speaking to read: The effects of continuous vs. discrete
speech recognition systems on the reading and spelling of children with learning disabilities.
Journal of Special Education Technology, 15(1), 19–30.

Koester, H.H. (2001). User performance with speech recognition: A literature review. *Assistive
Technology, 13,* 116–130.

How to Adapt Computer Access

with Christine L. Appert

Clinical computing competency #7: The clinician will demonstrate the ability to complete basic computer operations, troubleshoot common problems, and use various assistive technology options to provide adapted computer access.

Of the ten recommended clinical computing competencies, this one requires perhaps the most technical information and comprehension. The technical side includes understanding how computer input and output work, and familiarity with at least some of the devices and strategies available to change standard input and output. In addition, however, competent clinicians will also have enough experience with interdisciplinary teams and clients to successfully choose and implement adaptations that are well-suited to short-term or long-term individual needs.

The use of adaptive equipment to suit a wide variety of individuals requires extensive clinical experience and more than average technical expertise. This competency is the most "technical" of any typically sought by clinicians. Matching a client with an adapted or alternative system for computer access also requires common sense, good clinical judgment, and interdisciplinary collaboration. This topic introduces a range of software and hardware applications designed to facilitate computer access. Topic 41 will address issues related to working with other team members. As with biofeedback applications and computer-based diagnostics, clinicians should feel comfortable approaching adaptive access from the perspective of their professional experience and problem solving skills.

Many persons have cognitive, sensory, or motor impairments such that they cannot exercise functional control over a computer by conventional methods (e.g., keyboard and mouse). More than a thousand specialized devices are commercially available for modifying or adapting the way a computer is controlled. Topic 40 highlights adaptations that allow individuals to by-pass personal limitations and control the computer independently using specialized tools and strategies. Alternative keyboards, touch screens, "non-touch" devices, switch interfaces, modified screen displays and print output illustrate the wide variety of possible options. Information in subsequent topics will provide details about selection and management of adaptive devices.

LOW-TECH MODIFICATIONS TO STANDARD ACCESS

At times, individuals who are able to use a regular keyboard experience an access problem that can be resolved with a simple and relatively inexpensive solution. In terms of positioning, a wrist rest is a common tool used to provide ergonomic support of the hands and wrists for typing. A keyboard tray can also be helpful in positioning the keyboard at a comfortable angle. An extension bracket, mounted to the table or wall, can be used to place the monitor within view and at eye level for an individual with special seating arrangements.

For individuals with visual perceptual or acuity difficulties, the use of large-print, Braille, or color-coded key cap stickers can be helpful. A typing tool, such as a mouth stick, a head pointer, or a universal cuff (hand splint) with a stylus, is useful for individuals who want to use a regular keyboard but have limited or no hand use. A key guard is a custom-sized Plexiglas or metal plate that fits over a keyboard to isolate the keys.

Adapting a keyboard in this way enhances targeting for individuals with a hand tremor and for some individuals who input with typing tools or their toes. A keyboard moisture guard is a soft plastic skin that fits over the keyboard to protect it from dust, moisture, and liquids.

DIRECT SELECTION: A FIRST CHOICE

Whenever possible, *direct selection* or the option to select and enter information directly into the computer is preferred over methods of access that are indirect. Direct selection refers to the process of making a choice with a single response. Users take advantage of direct selection when they type a word on a computer keyboard, enter responses to prompts at an ATM, or choose a store description by pressing a picture on the electronic directory screen at a mall kiosk. In contrast, indirect selection involves a series of choices that are presented to the user, who must wait until choices are scanned and the desired item is available. For example, direct selection occurs when you reach toward a plate of cookies and grab the one you want. Indirect selection occurs when you are asked which cookie you prefer (this one? this one?), one cookie at a time until the desired cookie is offered and you confirm your selection. Clearly, direct selection has the benefit of a more efficient route to independent access. There are a variety of adaptive devices that allow computer users to control the computer by direct selection.

Alternative Keyboards

In addition to the standard keyboard that comes with computer systems, other special keyboards exist. Ergonomic or split keyboards are designed to improve hand position for more efficient typing. Specialized keyboards that plug directly into the computer's keyboard port and meet specific user needs are also commercially available. Some examples of alternative keyboards follow.

The USB *Mini Keyboard* (TASH International, Inc.) may be helpful for one-handed typists with limited range and strength or individuals using only one or two digits or a typing tool (stylus). Amazingly compact (about 5″ × 7″), the Mini Keyboard (TASH) features a configuration that places the most frequently used keys in the middle.

For maximum flexibility, the *Discover Board* (Madentec Limited) and *IntelliKeys* (Intelli-Tools) are somewhat larger than a standard keyboard and come with a variety of overlays that can be exchanged easily (see Figures 40.1 and 40.2). The standard overlays offer presentation of large, easy-to-read keys with different configurations (e.g., letters in alphabetical order, numbers only, simplified QWERTY). Accompanying software makes it possible to create customized overlays and add speech feedback. For the busy clinician, additional sets of pre-designed overlays, corresponding to popular educational programs, can be purchased.

A *chordic* keyboard provides a typist who has good dexterity in one hand with an efficient arrangement of keys configured for use in typing chord sets or combinations of keys that replicate all the functions of a standard keyboard. The *BAT Personal Keyboard* (Infogrip, Inc.) features seven color-coded keys and an ergonomic design that supports hand positioning and minimizes movement (see Figure 36.2).

Virtual or on-screen keyboards represent an alternative for an individual who is not able to use a keyboard but can use a mouse or other pointing tool. An image of a keyboard is displayed on the computer monitor and the user points to and selects the desired keys. The *Discover Screen* (Madentec Limited) software includes a selection of colorful on-screen keyboards, which display letters, words, or pictures. In addition, a software utility to modify or create custom keyboard presentations is available. *ScreenDoors 2000* (Madentec Limited) also offers a variety of on-screen keyboard layouts, including international keyboards. A special feature of *ScreenDoors 2000* is the availability of word prediction that can significantly expedite text entry.

Non-Touch Tools

Head-controlled mouse emulation devices offer a non-touch alternative for computer access. This access method is particularly well-suited for individuals who are paralyzed but have controlled head movement. Examples include *SmartNav* (R.J. Cooper), the *HeadMaster Plus* (Prentke Romich Co.), the *HeadMouse* (Origin Instruments) and *Tracker 2000* (Madentec Limited). The user wears a headset or small dot on the forehead that works with an infra-red computer interface to translate head movements into directly proportional movements of the computer mouse pointer. Mouse functions of clicking and dragging are managed by "dwell-clicking" or with a switch, such as a sip n' puff switch. Using a head-controlled mouse system, all mouse functions can be executed without physically touching the computer. Text entry can be accomplished using the head-controlled pointer with an on-screen keyboard.

Topic 39 highlighted speech recognition technology, an increasingly popular non-touch method for inputting text into the computer. With the appropriate hardware and software set up, it is possible to enter information solely by voice commands and dictation. Other technologies are currently under development which offer hands-free computer access by eye gaze and brain waves. For example, the *Cyberlink Hands-Free Controller* (Brain Activated Technologies, Inc.) makes use of muscle input or brainwave energy to simulate the computer access functions of a mouse. Persons with severe physical impair-

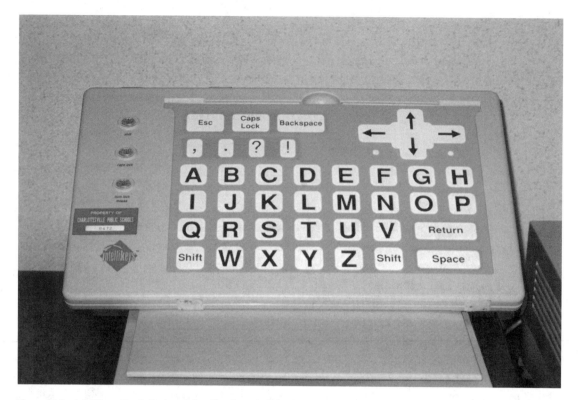

Figure 40.1.   Intellikeys Classic Keyboard (Intellitools, Inc.) with standard ABC overlay.

ment due to traumatic brain injury, cerebral palsy, and degenerative neurological disease can use this system to control a computer (Junker, 2002).

Touch Screen

A touch screen provides a straightforward and intuitive way to directly select an object on the screen. Some touch screens are imbedded in the monitor and others, such as the *TouchWindow* (Riverdeep/Edmark), are mounted over it. Touch screens are particularly appealing for work with young children and individuals with cognitive limitations because selection and feedback is direct and immediate (see Figure 8.1).

Cause-and-Effect with Switches

Software applications that offer a colorful visual display, animation, and sounds or music when a single button or switch is activated are called cause-and-effect or single-switch programs. For very young children and others with significant cognitive impairments, a keyboard or a touch screen with a display of multiple choices may be overwhelming. These individuals may be at a developmental stage in which they are learning that a purposeful action can cause a reaction or make something happen in the environment, and single-switch programs provide excellent opportunities to practice this. Alternatively, some clients require single-switch applications because it has been determined that a switch will be their access method of choice for physical reasons.

Switches, come in all shapes and sizes from a large round colorful button to a small, highly sensitive sensor switch (see Figures 40.3 and 40.4). Switches can be plugged into

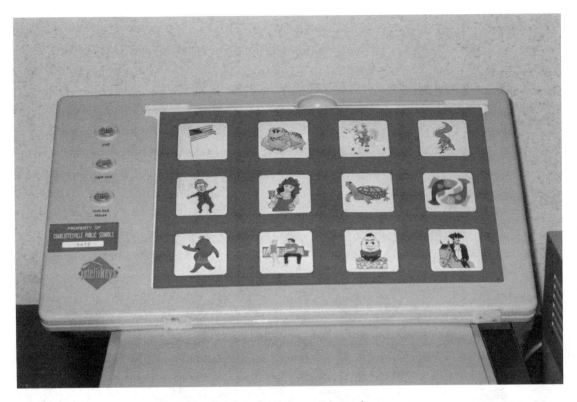

Figure 40.2.   Intellikeys Classic Keyboard (Intellitools, Inc.) with story activity overlay.

the computer using an interface box. The switch interface usually plugs into the computer like a mouse, with jacks that allow one or more switches to be attached. To the computer, clicking the switch is like clicking a mouse. Also, a "Touch-Free Switch" (Riverdeep) can trigger a mouse click when the user's movement is recognized by a digital video camera. Each time the switch is activated, the computer will respond with an appealing screen display and/or sounds. Besides learning to associate control of the switch with a pleasurable event, goals may include increasing attention span and visual tracking skill.

INDIRECT SELECTION (SCANNING): ACCESS AT THE PRICE OF EFFICIENCY

At times, individuals with severe physical impairments may need to rely on a single switch to control the computer, even though cognitively they are well beyond cause-and-effect applications. When an individual using a switch wishes to make choices to participate in an activity or produce text, indirect selection methods may be considered. With indirect selection, intermediate steps are involved in the choice-making process. Use of a switch to select from a scanning array presentation on the screen is the most common arrangement (see Figure 40.5).

A cursor moves sequentially through a set of items displayed on the screen. When the cursor is positioned on the user's choice, he generates a signal by activating the switch. The item is selected from the scanning array (the letter is printed on the screen,

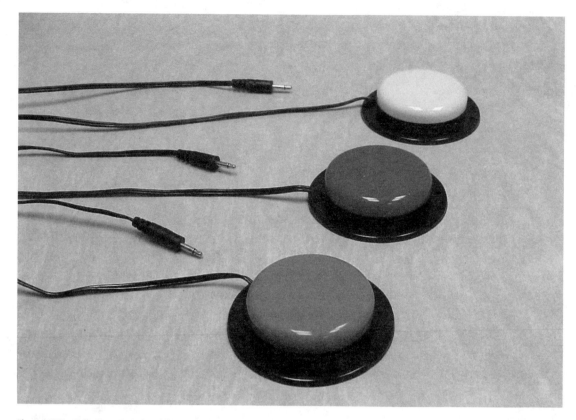

Figure 40.3. Jelly Bean Switches (Ablenet) are durable and popular for general purpose use (Courtesy of Truman State University Speech and Hearing Clinic).

the symbol is chosen, the action occurs, depending on what the scanning array included). Setting up the computer and user for scanning involves a number of details.

Setting Up the Computer for Scanning

Interface boxes are available for connecting a switch to a computer (see Figure 40.6). Some interface boxes have increasingly sophisticated options with correspondingly higher price tags. A simple interface box can be used with programs specifically written for switch use, such as the cause-and-effect programs described above.

Other applications, such as *Scan and Paint* (Judy Lynn Software, Inc.) are intended to train or reinforce choice-making and other requisite skills for scanning. Another option is to purchase switch utility software that provides scanning setups and customization features for accessing regular non-switch programs. This is helpful for giving a student access to the same software that other children in the class are using. For example, *ClickIt!* (IntelliTools, Inc.) provides a way to make "hot spots" for clickable areas on the screen in any software. Using a *ClickIt!* set up, an individual can scan menus or hot spots which would normally be accessed with a mouse.

Other interfaces, such as the *Discover Switch* (Madentec Limited), allow even greater flexibility by giving the user enhanced access to mouse and keyboard functions. For example, a word processor can be used with a corresponding onscreen alphabet-scanning array. The *Discover* software offers a number of generic scanning setups including letters

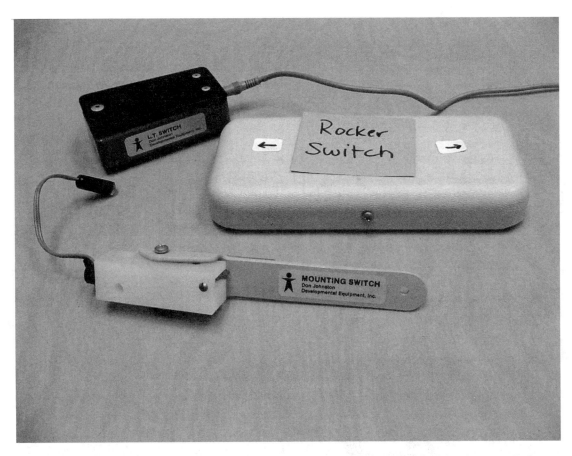

Figure 40.4. Switches (Don Johnston) come in many styles (Courtesy of Truman State University Speech and Hearing Clinic).

in alphabetical order, numbers, and an inclusive array with all keyboard characters. The package also includes pre-configured scanning setups for popular educational programs and a utility for creating customized arrays with alphanumeric characters, graphics, or symbols.

Setting Up the Switch for Scanning

Finding the appropriate switch for an individual requires careful assessment. The value of multidisciplinary expertise in this process should not be overlooked. For example, a speech-language pathologist may consult with physical and occupational therapists for assistance with decisions about control site, switch placement, and interface.

Switch selection begins with observing the individual's controllable movements and matching the most functional control site to appropriate switch characteristics. For example, if a client will activate the switch with her hand, a large and durable switch, such as the Big Red (Ablenet) might be appropriate. A highly sensitive P-Switch (Prentke Romich, Co.) might be a good choice for an individual who can only exhibit a small discrete muscle movement, such as raising an eyebrow, to activate the switch. After determining the control site and switch, a mounting system should be configured to position the switch for maximum independent access.

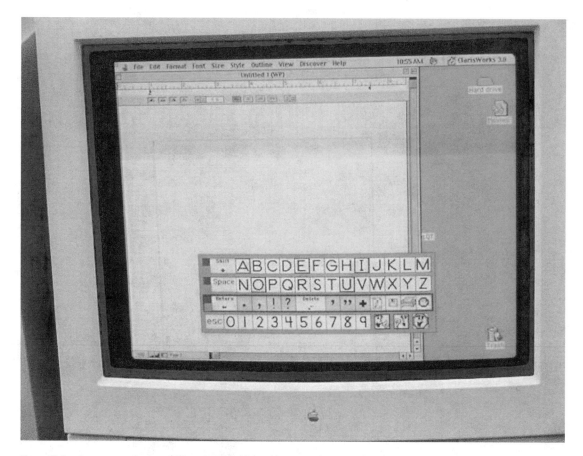

Figure 40.5. An on-screen keyboard (Discovery Switch) provides a scanning array that allows a person using a single switch to input letters and numbers, as if typing on the regular keyboard (Courtesy of Truman State University Speech and Hearing Clinic).

Setting Up the User for Scanning

Typically, when the decision is made to use a switch with scanning for computer input, it is because direct selection methods have been ruled out due to motor limitations. Indirect selection is considered a last resort because 1) it is much slower than direct select techniques and 2) no matter what technology is involved, the process of scanning requires the user to develop a complex set of skills. Specifically, an understanding of making a choice between two items must be firmly established. The individual must be able to demonstrate the visual and/or auditory attention, patience, and tracking skills to scan the entire set of choices and make a selection. Motor control to activate or press the switch for the amount of time required to send a signal to the computer and then release the switch is critical. The most difficult of all for many users is watching or listening to the choices and activating the switch in time to make a selection. Finally, an individual using a scanning method must persist and sustain attention and motivation to repeatedly carry out the steps necessary for choosing a desired target.

In some cases, individuals may also need to use scanning in multiple capacities, such as a way to access a computer, an augmentative communication device, and an environmental control system. Using the computer to practice and refine scanning skills is often recommended before considering an investment in an expensive communication system.

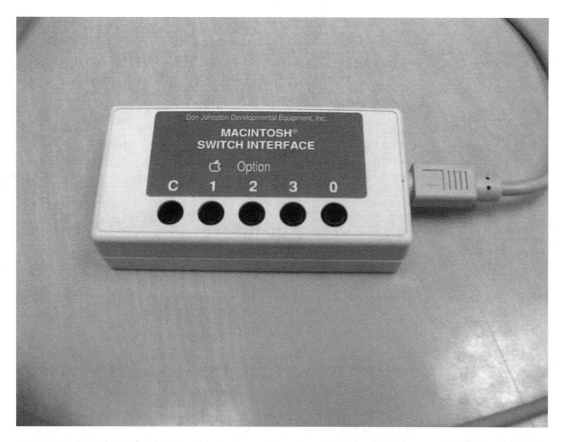

Figure 40.6. A switch interface box (Don Johnston) connects nearly any kind of switch to the computer (Courtesy of Truman State University Speech and Hearing Clinic).

A clinician can configure a scanning array with pictures, symbols, or words to simulate a flexible communication setup that can be easily modified as the individual's skills develop.

Adapted computer input includes diverse options ranging from inexpensive, simple, low-tech devices to devices that involve complex and sophisticated electronics and high prices. Table 40.1 provides an overview of adapted input options matched to the most common characteristics of users who require accommodation.

ADAPTED COMPUTER OUTPUT

Some computer users may require alternative options for visual display and printer output. Individuals with visual impairments are most likely to require some type of auditory or tactile support for computer output. Persons with hearing impairments may experience difficulties in recognizing auditory signals, such as a beep or alert.

System Control Panel Options

As discussed in Topic 38, the Windows and Macintosh operating systems offer control panel options for altering both input and output features.

Selection of "large icons" for desktop displays and menus is readily available, as are options for text enlargement or display magnification. The Mouse control panel in Win-

Table 40.1. Matching user needs to adapted computer access options.

User Profile	Access Solution	Description	Examples
Difficulty targeting keys on standard keyboard due to hand tremor or targeting difficulty	Keyguard	Plexiglass or metal plate that fits over the keyboard to facilitate access to individual keys	Snap-On Keyguards
Can not target and hit keys on standard keyboard but able to make direct selection with finger or pointing tool	Alternative or expanded keyboard	Typically a membrane-type surface, target areas (keys) size and location can be customized	*IntelliKeys, Discover Board, USB MiniKeyboard*
Minimal or no use of one hand but good use and dexterity with other hand, well-established literacy skills, and good memory and sequencing skills	One-handed chordic keyboard	Keyboard with seven keys that uses chord sets (combinations of keys) to replicate all the functions of a standard keyboard with one hand, ergonomic design minimizes hand movements	*BAT Personal Keyboard*
Cannot access a keyboard but able to make selections by pointing or touching with hand	Touch screen	Can be used for direct selection of objects on the screen or as a touch tablet for drawing and mouse emulation	*TouchWindow*
Cannot access a keyboard but able to use an on-screen keyboard, lack of upper extremity movement, but good head control and visual attention	Head controlled mouse emulation device	Head movements are translated into directly proportional movements emulating mouse movements, clicking and other button functions are managed with a switch (e.g., sip 'n puff switch)	*HeadMaster Plus, Tracker 2000, HeadMouse, Smart-Nav*
Does not have adequate controllable movement to access a direct selection device but has ability to activate, maintain and release switch closure, understands cause and effect	Single switch with specialized software developed for switch use	Switches are available in all shapes and sizes and different sensitivities from non-touch and light touch to switches designed for full force activation Switch communicates with computer through a simple switch interface Software applications must be specifically written for switch use	*TouchFree Switch, P-Switch, Bubble Switch, Jelly Bean Switch, Big Red* With simple switch interface box
Does not have adequate controllable movement to access a direct selection device but has ability to activate, maintain and release switch closure, wait for presentation of an array of choices, and activate switch on time to make selection	Indirect selection with switch and scanning	Switches are available in all shapes and sizes and different sensitivities from non-touch and light touch to switches designed for full force activation Switch in interfaced with computer through an interface box often bundled with scanning utility software	*Touch-Free Switch, P-Switch, Bubble Switch, Jelly Bean Switch, Big Red* With *Discover Switch* interface and software

dows offers features that adjust the size, appearance, and speed of the cursor (I Beam, pointer, or wristwatch). Macintosh users can purchase a product such as *Biggy* (R.J. Cooper & Associates) to install a control panel with a selection of cursors.

Similarly, sound and volume levels can be easily adjusted. The Windows Accessibility control panel provides options for visual alerts to signal auditory or spoken cues. The

Macintosh OS X control panel allows users to request that system alert messages be read aloud by a synthesized voice of choice.

Magnification, Screen Readers, and Read and Scan Systems

Magnification aids; screen readers; and scan, read, and write systems make the computer accessible to individuals with print impairment. Products such as *ZoomText Magnifier/ Screen Reader* (Ai Squared) and *SuperNova* (Dolphin Computer Access Group) offer integrated magnification and screen reading. Magnification enlarges and enhances the screen display and program settings allow customization of background and text color combinations to match user preferences. Screen reading features use synthesized speech to read everything on the screen including text, menus, dialogs, and controls. *Jaws* (Freedom Scientific, Inc.) and *Window-Eyes* (GW Micro) are examples of applications with advanced screen reading capabilities and the option of refreshable Braille output. Programs such as *Hal Screen Reader* (Dolphin Computer Access Group) also feature a multilingual speech synthesizer providing screen reading in a selection of languages such as Cantonese, Danish, Dutch, Finnish, French, German, Greek, Italian, Mandarin, Norwegian, Polish, and Portuguese.

Scan, read, and write tools, sometimes known as "reading machines," are designed for individuals with print impairments such as learning disabilities, reading difficulties, or low vision. These applications allow the user to scan printed documents or graphic-based text into an electronic text format using accurate optical character recognition (OCR). Once a document such as a book page or worksheet has been scanned, the user can utilize options for speech output, dictionary, word prediction, highlighting, and other study tools. *Kurzweil 3000* (Kurzweil Educational Systems) and *WYNN* (Freedom Scientific Learning Systems) are two of the most accurate and popular scan, read, and write applications.

Printers

Special printers capable of producing Braille and tactile graphics are often used in conjunction with screen readers. Using the latest technology it is possible to print out tactile maps, pictures, and even graphing calculator displays.

SUMMARY

Many persons with communication disorders also have the need for adapted access in order to make independent use of a computer. Whether for short-term needs during a therapy activity, or for long-term vocational or communicative needs, clients may require alternatives to the regular keyboard or mouse, and may depend on speech-language pathologists to help identify and resolve such needs. Adapted access approaches can be divided into two primary categories: direct selection and indirect selection, more commonly called scanning. Direct select methods are always considered first, because of their advantages in efficiency and simplicity of use. Scanning methods require the user to learn a complex set of skills that include making a choice, timing a selection appropriately, maintaining attention, acquiring automaticity in switch activation, and persisting even when making a choice or creating a message is a long and laborious process.

  Adapted output may be required for some clients. These may include speech output that assists with text editing or reading, and printer alternatives such as a Braille printer.

REVIEW FOR TOPIC 40

1. Describe the difference between *direct* and *indirect* selection methods.
2. Give two examples of direct and indirect selection that you might encounter in your everyday life (e.g., soda machines permit direct selection; setting your VCR probably requires scanning through available options then picking what you want). What would a "scanning" soda machine be like? Would you expect purchases to be faster or slower?
3. What are some ways that alternative keyboards enhance access for computer users?
4. Discuss reasons why indirect selection with scanning is often the option of "last resort" when deciding how a client will access the computer?
5. Describe the skills that an individual needs to develop to use a switch and scanning for computer input.

QUESTIONS FOR DISCUSSION

1. Have you known a computer user who made use of either low-tech or high-tech adapted access? Describe the modifications that were made. How successful was the adaptation in terms of speed and ease-of-use?
2. The devices and strategies available for adapting access to computers and other technologies are constantly changing and improving. How can clinicians to stay updated on such devices and strategies, and how important is it that they do so?
3. Using the continuum of low-tech to high-tech equipment introduced in Topic 40 consider any adaptive tools available to you. Explain which items you would consider to be "low tech" and which items would you consider to be "high tech."

RESOURCES FOR FURTHER STUDY

Cook, A.M., & Hussey, S.M. (2001). *Assistive technologies: Principles and practice* (2nd ed.). St. Louis: Elsevier Science.

Sweeney, J.P. (2002). *CIRCUIT: Model for assistive technology assessment.* Canton, CT: Onion Mountain Technology.

Choosing Assistive Technology and Making it Work

A Team Approach

with Christine L. Appert

Clinical computing competency #8: The clinician will demonstrate familiarity with legal and ethical considerations that apply to assistive technology and the use of computers in the management of communication disorders, and will adhere to appropriate standards.

Clinical computing competency #9: The clinician will demonstrate awareness of resources that provide continuing education, research results, technical support and information about availability, funding, efficacy, and efficiency of new clinical computing products as well as assistive technology devices and services.

The implication behind both of the competencies associated with Topic 41 is that there is more to assistive technology (AT) expertise than knowing which key to press or which switch to try. Just as success using computers as a context for therapy was not simply a matter of technical expertise, success with AT requires attention to philosophy and planning. Experts agree that both clinicians and clients benefit from a team approach to AT decisions and implementation in most settings. Contributing to a team requires that a competent clinician be aware of resources, including the expertise of her colleagues, and familiar with the best practices and legal considerations associated with AT.

The previous topics describe a range of standard and specialized access tools for computer input and output. Hundreds of low-tech and high-tech items are available that allow individuals to control computers or provide alternate forms of output. As discussed in Topic 36, short-term solutions to access may be adequate for brief educational or rehabilitative activities. When individuals need a permanent or full-time solution to computer access, however, many questions and issues need to be addressed beyond simply selecting a product or using a device that is already available. This is much the same situation as helping a client identify the best possible AAC system. Matching the features, options, and price tag of an access solution with individual characteristics and needs can be a complex and overwhelming responsibility for a speech-language pathologist working in isolation. Success is more likely with considerable special training in AT and an interdisciplinary team to rely on.

The process of evaluating and providing AT, including adapted computer access, begins with a partnership between the consumer and professionals. A collaborative team model that includes the client and family or caregivers is considered both best practice and implicit in the law. Decisions related to device selection should be predicated on desired outcomes as well as the client's goals, priorities, and preferences. Ongoing assessment of the individual's needs, the demands and supports available in the environment, and the tasks to be accomplished, are key to effective implementation (Zabala, 1996). This topic outlines the notion of quality assurance in AT service delivery, describes an AT team, provides an overview of the AT evaluation process, and raises issues related to effective service delivery and implementation.

QUALITY ASSURANCE IN ASSISTIVE TECHNOLOGY SERVICE DELIVERY

An initial interest in or search for an appropriate tool or technology solution may emanate from a variety of sources. A newspaper article or television story may prompt awareness of possible options. Recommendations from a friend, teacher, therapist, or physician may prompt further inquiry. In some instances a clinician may consider and suggest a simple adaptation, such as a trackball, to provide an alternate to computer mouse access. When a client's needs are more complicated, it is important to identify and consult with reliable individuals who have the established knowledge and qualifications.

Until recently, there have been few resources to guide consumers and professionals seeking quality and expertise in obtaining AT. RESNA, the Rehabilitation Engineering and Assistive Technology Society of North America, has actively worked with other organizations in promoting standards of quality assurance, outcome measures of AT interventions, and certification of individuals with preparation and qualifications in AT. A credentialing process has been established for assistive technology practitioners (ATP), assistive technology suppliers (ATS), and rehabilitation engineers (CRE/CRET). Certification is not a license to practice in a particular profession but indicates to consumers, payers, and peers that the certified individual demonstrates competence in foundation knowledge and skills.

Continuing education opportunities and certificate programs also promote development of skills and competencies in AT. For example, California State University at Northridge (CSUN) offers a sequential group of workshops designed to provide an in-depth study of AT. Consumers and family members are encouraged to enroll, along with professionals who can earn continuing education units (CEUs and ASHA CEUs). This

100-hour training program combines on-line and live (in-person) instruction with a culminating project that leads to an ATACP certificate. (Recall other examples of professional development opportunities and discussion of issues related to training addressed in Section I.)

Accreditation of clinical facilities that offer AT services is available through the Employment and Community Services division of the Rehabilitation Accreditation Commission (RAC). This nationally recognized accreditation organization has established standards of quality that focus on consumer expectations, provider credentials, and the results of services provided in terms of achieved goals and consumer satisfaction.

The Quality Indicators for Assistive Technology (QIAT) Consortium has piloted an effort to provide state and local education agencies with guidelines for improving and providing consistent quality in school-based AT service delivery. Although they are not intended to serve as professional competencies, adherence to the Quality Indicators for Assistive Technology requires the preparation and availability of competent service providers. The Quality Indicators can be used as a gauge for improving and nurturing service delivery within six areas including: 1) administrative support, 2) consideration of AT needs, 3) assessment of AT needs, 4) documentation in the IEP, 5) implementation, and 6) evaluation of effectiveness (Zabala, Blunt, Bowser, Carl, Davis, Deterding, et al., 2000).

ASSISTIVE TECHNOLOGY TEAM

The configuration of a client's treatment or education team varies considerably depending on the situation and purpose of intervention. A team for a preschool or school-age child will include parents, teachers, therapists, and others who plan and coordinate the individualized family service plan (IFSP) or individualized education program (IEP). Individuals in a medical or rehabilitation facility may have medical professionals, therapists, an educator or vocational counselor, and a social worker participating in their treatment or service plan. In cases when a client is primarily followed by a single provider, such as a speech-language pathologist, consultation with other professionals may be desirable if adapted computer access or other AT needs are being considered.

Each member of a team brings knowledge, skills, and experience that can contribute to the cumulative level of expertise. The group of individuals that comprises a team shares the responsibility of developing a system for effective collaboration. Relationships and interactions among team members, established guidelines for communication, development of a structure to promote effective meeting participation, and respect for individual priorities, beliefs, and time constraints are part of the team building process (Beukelman & Mirenda, 1998; Blackstone, 1995a). With combined knowledge and communication, team members are more likely to reach consensus and work together to address problems proactively. Depending on the technology solutions and objectives under consideration, one team member may take the lead in guiding decision making and planning.

Along with professionals and service providers, the client and parents or caregivers are critical and constant participants. As team members come and go, the client's input and historical perspective are integral to continuity and informed decision making. The law and common sense both advise that at least one team member should have specific training and competencies related to the AT under consideration. The following list includes individuals who may serve as potential AT team members:

1. Client
2. Parent or caregiver
3. Speech-language pathologist (SLP)
4. Occupational therapist (OT)
5. Physical therapist (PT)
6. Special educator
7. Rehabilitation engineer
8. Classroom teacher/employer representative
9. Computer coordinator
10. Vocational counselor, transition specialist, or job coach

CASE EXAMPLE: An Assistive Technology Team in Action

Gina, a second grader with beginning literacy skills, has significant motor impairments that affect mobility, speech intelligibility, handwriting, and self-help skills. Reinforcement of oral and written expressive language skills is a priority in Gina's education program. A talking word processor has been used effectively during speech-language therapy sessions, however, Gina demonstrated difficulty targeting and hitting desired letters on a regular keyboard. Adapted access for text entry has been suggested to provide more independence. A meeting is scheduled for Gina's team, including parents, general and special education teachers, and the SLP, OT, and PT. The PT and OT offer ideas related to setting up a work area to accommodate Gina's wheelchair and positioning of the computer monitor and other equipment. They also propose the use of a wheelchair lapboard to hold the new input device. The OT provides recommendations related to the use of an expanded keyboard with a keyguard and suggests a configuration for the keyboard layout (see Topic 40 for a description of special keyboards and keyguards). The SLP and teacher describe the skills that Gina needs to practice including spelling of words and sentences to communicate her spontaneous ideas and completion of simple written assignments related to the second grade curriculum. They discuss the content and arrangement of the keyboard layout with consideration for various instructional situations. For instance, Gina will not need numbers or punctuation, other than a period on her "writing" keyboard layout. Following the meeting Gina and the OT try out a variety of devices and overlays and Gina indicates preferences that concur with the parents' and professionals' observations.

A device is identified that improves the accuracy and efficiency of keyboard entry for Gina. With the adapted keyboard, Gina is better able to direct attention to the letter and words produced by the talking word processor. The team agrees on an action plan for purchasing and setting up the new equipment as well as training family members, the paraprofessional, and Gina in using the keyboard and word processor. Gina's IEP is modified to incorporate documentation of the evaluation process in the Present Level of Performance section and includes the adapted work area, keyboard, and word processor as auxiliary aids. By including application of the talking word processor in the annual goals and objectives for speech-language therapy and language arts instruction, Gina's parents and school team will be able to see measurable progress resulting from the use of the technology tools. In addition, the regular IEP updating process will ensure that Gina's AT needs are reconsidered and that accommodations are readjusted in a timely manner.

EVALUATION OF AT NEEDS

A primary focus of the evaluation process and subsequent recommendations for devices and services should be based on the individual's needs and consideration of the environments, activities to be performed, characteristics of the devices being considered, and the user's preferences. A thorough review of the client's records and the results of any standardized testing in areas such as visual or auditory acuity, cognition, speech and language development, motor skills, and academic achievement provide background details. Various checklists and data collection tools are available to aid AT teams in compiling information and conducting the evaluation. A selection of evaluation instruments is described in Table 41.1. The comprehensive information gathered during an initial evaluation should be used as part of a process that is followed by ongoing periodic review, modifications, and updates.

Maintaining a functional approach throughout the evaluation process is pivotal to the ultimate goal of using technology to perform a task or compensate for an obstacle posed by a disability. Key preliminary questions are:

1. What does the client need to do or accomplish?

2. What are the barriers or concerns prompting the consideration of AT as a solution?

Documentation of the client's skills and abilities is often available prior to the AT evaluation. In some cases, such as following a stroke or head injury, it may be necessary to assess current ability and skill levels. It is important to balance formal testing by surveying the perspectives of the therapy service providers, family members, and educators or employers. The effectiveness of interventions, strategies, or technologies already employed should also be factored into a needs appraisal.

The social and physical environment(s) in which the client will be performing the desired activities are critical variables in matching the technology to the user's needs. The spatial arrangement of furniture and people, lighting, ambient sound, and temperature represent the physical context to consider. The social context of a setting includes those people involved (e.g., peers, service providers, family), their attitudes, personalities, and culture. Clinicians must identify the expectations for an individual within a particular environment and which supports will be available. At times, a device will be appropriate and well-suited to a client's needs in one situation but ineffective in another setting. For instance, a speech recognition system may be used successfully in a quiet therapy room but may not work well in a noisy classroom or business office.

Given the number of available devices, matching the user's characteristics and needs with an optimal device is often a formidable task. To illustrate this process, it may be helpful to reference the tables in Topics 38 and 40, which highlight a selection of computer access alternatives and corresponding user abilities. As discussed in these sections, a con-

Table 41.1. Examples of assistive technology evaluation instruments

Evaluation instrument	Description	Source
CIRCUIT Evaluation Kit	CIRCUIT is a step-by-step training tool for evaluating the low-tech to high-tech assistive technology needs of students with learning and other mild disabilities. The kit includes a laminated color flow chart of the evaluation process, evaluation forms, and a copy of an AT Continuum Chart.	Developed by Judith Sweeney. Available from Onion Mountain Technology http://www.onionmountaintech.com
Wisconsin Assistive Technology Initiative (WATI) Assessment Packet	WATI offers a process-based, systematic approach to conducting a functional evaluation of a student's assistive technology needs in the individual's customary environment. Forms and instructions are provided for a three step process that includes information gathering, decision making, and trial use.	Available on-line http://www.wati.org
Matching Person and Technology Process	A description of the Matching Person and Technology (MPT) model and process for matching learners with the appropriate technologies and strategies is complemented by assessment forms and checklists for educational technology evaluation and selection.	Book available from Blackwell North America, Inc. Scherer, M. (2003). Connecting to learn: Educational and assistive technology for people with disabilities. Washington DC: American Psychological Association.
University of Kentucky Assistive Technology Toolkit	A comprehensive collection of tools intended to systematically guide IEP and AT teams in considering the use of AT from referral through implementation. Templates for seven tools, complete instructions, sample applications of the tools, and additional resources are provided for download.	Available on-line University of Kentucky Assistive Technology Project http://edsrc.coe.uky.edu/www/ukatii
Functional Evaluation for Assistive Technology (FEAT) Kit	FEAT is a systematic, comprehensive, multidimensional, and ecologically-based assessment protocol that can be used with people of all ages with learning and cognitive difficulties. The kit includes five scales that provide a method for examining an individual's unique set of abilities, experiences, and behavior and considering the specific tasks to be performed across settings.	Available from Psycho-Educational Services http://www.psych-educational.com Raskind, M. & Bryant, B. (2002) Functional evaluation for assistive technology kit. Austin, TX: Pscyho-Educational Services

tinuum of options should be considered from low-tech to high-tech. In most cases, important device attributes to consider include

- Convenience and ease of use offered by the device
- Size and portability
- Complex and multiple options versus simple but limited features
- Training demands
- Availability of technical support
- Compatibility or interface with other products
- Anticipated maintenance and repair
- Durability
- Cost

A variety of tools should be introduced and explored during a formal AT evaluation. As the choices are narrowed down, the best way to determine whether a good fit has been achieved is to arrange a trial for the client to use the proposed technology in the anticipated or natural environment. A trial with the selected solution in the milieu of everyday demands and situations can show if the right decision has been made and if adjustments need to be made or additional supports provided. Careful documentation of the outcomes and success achieved by the user with the technology is particularly important when funding justification is an issue.

IMPLEMENTATION OF AT

The initial evaluation and recommendations for particular options are only the first steps in implementing AT. Developing a plan and ongoing re-appraisal of device use and outcomes are critical to effective and sustained use.

As noted in Topic 37, the law requires that all IEP teams must consider whether AT is needed to support each student's ability to participate in the general education curriculum or benefit from special education. Not all students need AT, but the team developing the education plan must at least consider this option and document their decision. In cases in which AT is included in the plan, the results of a technology evaluation should be included in the Present Level of Performance section, and devices or services should be incorporated into the specific goals and objectives or supplementary aids and services. The formulation of IEP benchmarks must state the expected results of AT use in measurable and observable terms.

A vocational service plan, prepared for individuals served by a state vocational rehabilitation (VR) agency, must also consider provision of AT as a possible auxiliary aid or service. For clients enrolled in postsecondary institutions, state agencies are mandated to work together to devise a plan that determines which devices or services will be offered to a VR client and specify the agencies that will assume financial responsibility.

Beyond development of a formal education or service plan, it may be helpful for the client's team to meet and agree on an action plan that specifies what team members will do. Action plans facilitate case coordination and help to balance workloads for busy professionals and caregivers. Specifying team members' roles and responsibilities ensures that everyone contributes their fair share and protects individuals from being overwhelmed with coordinating all the details for one client.

Sarah Blackstone (1995b) outlined three fundamental elements of an AT action plan:

- What will be done?
- Who will do it?
- When will it be done?

The action plan delegates responsibilities and may also include details related to training, set-up and maintenance of equipment, and criteria for task completion. Time lines and shared objectives help to promote accountability and ensure that all team members, including the client, are working in tandem (Blackstone, 1995b).

SUMMARY

The process of evaluating, implementing, and monitoring AT provision is conducted by a team that includes the user and caregiver(s). It is essential that professionals involved in considering an individual's AT needs take the user's strengths and preferences into account and review desired tasks and anticipated settings. A variety of tools and checklists are available to help AT teams collaborate their efforts on evaluation and follow-up re-assessments of clients. Goals for training and implementation of AT devices and services should be incorporated into education or vocational service plans and supported by ongoing communication and development of an action plan by team members.

REVIEW FOR TOPIC 41

1. List two preliminary questions that are essential to consider before undertaking an AT evaluation.
2. Describe the physical (environmental) and social contexts that must be considered in an evaluation of AT needs.
3. Explain why an AT team would recommend that a client use a selected device on loan for a trial period of 3 months before actually purchasing the equipment.
4. Discuss the purpose, advantages, and fundamental elements of an action plan.

QUESTIONS FOR DISCUSSION

1. Describe the composition of an AT team for an adolescent in eleventh grade with a head injury. The student has adequate gross motor skills but demonstrates limited hand use, speech and breath support difficulties, and some cognitive impairments.
2. An AT team has conscientiously collected background and diagnostic information about a client. They have met as a group that included the client and her caregivers to discuss possible access solutions and try out various devices in an adapted lab setting. The client has indicated her preference for a specific device, which is not the first choice of other team

members. What are some strategies that might be used by this group to reach a decision and proceed with implementing a technology plan?

3. What steps and actions should a team take when a client is making a transition to a new setting? For example, what special considerations should be given to continuing the appropriate provision of AT as a child moves from elementary to middle school? What factors need to be reviewed in assessing the new environment, documenting the client's anticipated needs, and communicating with individuals who are assuming responsibility for case coordination?

RESOURCES FOR FURTHER STUDY

Beukelman, D.R., & Mirenda, P. (1998). *Augmentative and alternative Communication: Management of severe communication disorders in children and adults* (2nd ed.). Baltimore: Paul H Brookes Publishing Co.

Cook, A., & Hussey, S. (2001). *Assistive technologies: Principles and practices* (2nd ed.). St. Louis, MO: Elsevier Science.

Scherer, M. (Ed.). (2003). *Connecting to learn: Educational and assistive technology for people with disabilities.* Washington, DC: American Psychological Association.

Funding Assistive Technology

with Christine L. Appert

Clinical computing competency #9: The clinician will demonstrate awareness of resources that provide continuing education, research results, technical support and information about availability, funding, efficacy, and efficiency of new clinical computing products as well as assistive technology devices and services.

Clinical computing competency #8: The clinician will demonstrate familiarity with legal and ethical considerations that apply to assistive technology and the use of computers in the management of communication disorders, and will adhere to appropriate standards.

Clinicians who are knowledgeable about funding for assistive technology are well on their way to acquiring competencies #8 and #9. The process involved in actually obtaining assistive technology to meet the needs of clients goes beyond merely identifying and recommending it. This process entails expertise with the technology options that are available and skills in navigating the legal issues and community resources that may have bearing on a particular case. Competent clinicians will succeed in identifying a source to assist with purchasing assistive technology, understand the key vocabulary that funding sources expect to hear, and know how to prepare a successful funding request.

It is tempting to view the adoption of technology as a straightforward course of assessment, provision, and treatment resulting in a "fix" for the individual with an impairment. In reality, barriers abound that interfere with or completely sabotage effective technology acquisition and use.

In a comprehensive study related to this topic, the National Council on Disability found that the lack of funding and the intricacies of identifying financial resources to support assistive technology can represent a formidable barrier to acquiring needed tools and services (1993). Other obstacles, which are discussed in Topic 43, include the availability of expertise, lack of administrative support, inadequate communication and coordination, problems with the identification and maintenance of appropriate devices, and the concomitant issues associated with technology abandonment. In the present Topic, strategies and issues surrounding funding will be the point of focus.

FUNDING SOURCES

Costs associated with the provision of assistive technology go beyond the purchase of a device and may encompass evaluation, set-up of the device in the user's environment, training, follow-up, adjustments, maintenance, repairs, or upgrades. Arranging payment is further confounded by the fact that there is no single strategy or system for financing assistive technology in the United States. Dealing with multiple agencies and the lack of coordination between agencies contributes to the dilemmas faced by both technology users and providers. Consumers, clinicians, and suppliers need to be aware of various funding sources and how to tap into them.

There are three general categories of funding sources: public, private, and community based. Each has its own eligibility criteria, requirements for documentation of need, and definitions for the contexts in which assistive technology might be provided. Table 42.1 shows examples of typical funding sources for each classification.

Documenting a functional need for assistive technology and collecting detailed information about various financial resources are preliminary steps to making a funding request. In many instances, the best way to finance a package of technology needs is to put together a funding portfolio that takes advantage of multiple sources. In addition, a low-cost loan may be arranged. As part of the Tech Act projects, many states established low-cost loan programs to complement direct financial aid.

For example, a college student may need a computer with adaptive equipment. In addition, the student requires an evaluation, set-up of the system, training, and follow-up. A plan might be negotiated in which the vocational rehabilitation agency provides the evaluation and training, a local service organization supplies some of the equipment, the student's family purchases whatever else is needed, and the postsecondary institution agrees to provide follow-up and technical support. Families and clients must often rely on a competent professional to map out the details and coordinate resources.

Table 42.1.   Examples of funding sources for assistive technology

Public sources	Private sources	Community-based sources
Education-IDEA	Self-funded by consumer	Service organizations
Federal or state employers or public postsecondary institutions	Employers or private post-secondary institutions	Civic clubs
Vocational Rehabilitation	Worker's compensation	Equipment recycle programs
Medicaid and Social Security Insurance	Private insurance	Church groups
Children's Medical Services (CMS)	Low-interest loan program	Foundations
Veterans Affairs		

Table 42.2. Examples of concepts and key phrases associated with the priorities of various funding sources

Funding source	Concept	Key words
Education—IDEA and state special education funds: early intervention (Part C), preschool and school age (Part B)	Necessary for a free appropriate public education (FAPE)	Device or services required to implement an objective, allow the child to benefit from special education (related aid or service) or to support participation in the general education class
Government employer, agency, or educational institution—compliance with Section 504, Section 508, or ADA	Equal access, effective communication, consumer preference	Auxiliary aid or service required to ensure participation in programs and access to resources at least as effective as those offered to others
Vocational Rehabilitation	Preparing for or maintaining employment, increasing employability	Rehab technology devices or services to render individual with a disability employable
Medicaid	Reduction of physical or mental disability, restoration of the patient to his functional level	Medical necessity must be for use in the home NOTE: school or educational benefit should not be mentioned

From Rehabilitation Engineering Society of North America. (2000). *Fundamentals in assistive technology* (3rd ed.). Washington, DC: Author. Adapted by permission.

FUNDING PRIORITIES AND KEY PHRASES

When considering public funding streams, it is critical to understand the distinctions between agencies and services before developing a potential request and justification. In general, all funding sources want to know that the recommended technology will improve the individual's function in areas such as independence in daily living, decreased cost for care or treatment, performance in a training or pre-employment setting, or participation in a regular education class. Table 42.2 highlights the key concepts and phrases associated with public funding sources that clinicians are most likely to utilize.

Vocational rehabilitation agencies and independent living programs represent a primary federal/state funding source for individuals with disabilities needing adaptive devices for employment or as a means to enhance independence. Medicaid is a federal/state program of medical assistance for those who meet eligibility requirements based on income and individuals with disabilities who receive payments under the Supplemental Security Income (SSI) program. A durable medical equipment category under Medicaid provides funds for medically necessary devices. Financing through Medicaid involves extensive paperwork in order to acquire equipment such as aids for vision and hearing, wheelchairs, mobility aids, and augmentative communication devices. Typically, Medicaid does not fund computer equipment. However, the scope of devices and services varies from state-to-state.

Under the Individuals with Disabilities Education Act (IDEA), assistive technology must be considered in developing individualized family service or education programs (IFSP or IEP). The school system must provide assistive technology if it is needed to implement an IEP objective, allow the child to participate in the general education classroom, or benefit from special education for children receiving early intervention or preschool and school-age special education services. Cost may be considered in choosing the assistive technology device because the school district is not required to choose the most expensive item if a less expensive product or service will suffice.

In practice, disputes surrounding assistive technology and who will pay for it usually center around the determination of necessity and the provision of the best option versus an "appropriate" option. Because ownership of a device is usually retained by the school system, in some situations assistive technology is more suitably funded by other sources to provide exclusive use and possession by the child.

According to Section 504 of the Rehabilitation Act and the Americans with Disabilities Act (ADA), public postsecondary institutions and schools, and government employers must provide assistive technology to "qualified" individuals with disabilities when it is required for "equal access, effective communication, and consumer preference." As discussed in Topic 37, the financial backing for these legal mandates is non-existent. Institutions must be prepared to budget for the expenses of assistive technology when it is needed by a student or employee.

PREPARING A FUNDING REQUEST

In negotiating with both public and private sources, determination, knowledge, and preparation are the keys to success. The following steps, summarizing the points discussed in the previous section, may serve as a guide for clinicians preparing a funding request (Virginia Assistive Technology System, 2001).

1. Define and document the need for assistive technology. Know what is needed, why, and the anticipated functional outcomes.

2. Determine the appropriate technology through an assessment process conducted by a qualified professional or interdisciplinary team acquainted with assistive technology. Consider alternative technology options and document the reasons for deciding on the recommended selection. Collect as much documentation as possible to substantiate the specific request. Remember that consumer preferences should be considered.

3. Obtain purchasing information and associated costs for training, set-up, and device maintenance.

4. Investigate various funding resources and determine the most appropriate option to which to direct your request. Consider a funding portfolio that includes partial support from multiple resources and possibly a low-cost loan.

5. Submit the required paperwork and documentation. Be prepared to re-submit with additional information or changes.

6. If the request is approved, study the provisions of the authorization to determine the exact amount funded and any specific stipulations of the agreement.

7. If the request is not approved or only partially funded, consider other options to supplement the award. Particularly when dealing with public resources, consider re-submitting the request or challenging the decision. The appeals process is a common practice and expected by some agencies.

8. Be sure to acknowledge successful requests from private and community sources. All too often, recipients forget to directly express appreciation for such support.

SUMMARY

Competency managing the process of acquiring funding to support acquisition of assistive technology taps many other areas of clinical expertise. Clinicians should be aware of potential public and private funding streams as well as community-based sources. Clinicians who frequently assist with acquisition of assistive technology will need current information about each provider and how their funds are allocated. This requires understanding the priorities and procedures unique to each funding source, such as the key phrases and criteria for funding and the typical amounts and limits of funding awarded to individuals or agencies. Successful proposals are prepared with care, include complete information about how the money will be spent and why, and build-in a plan for documenting progress. Persistence and willingness to resubmit proposals are often the keys to success.

REVIEW FOR TOPIC 42

1. List the three general categories of funding sources and give two examples of each.
2. Other than the lack of available money, what other variables may contribute to funding dilemmas?

QUESTIONS FOR DISCUSSION

1. Why do you think that funding (not other problems) is considered the greatest deterrent to implementing assistive technology?
2. If you were submitting a funding request to provide an adapted keyboard for an elementary school student, which type of funding source might you approach? What key concepts would you convey in a justification statement?
3. Current funding alternatives may be difficult and time-consuming to pursue. Whether or not a person in need receives optimal or even minimal assistive technology devices and services may depend on the persistence of the professionals involved. In many cases, time spent seeking funds is not reimbursable to a clinician. Discuss the issues and dilemmas surrounding funding for assistive technology.

RESOURCES FOR FURTHER STUDY

Alliance for Assistive Technology (2001). Building a circle of support. In *Computer and web resources for people with disabilities* (Chapter 7). San Rafael, CA: Author.

Parette, H.P., & Hourcade, J.J. (1997). Family issues and assistive technology needs: A sampling of state practices. *Journal of Special Education Technology, 13*(3), 27–43.

Virginia Assistive Technology System. (2001). *A resource guide to assistive technology funding* (5th ed.). Richmond: Author.

Barriers to Implementation of Assistive Technology

with Christine L. Appert

Clinical computing competency #8: The clinician will demonstrate familiarity with legal and ethical considerations that apply to assistive technology and the use of computers in the management of communication disorders, and will adhere to appropriate standards.

Clinical computing competency #9: The clinician will demonstrate awareness of resources that provide continuing education, research results, technical support and information about availability, funding, efficacy, and efficiency of new clinical computing products as well as assistive technology devices and services.

Understanding the barriers to implementation of assistive technology requires that clinicians be familiar with legal and ethical perspectives as well as resources that might help clinicians and clients overcome such obstacles.

Although funding is cited as the number one deterrent to the use of assistive technology, other important barriers also exist. They include lack of training and availability of expertise, lack of administrative support, inadequate communication and coordination, problems with the identification and maintenance of appropriate devices and technologies, and the concomitant issues associated with technology abandonment. Clinicians should be aware of these barriers and be prepared to use available resources and strategies to navigate around them.

TECHNOLOGY ABANDONMENT

A device that is procured and then not used may be abandoned for a variety of reasons. In some instances, it is because newer and better technology is developed or because the user outgrows the system (e.g., a child who no longer fits in a wheelchair). Many times, however, equipment is purchased, used once or twice, and then retired to the back of a closet to collect dust. Hearing aids found in the dresser drawers of many senior citizens represents a good illustration of this phenomenon. Talk to any experienced SLP, OT, or PT, and he or she will probably be able to relate several tales of technology abandonment.

This problem is a frequent topic of concern and discussion among professionals heavily involved in augmentative and alternative communication (AAC). However, it is of equal concern in considering computer access or other purposes for assistive technology unrelated to communication. Clinicians may find themselves involved on teams that make assistive technology recommendations, even for clients who do not have speech or language impairments. As discussed in Topic 39, for example, the consideration of speech recognition as an alternative access method should usually involve the consultation of an SLP.

Matching individual needs to technology and supporting technology users is a complex process. The cycle of technology adoption and abandonment may lead to wasted money and other resources. A situation resulting in rejection or non-use of a device may contribute to an individual's feelings of frustration or lack of control. Although the identification and provision of assistive technology is a continuing process, it is a disappointment—for both clients and service providers—when much effort and time is invested in selecting and obtaining equipment that is never really put to use in satisfying the client's needs.

It is a clinician's professional responsibility to make an effort to avoid situations that lead to technology abandonment. The strategies recommended in Table 43.1 emanate from common sense and issues discussed throughout this book.

ADMINISTRATIVE SUPPORT, COORDINATION, AND AWARENESS

One of the most difficult aspects of introducing a new device or a different way of performing a task may be to gain the cooperation and consensus of everyone involved. As discussed in Topic 41, teamwork and collaboration among the key players is important, but there may be other individuals within an organization who play a less direct but important role. Resistance to technology, the notion that technology gives the person with a disability "special privileges," and a lack of administrative commitment may pose barriers for even the most enthusiastic technology user. In business and school settings, lack of awareness or knowledge about disabilities, the technology involved, or ignorance of legal implications may explain reticence on the part of administrators and peers. Of course, if communication and coordination are generally absent within an organization, the problems go well beyond adopting new technology for one person.

Administrative support can be significantly bolstered by written policies and guidelines related to equitable provision of assistive technology devices and services. Clearly

Table 43.1. Recommended strategies to help clinicians prevent technology abandonment by clients

Consider the opinions of the user, the caregiver, and direct service providers in making selections.

Assess the user's motivation and interest. It may be necessary to have some additional incentives to get a client started until he starts to achieve a level of success.

Determine expectations for what the client will be doing with the technology and the features of the environment where the technology will be used.

Include the necessary preparation, training, and follow-up in the "technology package."

Provide arrangements for adequate equipment set-up and on-going maintenance and repair.

Consider flexible device features which allow for changes in the user's functional abilities or activities.

Plan for continued follow-up and re-appraisal of technology use. It is often possible to promote sustained use by addressing the difficulties experienced by the client, caregivers or service providers. For example, addressing environmental variables that complicate or inhibit use may help. Gaining administrative support or reconfiguring support staff responsibilities may make a big difference.

defined procedures regarding assessment, implementation, and monitoring of assistive technology can significantly increase effective service delivery and reduce misunderstanding and controversy. Planning for assistive technology in a school or agency's technology budget, seeking alternate funding sources (as discussed in Topic 42) and complementing equipment purchases with training and technical support are additional ways that administrators can maximize institutional resources and comply with legal mandates.

CONSUMER TRAINING

Training for an individual who is learning to use a new device is indispensable. Ensuring that the client, direct caregivers, and service providers are familiar with the device and know how to resolve minor glitches is critical to the ultimate goals of independent, productive use. Provision of new technologies without training often results in inefficient use, inadvertent mishandling of the technology, and possible abandonment. In vocational settings, explanation and demonstration of assistive technologies to peers and co-workers can prevent anxiety and misunderstanding before they develop.

PROFESSIONAL TRAINING

The dilemma of adequate preparation in assistive technology for both preservice and practicing clinicians returns us to the beginning of this book. The possibilities change faster than organizations, curricula, and professional standards of practice can keep up. This book should serve as a helpful resource and inspiration for clinicians who are encountering the need for more clinical computing and assistive technology knowledge. Many opportunities for upgrading assistive technology skills exist for clinicians, but they may be hard to find in traditional venues, such as university programs in communication disorders. On-line workshops, on-line discussion groups, ASHA conferences, certificate programs, pre-conference workshops such as those sponsored by Closing the Gap, and interdisciplinary offerings from organizations such as Rehabilitation Engineering and

Assistive Technology Society of America (RESNA) can help clinicians continue their pursuit of clinical computing competency.

SUMMARY

In the real world, technology abandonment is an all-too-common occurrence. Determining an appropriate technology solution is only the first step in ensuring that a selected device or service will assist a client with communication, employment, and motivation to tackle other challenges of life. Some of the barriers to effective implementation of assistive technology include lack of professional expertise, lack of follow-up and long-term support, lack of administrative support, and lack of consumer understanding and training. Clinicians are encouraged to pursue professional training opportunities, using this book as a starting point.

REVIEW FOR TOPIC 43

1. Describe three barriers to implementing assistive technology. What is usually cited as the biggest problem?
2. Describe two situations that might lead to technology abandonment and what a clinician can do to prevent them.

QUESTIONS FOR DISCUSSION

1. Consult with a practicing clinician or think of a situation in your own experience, when a device or equipment was abandoned. If you have trouble thinking of an example, consider your abandoned kitchen gadgets! What factors do you think prompted selection of the device in the first place and why isn't it used any more?
2. What can clinicians do toward preventing technology abandonment?

RESOURCES FOR FURTHER STUDY

Alliance for Assistive Technology (2001). Developing your funding strategy. In *Computer and web resources for people with disabilities*. San Rafael, CA: Author.

Lesar, S. (1998). Use of assistive technology with young children with disabilities: Current status and training needs. *Journal of Early Intervention, 21*(2), 146–159.

Parette, H.P., & Hourcade, J.J. (1997). Family issues and assistive technology needs: A sampling of state practices. *Journal of Special Education Technology, 13*(3), 27–43.

Phillips, B., & Hongxin, Z. (1993). Predictors of assistive technology abandonment. *Assistive Technology, 5*(1), 36–45.

Conclusion
Embracing Change

One of the most frequently asked questions at technology workshops has to do with purchasing a computer. Clinicians want to know whether to buy now or wait until the next major changes in operating system or other functions occur. The underlying question is, "Will I get my money's worth if I invest in today's technology?" Everyone knows that technology is changing rapidly. It's not just personal computers and assistive technologies. Consider, for example, what has happened to telephones over the past few years.

Adapting to change is a continuing challenge for everyone. The standard answer to concerns about keeping up with new technologies is, "Well, we all have to do it" or, "It's just a part of life." This seems like a shallow and less than helpful answer to a clinician who is weighing the cost of clinical computing in terms of her own time and energy. The question of a financial investment in new versus older computers is important. But the issue of pursuing clinical computing competency now, knowing that things will change in the future, may be even more difficult for some clinicians to sort out.

Changes will happen—dramatic ones—in the clinical technologies that are discussed in this book. However, the underlying principles of effective clinical assessment and intervention, even those that incorporate technology, change much more slowly. The clinical computing competencies outlined and discussed in the present text have already lasted through dramatic technology evolution. They are not the kind of short-lived information and skills that we all learn and quickly have to re-learn. On the contrary, the information and skills involved in clinical computing competency are enduring and important to long-term clinical success.

Will it be enough to choose some of the competencies and applications described in this book and master them? What about all the new things that will keep coming? Just like other clinical competencies, expert use of technology will require continuing education. Ideally, the technology itself will make such expertise easier and easier to acquire and maintain. And some changes—such as easier, faster, and less expensive Internet access—will provide clinicians working alone or in remote settings with unprecedented access to the professional support of peers.

Peer interaction and support was fostered in the early days of clinical computing by such events as the Technology Leadership Conferences sponsored by the American Speech-Language-Hearing Foundation (ASHF). These conferences served as a meeting place for innovators to present and discuss ideas and possibilities. As has been mentioned in several places throughout this text, many of the most useful and successful clinical applications of computers were envisioned long before they were actually implemented in a dependable and cost-effective way. As we become accustomed to the omnipresence of computers in our lives, we must not take progress for granted. It will be important to continue to support the innovators and provide forums for dissemination of new advances in the clinical applications of technology.

It is anticipated that the competencies discussed and illustrated in this book will hold up well as new possibilities emerge in clinical technologies. Student clinicians may work on acquiring these competencies through their university training programs when possible. Working clinicians have several additional options for pursuing clinical computing competency, including self-study, individually designed CEU plans, and opportunities sponsored by employers and professional associations. Ideally, all of these approaches will be inspired and supported by the contents of this book.

References

Abberton, E., Hu, X., & Fourcin, A. (1998). Real-time speech pattern element displays for interactive therapy. *International Journal of Language and Communication Disorders, 33,* 292–297.

American Academy of Family Physicians (2003, September). *Why Get a PDA?* Retrieved 12/10/03 from http://www.aafp.org/x476.xml

American Speech-Language-Hearing Association. (1997). *Maximizing the provision of appropriate technology services and devices for students in schools: Technical report.* Rockville, MD: Author.

American Speech-Language-Hearing Association (2002). *2002 Omnibus survey caseload report: SLP.* Rockville, MD: Author.

Appert, C.L. (2002, June). *Power tools: Using assistive technology to support students' organizational and study skills.* A paper presented at the Rehabilitation Engineering and Assistive Technology Society of North America (RESNA) 25th annual conference on Technology and Disability: Research, Design, and Practice, Minneapolis, MN.

Axmear, E. & Poeschel, E. (2001, November). Part 1: Accuracy of beginning clinician's scoring techniques. Paper presented at the annual convention of the American Speech-Language-Hearing Association, New Orleans, LA.

Bahill, A.T., Bharathan, K., & Curlee, R.F. (1995). How the testing techniques for a decision support system changed over nine years. *IEEE Transactions on Systems, Man and Cybernetics, 25,* 1533–1542.

Baker-Van Den Goorbergh, L. (1994). Computers and language analysis: Theory and practice. *Child Language Teaching and Therapy, 10*(3), 329–348.

Bakker, K. (1999a). Clinical technologies for the reduction of stuttering and enhancement of speech fluency. *Seminars in Speech and Language, 20*(3), 271–280.

Bakker, K. (1999b). Technical solutions for quantitative and qualitative assessments of speech fluency. *Seminars in Speech and Language, 20,* 185–196.

Bakker, K., Ingham, R.J., & Netsell, R. (1997). The measurement of voice onset abruptness via acoustic, acceloerometric, electroglottographic and aerodynamic signal analysis. In W. Hulstijn & H.F.M. Peters & P.H.H.M. Van Lieshout (Eds.), *Speech production: Motor control, brain research, and fluency disorders.* New York: Elsevier.

Ball, L. (2002). *Computer-based feedback during articulation therapy.* A paper presented at annual convention of the Missouri Speech-Language-Hearing Association, Columbia, MO.

Ballanger, J. (1997). *A survey of public school clinician's consumer behaviors and use of commercial therapy materials.* Unpublished Master's Thesis, Truman State University, Kirksville, MO.

Bateman, B.D. (1998). *Better IEP's: How to develop legally correct and educationally useful programs* (3rd ed.). Longmont, CA: Sopris West.

Bauer, A.M., & Ulrich, M.E. (2002). "I've got a Palm in my pocket": Using handheld computers in an inclusive classroom. *TEACHING Exceptional Children, 35*(2), 18–22.

Baumann, J.F. (1986). The direct instruction of main idea comprehension ability. In J.F. Baumann (Ed.), *Teaching main idea comprehension* (pp. 133–193). Newark, DE: International Reading Association.

Bernstein, L.E., Goldstein, M.H., & Mahshie, J.J. (1988). Speech training aids for hearing-impaired individuals: Overview and aims. *Journal of Rehabilitative Research and Development, 25*(4), 53–62.

Beukelman, D., & Mirenda, P. (1998). *Augmentative and alternative communication: Management of severe communication disorders in children and adults* (2nd ed.). Baltimore: Paul H. Brookes Publishing Co.

Bishop, D.V.M., Carlyon, R.P., Deeks, J.M., & Bishop, S.J. (1999). Auditory temporal processing impairment: Neither necessary nor sufficient for causing language impairment in children. *Journal of Speech, Language, and Hearing Research, 42,* 1295–1311.

Blachman, B., Ball, E., Black, S., & Tangel, D. (1994). Kindergarten teachers develop phoneme awareness in low-income, inner city classrooms: Does it make a difference? *Reading and Writing: An Interdisciplinary Journal, 6,* 1–17.

Blackstone, S. (1995a). AAC Teams: How do we collaborate? *Augmentative Communication News, 8*(4), 1–3.

Blackstone, S. (1995b). Action planning. *Augmentative Communication News, 8*(4), 5.

Blischak, D.M. (1995). Thomas the writer: Case study of a child with severe physical, speech, and visual impairments. *Language, Speech, and Hearing Services in Schools, 26,* 11–20.

Blood, G. (1995). A behavioral-cognitive therapy program for adults who stutter: Computers and counseling. *Journal of Communication Disorders, 28,* 165–180.

Boone, D. (2004). Facilitator, Model 3500, Application Notes. Retrieved 6/29/04 from http://www.kayelemetrics.com/Product%20info/3500/3500appsec2.htm

Boothroyd, A., Archambault, P., Adams, R., & Storm, R. (1975). Use of a computer-based system of speech training for deaf persons. *Volta Review, 77,* 178–193.

Borden, G.J., & Harris, K.S. (1984). *Speech science primer* (2nd ed.). Baltimore: Williams & Wilkins.

Bouglé, F., Ryalls, J., & Le Dorze, G. (1995). Improving fundamental frequency modulation in head trauma patients: A preliminary comparison of speech-language therapy conducted with and without IBM's Speechviewer. *Folia Phoniatrica et Logopaedica, 47,* 24–32.

Brady, S., Scarborough, H., & Shankweiler, D. (1996). A perspective on two recent research reports. *Perspectives: International Dyslexia Association, 22*(3), 5–9.

Brody, D.M., Nelson, B.A., & Brody, J.F. (1975). The use of visual feedback in establishing normal vocal intensity in two mildly retarded adults. *Journal of Speech and Hearing Disorders, 40,* 502–507.

Broida, R. (June/July, 2003). Book-mobile: The best e-book reader on the planet is already in your pocket. *Handheld Computing, 6*(2), 47–48.

Brosch, S., Haege, A., & Johnson, H.S. (2002). Prognosis indicators for stuttering: The value of computer-based speech analysis. *Brain & Language, 82*(1), 75–86.

Buckleitner, W. (1999). The state of children's software evaluation – yesterday, today, and in the 21st century. *Information Technology in Childhood Education Annual* (pp. 211–220). Charlottesville, VA: Association for the Advancement of Computing in Education.

Bull, G., Bell, R., Garfalo, J., & Sigmon, T. (2002, Oct). The Case for Open Source Software. *Learning and Leading with Technology, 30*(2), 10–17.

Bull, G., Bull, G., Blasi, L., & Cochran, P. (2000). Electronic texts in the classroom. *Learning & Leading with Technology, 27*(4), 46–56.

Bull G., Bull, G., Cochran, P., & Bell, R. (2002). Learner-Based Tools Revisited. *Learning and Leading with Technology, 30*(1), 11–17.

Bull, G., Bull, G., & Dawson, K. (1999). The universal solvent. *Learning & Leading with Technology, 27*(2), 36–41.

Bull, G., Bull, G., Thomas, J., & Jordon, J. (2000). Incorporating imagery into instruction. *Learning & Leading with Technology, 27*(6), 46–56.

Bull, G., & Cochran, P. (1985). Creating tools for clinicians and teachers. *Journal for Computer Users in Speech and Hearing, 1*(1), 45–49.

Bull, G., & Cochran, P. (1987). Logo and exceptional individuals. In J.D. Lindsey (Ed.), *Computers and Exceptional Individuals* (pp. 169-187). Columbus, OH: Charles Merrill.

Bull, G.L., Cochran, P.S., & Snell, M.E. (1988). Beyond CAI: Computers, language, and persons with mental retardation. *Topics in Language Disorders, 8*(4), 55–76.

Carmein, S. & Hudak, G. (2003). MAPS: PDA scaffolding for independence for persons with cognitive impairment. In *Proceedings of the 2003 Convention of the Rehabilitation Engineering and Assistive Technology Society of North America.* Arlington, VA: RESNA. Retrieved 1/11/04 from http://www.resna.org/ProfResources/Publications/Proceedings/2003/Papers/TSP/Carmien_TSP.php

Case, J.L. (1999a). Technology in the assessment of voice disorders. *Seminars in Speech and Language, 20*(2), 169–196.

Case, J. L. (1999b). Technology in the treatment of voice disorders. *Seminars in Speech and Language, 20*(3), 281–295.

Catts, H. (1993). The relationship between speech-language impairments and reading disabilities. *Journal of Speech and Hearing Research, 36,* 948–958.

Channell, R.W., & Johnson, B.W. (1999). Automated grammatical tagging of child language samples. *Journal of Speech, Language, and Hearing Research, 42,* 727–734.

Clements, D.H. (1987). Computers and young children: A review of research. *Young Children, 43,* 34–44.

Clements, D.H., Nastasi, B.K., & Swaminatha, W. (1993). Young children and computers: Crossroads and directions from research. *Young Children, 48,* 56–64.

Cochran, P.S. (1989). Clinical computing in the 1990's: There's more to it than which key to press. *Journal for Computer Users in Speech and Hearing, 5*(2), 110–113.

Cochran, P.S. (2000). Technology for individuals with speech and language disorders. In J.D. Lindsey (Ed.), *Technology and exceptional individuals 3rd Ed.* (pp. 303–325). Austin: PRO-ED.

Cochran, P.S., & Bull, G.L. (1985). *Creating a shared context: Using a computer in language therapy*. A paper presented at the annual convention of the American Speech-Language-Hearing Association, Washington, D.C.

Cochran, P.S., & Bull, G.L. (1991). Integrating word processing into language intervention. *Topics in Language Disorders, 11*(2), 31–48.

Cochran, P.S., & Bull, G.L. (1992). Computer-assisted learning and instruction. In J. Rassi & M. McElroy (Eds.), *The Education of Audiologists and Speech-Language Pathologists* (pp. 363–386). Timonium, MD: York.

Cochran, P.S., & Masterson, J.J. (1995). NOT using a computer in language assessment / intervention: In defense of the reluctant clinician. *Language, Speech, and Hearing Services in Schools, 26*(3), 213–222.

Cochran, P.S., Masterson, J.J., Long, S.H., Katz, R., Seaton, W., Wynne, M., Lieberth, A., & Martin, D. (1993). Computer competencies for clinicians. *Asha, 35*(8), 48–49.

Cochran, P.S., & Nelson, L.K. (1999). Technology applications in intervention for preschool-age children with language disorders. *Seminars in Speech and Language, 20*(3), 203–218.

Collis, B. (1988, February). Research windows. *The Computing Teacher,* 15–16, 61.

Collis, B. (1989). *Research in the application of computers in education: Trends and issues.* Paper presented at the the National Educational Computing Conference, Boston, MA.

Conant, S., Budhoff, M., & Hecht, B. (1983). *Teaching language-disabled children: A communication games intervention.* Cambridge, MA: Brookline Books.

Conture, E.G., & Yaruss, J.S. (1993). *A Handbook for Childhood Stuttering: A Second Opinion.* Tucson, AZ: Bahill Intelligent Computer Systems.

Cook, A.M., & Hussey, S.M. (2001). *Assistive technology: Principles and practice* (2nd Ed). St. Louis, MO: Elsevier Science.

Cooper, M. (1971). Modern techniques of vocal rehabilitation for functional and organic dysphonias. In L. Travis (Ed.), *Handbook of speech pathology and audiology* (pp. 585–616). Englewood Cliffs: Prentice-Hall.

Cooper, R., & Neilson, H. (1986). *Computer-aided speech production.* Los Angeles, CA: Voice Learning Systems.

Council for Exceptional Children. (2000). *Developing educationally relevant IEP's: A technical assistance document for speech-language pathologists.* Reston, VA: Author.

Council for Exceptional Children. (2004). *Professional standards: knowledge and skills base for beginning teachers.* Retrieved 1/08/04 from http://www.cec.sped.org/ps/perf_based_stds/knowledge_standards.html

Council for Exceptional Children. (2002). New report calls for reform of teacher preparation programs, *CEC TODAY, 9*(2), 7.

Cradler, J., Freeman, M., Cradler, R., & McNabb, M. (2002). Research implications for preparing teachers to use technology. *Learning and Leading with Technology, 30*(1), 50–54.

Crary, M.A. (1995). A direct intervention program for chronic neurogenic dysphagia secondary to brainstem stroke. *Dysphagia, 10,* 6–18.

Crary, M.A., & Baldwin, B.O. (1997). Surface electomyographic characteristics of swallowing in dysphagia secondary to brainstem stroke. *Dysphagia, 12,* 180–187.

Crary, M.A., & Groher, M.E. (2000). Basic concepts of surface electromyographic feedback in the treatment of dysphasia: A tutorial. *American Journal of Speech-Language Pathology, 9,* 116–125.

Dagenais, P. (1995). Electropalatography in the treatment of articulation/phonological disorders. *Journal of Communication Disorders, 28,* 303–329.

Dagenais, P.A., Costello-Ingham, J., & Powell, T. (1999, November). *Treatment research on articulation/phonological disorders: Past, present, and future.* A paper presented at the annual convention of the American Speech-Language-Hearing Association, San Francisco, CA.

Dalston, R.M., & Seaver, E.J. (1992). Relative values of various standardized passages in the nasometric assessment of patients with velopharyngeal impairment. *Cleft Palate-Craniofacial Journal, 29*(1), 17–21.

Dalston, R.M., Warren, D.W., & Dalston, E.T. (1991). A preliminary investigation concerning the use of nasometry in identifying patients with hyponasality and/or nasal airway impairment. *Journal of Speech and Hearing Research, 34*(1), 8–11.

Day, P. (2001, Feb 5). Telehealth in stuttering treatment. *Express News* [online newsletter, University of Alberta, Canada]. Retrieved 1/10/04 from http://www.expressnews.ualberta.ca/ExpressNews/articles/printer.cfm?p_ID=307

De La Plaz, S. (1999). Composing via dictation and speech recognition systems: Compensatory strategies for students with learning disabilities. *Learning Disability Quarterly, 22*(3), 173–182.

Dudding, C.C., & Purcell-Robertson, R.M. (2003, June 10). Beyond the technology: How to navigate distance education. *The ASHA Leader , 8*(11), 6–7, 16.

Eisenberg, S.L., Fersko, T.M., & Lundgren, C. (2001). The use of MLU for identifying language impairment in preschool children: A review. *American Journal of Speech-Language Pathology, 10,* 323–342.

Electromechanical Transducer. *Encyclopædia Britannica.* Retrieved January 18, 2004, from http://www.britannica.com/eb/article?eu=117556

Evans, J.L., & Miller, J.F. (1999). Language sample anaylsis in the 21st century. *Seminars in Speech and Language, 20*(2), 101–116.

Fallon, M.A., & Sanders Wann, J.A. (1994). Incorporating computer technology into activity-based thematic units for young children with disabilities. *Infants and Young Children, 6,* 64–69.

Fazio, B.B., & Rieth, H.J. (1986). Characteristics of pre-school handicapped children's microcomputer use during free-choice periods. *Journal of the Division for Early Childhood, 10*(3), 247–254.

Fitch, J.J. (1984). Computer managed articulation diagnosis [computer program]. Tuscon: AZ: Communication Skill Builders.

Fitch, J.L. (1989). Computer recognition of correct sound productions in articulation treatment. *Journal for Computer Users in Speech and Hearing, 5*(1), 8–18.

Friel-Patti, S., DesBarres, K., & Thibodeau, L.M. (2001). Case studies of children using Fast ForWord. *American Journal of Speech-Language Pathology, 10*(3), 203–216.

Frome Loeb, D., Stoke, C., & Fey, M. (2001). Language changes associated with Fast ForWord: Language evidence from case studies. *American Journal of Speech-Language Pathology, 10*(3), 216–230.

Gardner, J.E., Taber-Brown, F., & Wissick, C. (1992). Selecting age-appropriate software for adolescents and adults with developmental disabilities. *Teaching Exceptional Children, 24*(3), 60–63.

Gardner, J.E., Wissick, C.A., Schweder, W., & Canter, L.S. (2003). Enhancing interdisciplinary instruction in general and special education: Thematic units and technology. *Remedial and Special Education, 24*(3),161–72.

Gayton, D. & Ferrel, S. (2001). *Palm Pilots in practice.* A paper presented at the annual convention of the Rehabilitation Engineering and Assistive Technology Society of North America, Reno, NV.

Gillam, R., Crofford, J.A., Gale, M.A., & Hoffman, L.M. (2001). Language change following computer-assisted language instruction with Fast ForWord or Laureate Learning Systems software. *American Journal of Speech-Language Pathology, 10*(3), 231–247.

Gillam, R., Frome Loeb, D., & Friel-Patti, S. (2001). Looking back: A summary of five exploratory studies of Fast ForWord. *American Journal of Speech-Language Pathology, 10,* 269–273.

Golden, D. (1998). *Assistive technology in special education: Policy and practice.* Reston, VA: CASE/TAM of the Council for Exceptional Children.

Grott, R. (June, 2000). *Microphones for speech recognition.* A paper presented at the annual convention of the Rehabilitation Engineering and Assistive Technology Society of North America (RESNA), Orlando, FL.

Haaf, R., Duncan, B., Skarakis-Doyle, E., Garew, M., & Kapitan, P. (1999). Computer-based language assessment software: The effects of presentation and response format. *Language, Hearing, Speech Services in Schools, 30,* 68–74.

Hallowell, B., & Katz, R.C. (1999). Technology applications in the assessment of acquired neurogenic communication and swallowing disorders in adults. *Seminars in Speech and Language, 20*(2), 149–168.

Hammel, J. & Angelo, J. (1996). Technology competencies for occupational therapy practitioners. *Assistive Technology, 8,* 34–42.

Haugland, S.W. (1992). The effect of computer software on preschool children's developmental gains. *Journal of Computing in Childhood Education, 3,* 15–30.

Haugland, S.W., & Shade, D. (1988). Developmentally appropriate software. *Young Children, 43,* 37–43.

Haugland, S.W., & Wright, J.L. (1997). *Young children and technology: A world of discovery.* Boston, MA: Allyn and Bacon.

Healey, C.H., & Scott, L.A. (1995). Stratagies for treating elementary school-age children who stutter: An integrative approach. *Language, Hearing, Speech Services in Schools, 26,* 151–161.

Higgens, E., & Raskind, M. (Spring 1995). Compensatory effectiveness of speech recognition on the written composition performance of postsecondary students with learning disabilities. *Learning Disability Quarterly, 18,* 159–174.

Higgins, M.B., McCleary, E.A., & Schulte, L. (2000). Use of visual feedback to treat negative intraoral air pressure of preschoolers with cochlear implants. *American Journal of Speech-Language Pathology, 9,* 21–35.

Holder-Brown, L., & Parette Jr., H.P. (1992). Children with disabilities who use assistive technology: Ethical considerations. *Young Children, 47*(6), 73–77.

Hoon, P. (Ed.)(1997). *Guidelines for educational use of copyrighted materials.* Pullman: Washington State University Press.

Hunt-Berg, M., Rankin, J.L., & Beukelman, D. (1994). Ponder the possibilities: Computer-supported writing for struggling writers. *Learning Disabilities Research and Practice, 9,* 169–178.

Ingram, D., & Ingam, K.D. (2001). A whole-word approach to phonological analysis and intervention. *Language, Hearing, Speech Services in Schools, 32,* 271–283.

International Society for Technology in Education (2000). *National educational technology standards for teachers.* Eugene, OR: Author. Available: http://cnets.iste.org/.

Jacobs, E.L. (2001). The effects of adding dynamic assessment components to a computerized preschool language screening test. *Communication Disorders Quarterly, 22,* 217–226.

Johnson, D., & Broida, R. (2001). *How to do everything with your Palm Handheld* (2nd Edition). New York: McGraw-Hill Osborne Media.

Judge, S.L. (2001). Integrating computer technology within early childhood classrooms. *Young Exceptional Children, 5*(1), 20–26.

Junker, A. (2002, October). *Providing access for people with changing neuromuscular control abilities using the Cyberlink Hands-Free Controller.* A presentation given at the annual Closing the Gap Technology Conference, Minneapolis, MN.

Kamhi, A., & Catts, H. (1986). Toward an understanding of developmental language and reading disorders. *Journal of Speech and Hearing Disorders, 51,* 337–347.

Katims, D.S. (1991). Emergent literacy in early childhood special education: Curriculum and instruction. *Topics in Early Childhood Special Education, 11*(1),69–84.

Katz, R.C. (1984). Using microcomputers in the diagnosis and treatment of chronic aphasic adults. *Seminars in Speech and Language, 5,* 11–22.

Katz, R.C. (1986). *Aphasia treatment and microcomputers.* San Diego, CA: College-Hill.

Katz, R.C., & Hallowell, B. (1999). Technological applications in the treatment of acquired neurogenic communication and swallowing disorders in adults. *Seminars in Speech and Language, 20*(3), 251–269.

Katz, R.C., & Wertz, R.T. (1997). The efficacy of computer-provided reading treatment for chronic adult aphasics. *Journal of Speech and Hearing Research, 40,* (493-507).

Kay Elemetrics Corporation, (1999). *Multi-speech, Model 3700 CSL for Windows, Models 4100, 4300B: Software instruction manual Version 2.3.* Lincoln Park, NJ: Author.

Kemp, K., & Klee, T. (1997). Clinical language sampling practices: Results of a survey of speech-language pathologists in the United States. *Child Language Teaching and Therapy, 13,* 161–176.

Kent, R.D. (1997). *Speech Science.* San Diego: Singular Publishing Group.

Kewley-Port, D. (1994). Speech technology and speech training for the hearing impaired. *The Journal of the Academy of Rehabilitative Audiology* (XXVII), 251–265.

Kewley-Port, D., Watson, C.S., Elbert, M., Maki, D., & Reed, D. (1991). The Indiana Speech Training Aid (ISTRA) II: Training curriculum and selected case studies. *Clinical Linguistics & Phonetics, 5,* 13–38.

King, J.M., & Hux, K. (1995). Intervention using talking word processing software: An aphasia case study. *Augmentative and Alternative Communication, 11,* 187–192.

Kinsey, C. (1986). Microcomputer speech therapy for dysphasic adults: A comparison with two conventionally administered tasks. *British Journal of Disorders of Communication, 21,* 125–133.

Kinsey, C. (1990). Analysis of dysphasics' behaviour in computer and conventional therapy environments. *Aphasiology, 4*(3), 281–291.

Koester, H.H. (2001). User performance with speech recognition: A literature review. *Assistive Technology, 13,* 116–130.

Koppenhaver, D.A., Coleman, P.P., Kalman, S.L., & Yoder, D.E. (1991). The implications of emergent literacy research for children with developmental disabilities. *American Journal of Speech-Language Pathology, 1,* 38–44.

Kuntz, T., & Bakker, K. (1997). Doctor Fluency: A computerized system for precision fluency shaping. *Clinical Connection, 10*(4), 21.

Lambert, J. (2003). *Digital storytelling: Capturing lives, creating community.* Berkeley, CA: Digital Diner Press.

Lancioni, G.E., Brouwer, J.A., & Markus, S. (1995). A portable visual-feedback device for reducing vocal loudness in persons with mental retardation. *Perceptual and Motor Skills, 81,* 851–857.

Lancioni, G.E., Van Houten, K., & Ten Hoopen, G. (1997). Reducing excessive vocal loudness in persons with mental retardation through the use of a portable auditory-feedback device. *Journal of Behavior Therapy and Experimental Psychiatry, 28*(2), 123–128.

Langmore, S.E., Schatz, K., & Olson, N. (1988). Fiberoptic endoscopic examination of swallowing safety: a new procedure. *Dysphagia, 2,* 216–219.

Leadholm, B.J., & Miller, J.F. (1992). *Language sample analysis: The Wisconsin guide.* Madison, WI: Wisconsin Department of Public Instruction.

Lee, L. (1974). *Developmental sentence analysis.* Evanston, IL: Northwestern University Press.

Lent, J.R. (1982). Intellectual prosthesis: Reality or dream for the severely/profoundly retarded person. *Journal of Special Education Technology, 5*(4), 22–24.

Lepper, M.R. (1985). Microcomputers in education: Motivational and social issues. *American Psychologist, 40,* 1–18.

Lesar, S. (1998). Use of assistive technology with young children with disabilities: Current status and training needs. *Journal of Early Intervention, 21*(2), 146–159.

Lieberth, A.K., & Martin, D.R. (1995). Authoring and hypermedia. *Language, Hearing, Speech Services in Schools, 26*(3), 241–250.

Logemann, J.A., & Kahrilas, P.J. (1990). Relearning to swallow after stroke–application of maneuvers and indirect biofeedback: A case study. *Neurology, 40,* 1136–1138.

Long, S. (2001). About time: a comparison of computerized and manual procedures for grammatical and phonological analysis. *Clinical Linguistics & Phonetics, 15*(5), 399–426.

Long, S., & Masterson, J.J. (1993, September). Computer technology: Use in language analysis. *Asha, 35,* 40–41, 51.

Long, S.H. (1991). Integrating microcomputer applications into speech and language assessment. *Topics in Language Disorders, 11*(2), 1–17.

Long, S.H. (1999). Technology applications in the assessment of children's language. *Seminars in Speech and Language, 20*(2), 117–132.

Long, S.H., & Channell, R.W. (2001). Accuracy of four language analysis procedures performed automatically. *American Journal of Speech-Language Pathology, 10,* 180–188.

Lynch, W. (1993). Update on a computer-based language prosthesis for aphasia therapy. *Journal of Head Trauma Rehabilitation, 8,* 107–109.

Macaruso, P., & Hook, P.E. (2001). Auditory processing: Evaluation of Fast ForWord for children with dyslexia. *Perspectives: International Dyslexia Association, 27*(3), 5–8.

Manasse, N.J., Hux, K., & Rankin-Erickson, J.L. (2000). Speech recognition training for enhancing written language generation by a traumatic brain injury survivor, *Brain Injury, 14*(11), 1015–1034.

Marler, J., Champlin, C., & Gillam, R. (2001). Backward and simultaneous masking measured in children with language-learning impairments who recieved intervention with Fast ForWord or Laureate Learning Systems software. *American Journal of Speech-Language Pathology, 10*(3), 28–37.

Martin, B.J.W., Logemann, J.A., Shaker, R., & Dodds, W.J. (1994). Coordination between respiration and swallowing: Respiratory phase relationships and temporal integration. *Journal of Applied Physiology, 76*(2), 714–723.

Masterson, J.J. (1995). Computer applications in the schools: What we can do - what we should do. *Language, Speech and Hearing Services in Schools, 26*(3), 211–212.

Masterson, J.J. (1999a). Clinical applications of *Earobics, P.B. Bear's Birthday*, and *Let's Explore the Jungle with Buzzy. Clinical Connection, 12*(15–16).

Masterson, J.J. (1999b). Preface: Technical advances for speech-language interventions. *Seminars in Speech and Language, 20*(3), 201–202.

Masterson, J.J., Long, S., & Buder, E. (1998). Instrumentation in clinical phonology. In J.B. Bernthal & N. Bankson, (Eds.), *Articulation and phonological disorders* (4th Ed.), (pp. 378–406). Des Moines, IA: Allyn and Bacon.

Masterson, J.J., & Oller, D.K. (1999). Use of technology in phonological assessment: Evaluation of early meaningful speech and prelinguistic vocalizations. *Seminars in Speech and Language, 20*(2), 133–148.

Masterson, J.J., & Pagan, F. (1989). *Interactive system for phonological analysis (ISPA)* [computer program]. San Antonio, TX: Psychological Corporation.

Masterson, J.J., & Rvachew, S. (1999). Use of technology in phonological intervention. *Seminars in Speech and Language, 20*(3), 233–250.

McGuire, R.A. (1995). Computer-based instrumentation: Issues in clinical applications. *Language, Hearing, Speech Services in Schools, 28*(3), 223–231.

McPherson, F. (2002). *How to do everything with your Pocket PC,* (2nd ed.). New York: McGraw-Hill Osborne Media.

McRay, L.B., & Fitch, J.L. (1996). A survey of computer use by public school speech-language pathologists. *Language, Speech, and Hearing Services in Schools, 27*(1), 40–7.

Merzenich, M.M., Jenkins, W.M., Miller, S.L., Schreiner, C., & Tallal, P. (1996). Temporal processing deficits of language-learning impaired children ameliorated by training. *Science, 271,* 77–81.

Merzenich, M.M., Tallal, P., Peterson, B., Miller, S., & Jenkins, W.M. (1999). Some neurological principles relevant to the origins of - and the cortical plasticity based remediation of - developmental language impairments. In J. Grafman & T. Christen (Eds.), *Neuronal plasticity: Building a bridge from the laboratory to the clinic* (pp. 169-187). New York: Springer-Verlag.

Metz, S.M., & Hoffman, B. (1997). Mind operated devices. *Cognitive Psychology, 2,* 69–74.

Meyers, L.F. (1984). Unique contributions of microcomputers to language intervention with handicapped children. *Seminars in Speech and Language, 5,* 23–24.

Miller, J.F. (2000). Innovations in language sample analysis in the schools. A paper presented at the annual convention of the American Speech-Language-Hearing Association, Washington, DC.

Miller, J.F. (1981). *Assessing language production in children: Experimental procedures.* Baltimore: University Park Press.

Miller, J.F., & Chapman, R.S. (1984–2000). *Systematic Analysis of Language Transcripts (SALT)* [computer program]. Madison, WI: University of Wisconsin Waisman Center, Language Analysis Laboratory.

Miller, J.F., & Chapman, R.S. (1981). The relation between age and mean length of utterance in morphemes. *Journal of Speech and Hearing Research, 24,* 154–161.

Miller, J.F., & Chapman, R.S. (1988). *Basic SALT program for Windows Version 5.0.* Madison, WI: University of Wisconsin Waisman Center, Language Analysis Laboratory.

Miller, J.F., Freiberg, C., Rolland, M.B., & Reeves, M.A. (1992). Implementing computerized language sample analysis in the public school. *Topics in Language Disorders, 12*(2), 69–82.

Mills, R.H. (1986). Computerized management of aphasia. In R. Chapey (Ed.), *Language intervention strategies in adult aphasia* (pp. 333–344). Baltimore: William & Wilkins.

Moats, L.C. (2000). *Speech to print: Language essentials for teachers.* Baltimore: Paul H. Brookes Publishing Co.

Morawej, A., Jackson, A.T., & McLeod, R.D. (1999). Fonetix: Building virtual speech therapy practicum over the Internet. *Studies in Health Technology and Informatics, 64,* 253–261.

Morrison, J., & Shriberg, L.D. (1992). Articulation testing versus conversational speech sampling. *Journal of Speech and Hearing Research, 35*(2), 259–273.

Musselwhite, C., & King-DeBaun, P. (1997). *Emergent literacy success: Merging technology with whole language for students with disabilities.* Park City, UT: Creative Communicating.

Naremore, R.C., Densmore, A.E., & Harman, D.H. (2001). *Assessment and treament of school-age language disorders.* San Diego: Singular.

National Association for the Education of Young Children. (1996). *Position statement on technology and young children-Ages 3 through 8* (position statement). Washington, DC: Author.

National Council on Disability. (1993). *Study on the financing of assistive technology devices and services for individuals with disabilities.* Washington DC.: Author.

Nellis, J.L., Neiman, G.S., & Lehman, J.A. (1992). Comparison of nasometer and listener judgments of nasality in the assessment of velopharyngeal function after pharyngeal flap surgery. *Cleft Palate-Craniofacial Journal, 29*(2), 157–163.

Nelson, N. (1981). An eclectic model of language intervention for disorders of listening, speaking, reading, and writing. *Topics in Language Disorders, 1*(2), 1–23.

Nelson, N.W., Bahr, C.M., & Van Meter, A.M. (2004). *The writing lab approach to language instruction and intervention.* Baltimore, MD: Paul H. Brookes Publishing Co.

Nickerson, R.S., Kalikow, D.N., & Stevens, K.N. (1976). Computer-aided speech training for the deaf. *Journal of Speech and Hearing Disorders, 41,* 120–132.

Nippold, M.A., Schwarz, I.E., & Lewis, M. (1992). Analyzing the potential benefit of microcomputer use for teaching figurative language. *American Journal of Speech-Language Pathology, 1*(2), 36–43.

Oller, D.K. (1991). Computational approaches to transcription and analysis in child phonology. *Journal for Computer Users in Speech and Hearing, 7,* 44–59.

Onslow, M., Costa, L., Andrews, A., Harrison, E., & Packman, A. (1996). Speech outcomes of a prolonged-speech treatment for stuttering. *Journal of Speech and Hearing Research, 39,* 734–749.

Ott-Rose, M., & Cochran, P.S. (1992). Teaching action verbs with computer-controlled videodisc vs. traditional picture stimuli. *Journal for Computer Users in Speech and Hearing, 8*(2), 15–32.

Palacio, M. (2001). Computer applications in therapy. *ADVANCE for Speech-Language Pathologists and Audiologists, 11*(12), 10–11.

Palacio, M. (2001). Take a picture, it lasts longer: Novel use of digital cameras enhances therapy in schools. *ADVANCE for Speech-Language Pathologists and Audiologists,* 6–7.

Papert, S. (1980). *Mindstorms: Children, computers, and powerful ideas.* NY: Basic Books.

Parette, H.P., & Hourcade, J.J. (1997). Family issues and assistive technology needs: A sampling of state practices. *Journal of Special Education Technology, 13*(3), 27–43.

Pascarelli, E.F. (1994). *Repetitive strain injury: A computer user's guide.* NY: John Wiley & Sons.

Petheram, B. (1992). A survey of therapists' attitudes to computers in the home-based treatment of adult aphasics. *Aphasiology, 6*(2), 207–212.

Phillips, B., & Hongxin, Z. (1993). Predictors of assistive technology abandonment. *Assistive Technology, 5*(1), 36–45.

Pierce, P.L., & McWilliam, P.J. (1993). Emerging literacy and children with severe speech and physical impairments (SSPI): Issues and possible intervention strategies. *Topics in Language Disorders,13*(2), 47–57.

Pogue, D. (1998). *PalmPilot: The ultimate guide.* Sebastopol, CA: O'Reilly & Associates.

Potter, R., Kopp, G., & Green, H. (1947). *Visible speech.* New York: NY: D. Van Nostrand.

Povel, D., & Wansink, M. (1986). A computer-controlled vowel corrector for the hearing impaired. *Journal of Speech and Hearing Research, 29,* 99–105.

Pownell, D., & Bailey, G.D. (2002). Are you ready for handhelds? *Learning and Leading with Technology, 30*(2), 50–57.

Pratt, S.R., Heintzelman, A.T., & Deming, S.E. (1993). The efficacy of using IBM Speechviewer vowel accuracy module to treat young children with hearing impairment. *Journal of Speech and Hearing Research, 36,* 1063–1074.

Rehabilitation Engineering Society of North America (2000). *Fundamentals in assistive technology* (3rd ed.). Washington DC: Author.

Rice, M.L. (1997). Speaking out: Evaluating new training programs for language impairment. *Asha, 39*(3), 13.

Rogers, E.M. (1995). *Diffusion of innovations* (4th ed.). NY: Free Press.

Rose, D., & Meyer, A. (2002) *Teaching every student in the digital age: Universal Design for Learning.* Alexandria, VA: Association for Supervision and Curriculum Development.

Rosegrant, T.J. (1984). Use of microprocessors to remediate speech through literacy. In W.H. Perkins (Ed.), *Current therapy for communication disorders: Language handicaps in children.* (pp. 57–62). New York: Thieme-Stratton.

Rosegrant, T.J. (1985). Using the microcomputer as a tool for learning to read and write. *Journal of Learning Disabilities, 18*(2), 113–115.

Ruscello, D. (1995). Visual feedback in treatment of residual phonological disorders. *Journal of Communication Disorders, 28,* 279–302.

Rushakoff, G.E. (1984). A clinician's model for the review of speech, language, and hearing microcomputer software. *Asha,* 78–79.

Rushakoff, G.E., & Edwards, W. (1982, November). *The /s/ meter: A beginning for microcomputer assisted articulation therapy.* A paper presented at the American Speech-Language-Hearing Association, Toronto, Canada.

Russell, S.J. (1986, Spring). But what are they learning? The dilemma of using microcomputers in special education. *Learning Disability Quarterly, 9,* 100–104.

Russell, S.J., Corwin, R., Mokros, J.R., & Kapisovsky, P.M. (1989). *Beyond drill and practice: Expanding the computer mainstream.* Reston, VA: Council for Exceptional Children.

Scherer, M.J. (1991). *Matching person and technology (MPT).* Rochester, NY: Author.

Scherer, M.J., & Galvin, J.C. (1996). An outcome perspective of quality pathways to the most appropriate technology. In J.C. Galvin & M.J. Scherer (Eds.), *Evaluating, selecting and using appropriate assistive technologies.* Gaithersburg, MD: Aspen.

Schetz, K.F. (1989). Computer-aided language /concept enrichment in kindergarten. *Language, Hearing, Speech Services in Schools, 20,* 2–10.

Schwartz, A.H. (1986). Microcomputer applications: What changes hath this tool wrought? *Texas Journal of Audiology and Speech Pathology, 12*(1), 4–9.

Schwartz, A.H., Brogan, V.M., Emond, G.A., & Oleksiak, J.F. (1993). Technology-enhanced accent modification. *Asha, 35*(8), 44–45, 51.

SEEDS: Rural Assistive Technology Project (Southwest Educational Development Laboratory). (1996). *So What's a Rural School Leader to Do?* Retrieved 3/5/00 from http://www.sedl.org/rural/seeds/assistivetech/leader.html

Sharp, P., Kelly, S., Main, A., & Manley, G. (1999). An instrument for the multiparameter assessment of speech. *Medical Engineering & Physics, 21,* 661–671.

Shriberg, L.D. (1993). Four new speech and prosody-voice measures for genetics research and other studies in developmental phonological disorders. *Journal of Speech and Hearing Research, 36,* 105–140.

Shriberg, L.D., & Kwiatkowski, J. (1982). Phonological disorders III: A procedure for assessing severity of involvement. *Journal of Speech & Hearing Disorders, 47,* 256–270.

Shriberg, L.D., Kwiatkowski, J., & Snyder, T. (1986). Articulation testing by microcomputer. *Journal of Speech and Hearing Disorders, 51,* 309–324.

Shriberg, L.D., Kwiatkowski, J., & Snyder, T. (1989). Tabletop versus microcomputer-assisted speech management: Stabilization phase. *Journal of Speech and Hearing Disorders, 54*(2), 233–248.

Shuster, L.I., Ruscello, D.M., & Toth, A.R. (1995). The use of visual feedback to elicit correct /r/. *American Journal of Speech-Language Pathology, 4,* 37–44.

Siemsen, R.L. (1993). *The effects of word processing with speech output on the literacy skills of language-disabled adolescents.* Unpublished master's thesis. Northeast Missouri State University, Kirksville, MO (OCLC# 28887113).

Silverman, F.H. (1997). *Computer applications for augmenting the management of speech-language, and hearing disorders.* Des Moines, IA: Allyn & Bacon.

Smit, A.B., Hand, L., Freilinger, J., Bernthal, J.E., & Bird, A. (1990). The Iowa articulation norms project and its Nebraska replication. *Journal of Speech & Hearing Disorders, 55,* 779–798.

Snow, C., Midkiff-Borunda, S., Small, A., & Proctor, A. (1984). Therapy as social interaction: Analyzing the contexts for language remediation. *Topics in Language Disorders, 4*(4), 72–85.

Software & Information Industry Association (SIIA).(2000). *SIIA's Report on Global Software Piracy 2000.* Retrieved May 29, 2004 from http://www.siia.net/estore/10browse.asp.

Software Publisher's Association. (1998). Software piracy: Is it happening in your school or university. *T.H.E. Journal, 25*(9), 66–67.

Stahl, S., & Murray, B. (1994). Defining phonological awareness and its relationship to early reading. *Journal of Educational Psychology, 86,* 221–234.

Steelman, J.D., Pierce, P.L., & Koppenhaver, D.A. (1993). The role of computers in promoting literacy in children with severe speech and physical impairments. *Topics in Language Disorders, 13*(2), 76–88.

Steiner, S., & Larson, V.L. (1991). Integrating microcomputers into language intervention with children. *Topics in Language Disorders, 11*(2), 18–30.

Steinfeld, E. (1994). *The concept of universal design.* Paper presented at the Sixth Ibero-American Conference on Accessibility, Center for Independent Living, Rio de Janeiro. Retrieved 10/10/03 from http://www.ap.buffalo.edu/idea.

Stevenson, D. & Kenny, K. (2003, August/September). Ergonomics: It's not just for your clients. *Closing the Gap, 21*(3). Retrieved 1/10/04 from http://www.closingthegap.com/ctg2/members2/detailsInline.lasso

Sturm, J.M., Rankin, J.L., Beukelman, D., & Schutz-Meuhling, L. (1997). How to select appropriate software for computer-assisted writing. *Intervention in School & Clinic, 32,* 148–162.

Swan, R. (1996). "Port-O-Tech": Technology on the home-health front. *Phi Kappa Phi National Forum, 76*(3), 6–7.

Sweeney, J.P. (2002). *CIRCUIT: Model for assistive technology assessment.* Canton, CT: Onion Mountain Technology.

Tackett, S.L., Rice, D.A., Rice, J.C., & Butterbaugh, G. J. (2001). Using a Palmtop PDA for reminding in prospective memory deficit. In *Proceedings of the 2001 Convention of the Rehabilitation Engineering and Assistive Technology Society of North America* (pp. 23–25). Arlington, VA: RESNA.

Tallal, P. (2000). Experimental studies of language learning impairments: From research to remediation. In D.V.M. Bishop & L.B. Leonard (Eds.), *Speech and language impairments in children: Causes, characteristics, intervention and outcomes* (pp. 131–155). Philadelphia: Psychological Press.

Tallal, P., Miller, S.L., Bedi, G., Byma, G., Wang, X., Nagarajan, S., Schreiner, C., Jenkins, W.M., & Merzenich, M.M. (1996). Fast-element enhanced speech improves language comprehension in language-learning impaired children. *Science, 271,* 81–84.

Tam, C., & Stoddart, P. (1997, October). *Selecting voice recognition systems: Considerations in making an informed choice.* A paper presented at the Closing the Gap Technology Conference, Minneapolis, MN.

Tanner, D.C. (2001). The brave new world of the cyber speech and hearing clinic. *The Asha Leader, 6*(22), 6–7.

Templin, M. (1957). *Certain language skills in children: Their development and relationships.* Minneapolis, MN: University of Minnesota Press.

Thibodeau, L.M., Friel-Patti, S., & Britt, L. (2001). Psychoacoustic performance in children completing Fast ForWord training. *American Journal of Speech-Language Pathology, 10,* 248–257.

Thomas-Stonell, N., McLean, M., Dolman, L., & Oddson, B. (1992). Development and preliminary testing of a computer-based program for training stop consonants. *Journal of Speech-Language Pathology and Audiology, 16*(1), 5–9.

Tinker, B., Staudt, C., & Walton, D. (2002). The handheld computer as field guide. *Learning & Leading with Technology, 30*(1), 36–41.

Torgesen, J.K., & Barker, R.A. (1995). Computers as aids in the prevention and remediation of reading disabilities. *Learning Disability Quarterly, 18*(76–87).

Turnbull, A., Turnbull, R., Shank, M., & Leal, D. (1999). *Exceptional lives: Special education in today's schools* (2nd ed.). Upper Saddle River, NJ: Prentice-Hall.

Vanderheiden, G.C. (1990). Thirty-something million: should they be exceptions? *Human Factors, 32*(4), pp. 383–396.

Ventkatagiri, H.S. (1987). Writing your own software: What are the options? *Asha, 29*(6), 27–29.

Ventkatagiri, H.S. (1996). The quality of digitized and synthesized speech: What clinicians should know. *American Journal of Speech-Language Pathology, 5,* 31–42.

Virginia Assistive Technology System (1997). *A resource guide to assistive technology funding.* Richmond, VA: Author.

Voelkerding, K.A. (2002, Feb-Mar). PowerPoint as an assistive technology tool. *Closing the Gap: Computer Technology in Special Education and Rehabilitation* Retrieved June 1, 2003 from http://www.closingthegap.com/ctg2/members2/search.lasso

Volin, R.A. (1991). Microcomputer-based systems providing biofeedback of voice and speech production. *Topics in Language Disorders, 11*(2), 65–79.

Volin, R.A. (1998). A relationship between stimulability and the efficacy of visual feedback in the training of a respiratory control task. *American Journal of Speech-Language Pathology, 7,* 81–90.

Wallace, J. (1995). Creative financing of assistive technology. In K.F. Flippo & I.K.J. & B.M.J. (Eds.), *Assistive technology: A resource for school, work, and community.* Baltimore, MD: Paul H. Brookes Publishing Co.

Watson, C.S., & Kewley-Port, D. (1989). Advances in computer-based speech training (CBST): Aids for the profoundly hearing impaired. *Volta Review, 91*(5), 29–45.

Watson, C.S., Reed, D., Kewley-Port, D., & Maki, D. (1989). The Indiana Speech Training Aid (ISTRA) I: Comparisons between human and computer-based evaluation of speech quality. *Journal of Speech & Hearing Research, 32,* 245–251.

Weston, A.D., Shriberg, L.D., & Miller, J.F. (1989). Analysis of language-speech samples with SALT and PEPPER, *Journal of Speech and Hearing Research, 32*(4), 755–766.

Wiig, E.H., Jones, S.S., & Wiig, E.D. (1996). Computer-based assessment of word knowledge in teens with learning disabilities. *Language, Speech, and Hearing Services in Schools, 27*(1), 21–28.

Windham, T. (2000). *Preschoolers' exploration of word processing with and without speech output.* Unpublished master's thesis, Truman State University, Kirksville, MO.

Witzel, M.A., Tobe, J., & Salyer, K.E. (1989). The use of videonasopharyngoscopy for biofeedback therapy in adults after pharyngeal flap surgery. *The Cleft Palate Journal, 26,* 129–135.

Wood, L.A., & Masterson, J.H. (1999). The use of technology to facilitate language skills in school-age children. *Seminars in Speech and Language, 20*(3), 219–232.

Wood, L.A., Rankin, J.L., & Beukelman, D. (1997). Word prompt programs: Current uses and future possibilities. *American Journal of Speech-Language Pathology, 6*(3), 57–65.

Woods, S.A. (2000). *Designing single-subject articulation treatment studies using computer-based biofeedback.* Unpublished master's thesis. Truman State University, Kirksville, MO.

Wright, P, Rogers, N., Hall, C., Wilson, B., Evans, J., Emslie, H., & Bartram, C. (2001). Comparison of pocket-computer memory aids for people with brain injury. *Brain Injury, 15*(9), 787–800.

Wright, P., Rogers, N., Hall, C., Wilson, B., Evans, J., & Emslie, H. (2001). Enhancing an appointment diary on a pocket computer for use by people after brain injury. *International Journal of Rehabilitation Research, 24*(4), 299–308.

Wynne, M.K. (August 7, 2001). The shape of things to come and those that are here today. *Asha Leader.* Retrieved 1/11/04 from http://www.asha.org/about/publications/leaderonline/archives/2001/things_to_come.htm

Wynne, M.K., & Hurst, D.S. (1995). Legal issues and computer use by school-based audiologists and speech-language pathologists. *Language, Hearing, Speech Services in Schools, 28*(3), 251–259.

Yell, M.L. (1998). *The law and special education.* Upper Saddle River, NJ: Prentice-Hall.

Yorkston, K., Beukelman, D., & Traynor. (1984). *Computerized assessment of intelligibility of dysarthric speech* [computer program]. Tuscon, AZ: Communication Skill Builders.

Zabala, J. (1996). *SETTing the stage for success.* Paper presented at the Seventeenth Annual Southeast Augmentative Communication Conference, Birmingham, AL.

Zabala, J., & Lavadure, M. (2000). *Quality indicators for assistive technology services in school settings: Sharing the ongoing work of the QIAT consortium.* Paper presented at the RESNA 2000 Annual Conference: Technology for the New Millennium, Orlando, FL.

Zabala, J., Blunt, M., Bowser, G., Carl, D., Davis, S., Deterding, C., et. al. (Fall 2000). Quality indicators for assistive technology services in school settings. *Journal of Special Education Technology, 15*(4), 25–35.

Appendix

Software and Hardware Sources

Title	Publisher/Source	Web Site
A Whale of a Tale: Leap into Language 1	Innova Multimedia	www.innovamultimedia.com
A.D.A.M. The Inside Story	A.D.A.M. Software, Inc.	www.adam.com
Aphasia 4: Reading Comprehension	Parrot Software	www.parrotsoftware.com
Aphasia Tutor	Bungalow Software	www.bungalowsoftware.com
Articulation I, II, III	LocuTour Multimedia	www.locutour.com
ArtMatic Pro	U&I Software	www.uisoftware.com
Aurora 3 for Windows	Aurora Systems	www.aurora-systems.com
Automatic Articulation Analysis Plus	Parrot Software	www.parrotsoftware.com
Bailey's Book House	Riverdeep/Edmark	www.riverdeep.com
Bake & Taste	MindPlay	www.mindplay.com
Barbie Software: Kelly Club	Mattel/Vivendi	www.vugames.com
BAT Personal Keyboard	Infogrip, Inc.	www.infogrip.com
Big Red Switch	Ablenet	www.ablenetinc.com
Biggy (cursor utility)	R.J. Cooper and Associates	www.rjcooper.com
Boardmaker (1993)	Mayer-Johnson	www.mayer-johnson.com
Bob the Builder	THQ	www.thq.com
Brubaker on Disk	Parrot Software	www.parrotsoftware.com
BuildAbility	Don Johnston, Inc.	www.donjohnston.com
Child Language Data Exchange System (CHILDES)	MacWhinney and Snow (1986)	http://childes.psy.cmu.edu
Childhood Stuttering: A Second Opinion (ASO)	Bahill Intelligent Computer Systems	http://tucson.sie.arizona.edu/sysengr/2op/
Click It!	IntelliTools	www.intellitools.com
Clicker 4	Crick Software, LTD.	www.cricksoft.com
Co:Writer 4000	Don Johnston, Inc.	www.donjohnston.com
Community Exploration	Jostens Home Learning	www.compasslearning.com
Computer Aided Fluency Establishment Trainer (CAFET)	Martha Goebel	Not commercially available
Computer Managed Articulation Diagnosis (1984)	Communication Skill Builders	Not commercially available
Computerized Articulation and Phonology Evaluation System (2001) (CAPES)	Masterson and Berhnardt / The Psychological Corp.	www.PsychCorp.com
Computerized Assessment of Intelligibility of Dysarthric Speech (1984)	Yorkston, Beukelman, Traynor	Not commercially available– see listing for SIT

Title	Publisher/Source	Web Site
Computerized Profiling v. 9 (CP) (PROPHecy, PROPHet, PROPHer) (free download)	Long, Fey, & Channell (1998)	www.computerizedprofiling.org
Computerized Scoring of Stuttering Severity (CSSS)	Pro-Ed	www.proedinc.com
Computerized Speech Lab (CSL)	Kay Elemetrics	www.kayelemetrics.com
Computerized Speech Research Environment (CSRE)	AVAAZ Innovations	www.avaaz.com
Cyberlink Hands-Free Computer Controller	Brain Actuated Technologies, Inc.	www.brainfingers.com
Digital Swallowing Workstation and Fiberoptic Endoscopic Evaluation of Swallowing (FEES)	Kay Elemetrics	www.kayelemetrics.com
Discover Board	Madentec Limited	www.madentec.com
Discover Screen Software	Madentec Limited	www.madentec.com
Discover Switch	Madentec Limited	www.madentec.com
Disney Bundle	Educational Resources	www.educationalresources.com
Dr. Fluency	Speech Therapy Systems, Ltd.	www.drfluency.com
Dr. Seuss ABC's	Riverdeep/Broderbund	www.riverdeep.com
Dragon Tales Dragon Land Festival	Encore Software, Inc.	www.encoresoftware.com
Dreamweaver	Macromedia	www.macromedia.com
Earobics	Cognitive Concepts, Inc.	www.earobics.com
Earobics for Adolescents and Adults	Cognitive Concepts	www.earobics.com
Easy Voice	E-Press Corp.	www.e-press.com
E-Z Voice	Parrot Software	www.parrotsoftware.com
Facilitator	Kay Elemetrics	www.kayelemetrics.com
Fall Fun	SoftTouch, Inc.	www.softtouch.com
Fast ForWord	Scientific Learning	www.fastforword.com
Frenchay Dysarthria Assessment: Computer Differential Analysis (1983)	Enderby	Not commercially available
Fripple Town	Riverdeep/Edmark	www.riverdeep.com
Functional Living and Behavioral Rules	Silver Lining Multimedia, Inc.	www.silverliningmm.com
Functional Vocabulary Plus	Parrot Software	www.parrotsoftware.com
GamePak Interactive	FTC Publishing	www.ftcpublishing.com
Green Eggs and Ham	Riverdeep/Broderbund	www.riverdeep.com
HAL (screen reader)	Dolphin Computer Access Group	www.dolphinuk.co.uk
Head Master Plus (mouse emulator)	Prentke Romich Co.	www.prentrom.com
Head Mouse (mouse emulator)	Origin Instruments	www.orin.com
HearSay for All or HearSay	Communication Disorders Technology, Inc.	www.comdistec.com
Hot Dog Stand	Sunburst Technology	www.sunburst.com
Hyper Studio 4	Sunburst/Knowledge Adventure	www.sunburst.com
HyperCard (1987)	Apple Computer	Not commercially available
I KNOW American History	SoftTouch, Inc.	www.softtouch.com
Ice Cream Truck	Sunburst Technology	www.sunburst.com
Imagination Express Series: Castle, Neighborhood, Ocean, Pyramid, Rainforest	Riverdeep/Edmark	www.riverdeep.com

Title	Publisher/Source	Web Site
Indiana Speech Training Aid (ISTRA)	Communication Disorders Technology, Inc.	www.comdistec.com
Inspiration	Inspiration, Inc.	www.inspiration.com
IntelliKeys Classic Keyboard	IntelliTools, Inc.	www.intellitools.com
IntelliPics Studio	IntelliTools, Inc.	www.intellitools.com
IntelliTalk 3	IntelliTools, Inc.	www.intellitools.com
Interactive System for Phonological Analysis (ISPA) (No longer available)	Masterson and Pagan (1993)	Not commercially available
Interactive Voice Analysis System (IVANS) software	AVAAZ Innovations	www.avaaz.com
JAWS (screen reader)	Freedom Scientific	www.freedomscientific.com
Joystick SAM	R.J. Cooper and Associates	www.rjcooper.com
Joystick-To-Mouse (software utility)	Innovation Management Group, Inc.	www.imgpresents.com
Jump Start Animal Adventures	Sunburst/Knowledge Adventures	www.sunburst.com
Just Grandma and Me	Riverdeep/Broderbund	www.riverdeep.com
KidPix Deluxe	Riverdeep/Broderbund	www.riverdeep.com
Kidspiration	Inspiration Software, Inc.	www.inspiration.com
Kurtzweil 3000 (talking word processing, screen reader, study tools)	Kurtzweil Education Systems	www.kurtzweiledu.com
Leaps & Bounds 3	Tool Factory	www.sunburst.com
Lingquest 1: Language Sample Analysis (1982)	Mordecai, Palin, Palmer	Not commercially available
Literacy Phonemic Awareness	Locutour/Learning Fundamentals	www.locutour.com
Logical International Phonetic Programs (LIPP) and THINLIPP	Intelligent Hearing Systems of Miami	www.ihsys.com
MAGic (screen magnifier)	Freedom Scientific	www.freedomscientific.com
Microworlds Pro	Logo Computer Systems Incorporated	www.microworlds.com
Mini Keyboard	TASH International, Inc.	www.tashinc.com
Monkeys Jumping on a Bed	SoftTouch, Inc.	www.softtouch.com
MultiWare media CD	Beachware, available from Don Johnston, Inc.	www.donjohnston.com
My Town	Laureate Learning Systems, Inc.	www.LaureateLearning.com
Nasometer	Kay Elemetrics Corp.	www.kayelemetrics.com
Naturally Speaking v.7	ScanSoft, Inc.	www.scansoft.com
NetLogo	Center for Connected Learning	www.ccl.sesp.northwestern.edu/netlogo
Old MacDonald's Farm Deluxe	SoftTouch, Inc.	www.softtouch.com
Ollo in Sunny Valley Fair	Plaid Banana Hulabee Enter.	www.hulabee.com
OpenBook (OCR & screen reader)	Freedom Scientific	www.freedomscientific.com
Opposites and Similarities	Parrot Software	www.parrotsoftware.com
Oregon Trail	Riverdeep/Broderbund	www.riverdeep.com
OroNasal System	AVAAZ Innovations, Inc.	www.avaaz.com
Overlay Maker	IntelliTools, Inc.	www.intellitools.com
P.B. Bear's Birthday Party	Dorling Kindersly Multimedia	www.amazon.com
Pacer/Tally for Windows by Robert Tice	Madonna Rehabilitation Hospital	www.madonna.org/res_software.htm

Title	Publisher/Source	Web Site
Parrot Easy Language Sample Analysis Plus (PELSA)	Parrot Software	www.parrotsoftware.com
Penny and Giles Joystick	Don Johnston, Inc.	www.donjohnston.com
Phoneme Intelligibility Test (PIT)	Madonna Rehabilitation Hospital, Lincoln, NE	www.madonna.org=res_software.htm
Phonetic Font Plus	Parrot Software	www.parrotsoftware.com
Phonology I, II	Locutour	www.locutour.com
Photo-Objects Collections	Mayer-Johnson, Inc.	www.mayer-johnson.com
Picture Categories	Parrot Software	www.parrotsoftware.com
Picture Express	Picture Express	http://www.pictureexpresssoftware.com/
Picture This! And Picture This Pro!	Silver Lining Multimedia, Inc.	www.silverliningmm.com
PixReader, PixWriter	Slater Software, Inc.	www.slatersoftware.com
Print Shop	Riverdeep/Broderbund	www.riverdeep.com
PROPH, PROPHecy, PROPHet, PROPHer (free download)	Steven Long	www.computerizedprofiling.org
ProTrain I	AVAAZ Innovation	www.avaaz.com
P-Switch	Prentke Romich, Co.	www.prentrom.com
Read & Write v.6: textHELP	Global Adaptive Technologies, Inc.	www.globaladaptive.com
Reader's Quest I, II	Sunburst Technology	www.sunburst.com
Road Adventures USA	Riverdeep/The Learning Company	www.riverdeep.com
Scanware for SCAN, SCAN-A	Parrot Software	www.parrotsoftware.com
School Routines and Rules	Silver Lining Multimedia, Inc.	www.silverliningmm.com
Screen Doors II	Madentec Limited	www.madentec.com
Sentence Intelligibility Test (SIT) for Windows by Robert Tice	Madonna Rehabilitation Hospital, Lincoln NE	www.madonna.org/res_software.htm
Sesame Street Baby	Encore Software, Inc.	www.encoresoftware.com
Shop 'Til You Drop	SoftTouch, Inc.	www.softtouch.com
SIL Encore IPA Fonts (free download)	International Publishing Services	www.sil.org
Simon Sounds It Out	Don Johnston, Inc.	www.donjohnston.com
SimTown	Maxis Software, Inc.	www.maxis.com
Sky Island Mysteries	Riverdeep/Edmark	www.riverdeep.com
SmartNav (mouse emulator)	R.J. Cooper & Associates	www.rjcooper.com
Sona-Speech	Kay Elemetrics Corp.	www.kayelemetrics.com
Sorting By Category	Parrot Software	www.parrotsoftware.com
SoundScope I and II	G.W. Instruments	www.gwinst.com
Speech Assessment and Interactive Learning System (SAILS) (1994)	Rvachew	www.avaaz.com
SpeechEasy	Janus Development Group, Inc.	www.speecheasy.com
SpeechPrism, Speech Prism Pro	Language Vision, Inc.	www.langvision.com
SpeechViewer III	Psychological Corp.	www.PsychCorp.com
Spider in the Kitchen	Encore Software, Inc.	www.encoresoftware.com
Stanley's Sticker Stories	Riverdeep/Edmark	www.riverdeep.com
Start-to-Finish Books	Don Johnston, Inc.	www.donjohnston.com
Stuttering Measurement Module (free download)	Richard Moglia Univ of CA Santa Barbara	www.speech.ucsb.edu
Sunbuddy Writer	Sunburst Technology	www.sunburst.com
Super Nasal Oral Ratiometry System (SNORS+)	Medical Electronics University of Kent (U.K.)	www.cstr.ed.ac.uk/artic/airflow.html

Title	Publisher/Source	Web Site
SuperScope II	G.W. Instruments,	www.gwinst.com
Systematic Analysis of Language Transcripts (SALT)	Miller & Chapman, Waisman Center	www.languageanalysislab.com
TalkTime with Tucker	Laureate Learning Systems	www.LaureateLearning.com
Teddy Games	Inclusive TLC	www.inclusiveTLC.com
Teen Tunes Plus	SoftTouch, Inc.	www.softtouch.com
Terrapin Logo	Terrapin Software	www.terrapinlogo.com
The Big Box of Art	Mayer-Johnson, Inc.	www.mayer-johnson.com
The Cat in the Hat	Riverdeep/Broderbund Living Book Series	www.riverdeep.com
The Deciders Take on Concepts (2000)	Thinking Publications	www.thinkingpublications.com
The Playroom	Riverdeep/Broderbund	www.riverdeep.com
The Sims	Maxis Software, Inc.	www.maxis.com
ThemeWeaver	Riverdeep	www.riverdeep.com
Thinking Out Loud	Sunburst Technology	www.sunburst.com
Thinking Things Series: Collection 1, 2, or 3	Riverdeep/Edmark	www.riverdeep.com
Tiger Tales	Laureate Learning Systems	www.LaureateLearning.com
Touch Window (touch screen)	Riverdeep/Edmark	www.riverdeep.com
Touch-Free Switch	Riverdeep/Edmark	www.riverdeep.com
Tracker 2000 (mouse emulator)	Madentec Limited	www.madentec.com
Transcription Builder	Thinking Publications	www.thinkingpublications.com
True Friends: A Coloring Experience	Judy Lynn Software, Inc.	www.judylynn.com
Usborne's Animated First Thousand Words	Scholastic, Inc.	www.scholastic.com
Using a Television Schedule	Parrot Software	www.parrotsoftware.com
Via Voice	IBM	www.ibm.com/us
Video Voice Speech Training System	Micro Video	www.videovoice.com
Visi-Pitch (II and III)	Kay Elemetrics Corp.	www.kayelemetrics.com
Visivox (voice activated light box)	RSQ	www.visivox.com
Visual Voice Tools	Riverdeep/ Interactive Learning Limited	www.riverdeep.com
Voice Xpress	Lernout & Hauspie	Not commercially available
Vowel Target	Language Vision, Inc.	www.langvision.com
Where in the USA is Carmen Sandiego?	Riverdeep/Broderbund	www.riverdeep.com
Window Eyes (screen reader/ Braille output)	GW Micro	www.gwmicro.com
Write: Outloud	Don Johnston, Inc.	www.donjohnston.com
WriteAway 2000	Information Services, Inc.	www.is-inc.com
WYNN (literacy, screen reader, study tools pkg)	Freedom Scientific, Inc./ Learning Systems Group	www.freedomscientific.com
ZoomText (screen magnifier/ screen reader)	AI Squared	www.aisquared.com

Index

Page numbers followed by *f* indicate figures; those followed by *t* indicate tables.